The ASMBS Textbook of Bariatric Surgery

Christopher Still • David B. Sarwer
Jeanne Blankenship
Editors

The ASMBS Textbook of Bariatric Surgery

Volume 2: Integrated Health

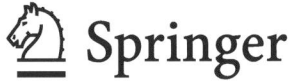

Editors
Christopher Still
Department of GI and Nutrition
Geisinger Obesity Institute
Geisinger Medical Center
Danville, PA, USA

Jeanne Blankenship
Policy Initiatives and Advocacy
American Dietetic Association
Falls Church, VA, USA

David B. Sarwer
Professor of Psychology
Departments of Psychiatry
Director of Clinical Services
Center for Weight and Eating Disorders
Perelman School of Medicine
  at the University of Pennsylvania
Philadelphia, PA, USA

ISBN 978-1-4939-1196-7   ISBN 978-1-4939-1197-4 (eBook)
DOI 10.1007/978-1-4939-1197-4
Springer New York Heidelberg Dordrecht London

Library of Congress Control Number: 2014945755

© Springer Science+Business Media New York 2014
This work is subject to copyright. All rights are reserved by the Publisher, whether the whole or part of the material is concerned, specifically the rights of translation, reprinting, reuse of illustrations, recitation, broadcasting, reproduction on microfilms or in any other physical way, and transmission or information storage and retrieval, electronic adaptation, computer software, or by similar or dissimilar methodology now known or hereafter developed. Exempted from this legal reservation are brief excerpts in connection with reviews or scholarly analysis or material supplied specifically for the purpose of being entered and executed on a computer system, for exclusive use by the purchaser of the work. Duplication of this publication or parts thereof is permitted only under the provisions of the Copyright Law of the Publisher's location, in its current version, and permission for use must always be obtained from Springer. Permissions for use may be obtained through RightsLink at the Copyright Clearance Center. Violations are liable to prosecution under the respective Copyright Law.
The use of general descriptive names, registered names, trademarks, service marks, etc. in this publication does not imply, even in the absence of a specific statement, that such names are exempt from the relevant protective laws and regulations and therefore free for general use.
While the advice and information in this book are believed to be true and accurate at the date of publication, neither the authors nor the editors nor the publisher can accept any legal responsibility for any errors or omissions that may be made. The publisher makes no warranty, express or implied, with respect to the material contained herein.

Printed on acid-free paper

Springer is part of Springer Science+Business Media (www.springer.com)

Preface

The American Society for Metabolic and Bariatric Surgery (ASMBS) is comprised of a dynamic group of surgeons, physicians, and integrated health members, all of whom are constantly challenged to improve the care of obese patients. As acknowledged in a landmark 2013 decision by the American Medical Association, clinically severe obesity is a disease process that is associated with multiple life-threatening conditions that may lead to premature death. As repeatedly and consistently demonstrated by literature evidence, bariatric surgery has shown to be the only long-lasting effective treatment for obesity and its related comorbidities.

Due to the development of videoscopic instrumentation, critical care, modern stapling devices, and laparoscopy, the field of bariatric surgery has changed tremendously over that past three decades since ASMBS's founding in 1983. Until 1998, only 10,000–12,000 bariatric operations were being performed yearly in the United States, with high rates of morbidity and mortality. This number of operations has increased exponentially over the subsequent years and eventually peaked at more than 140,000 operations in 2004. This growth directly correlates with the development and transition from open to laparoscopic Roux-en-Y gastric bypass. Additionally in 2001, following the US Food and Drug Administration's approval of the laparoscopic adjustable gastric band, the number of bariatric procedures experienced a significant increase. By 2005, the number of laparoscopic Roux-en-Y gastric bypass cases being performed in the United States surpassed the number of open Roux-en-Y gastric bypass cases. Most recently, the laparoscopic sleeve gastrectomy has proven to be an additional effective bariatric surgical option, with a risk and benefit profile between that of laparoscopic gastric bypass and laparoscopic adjustable gastric banding.

Along with those utilization changes, technological advancement, surgical technique, and quality improvement all required our society to respond to and accommodate the educational needs of our members. This dynamic field of surgery will continue to grow with enhanced understanding of the mechanisms of action of the procedures we can offer and the development of innovative and complementary treatment of obesity. As the needs of the society and its members evolve, the ASMBS is committed to continuing to serve the educational needs of our members and expanding public education. Our annual meeting is the primary venue to disseminate new information and educational materials to clinical professionals. To enhance and augment these educational offerings, we are excited to present this comprehensive ASMBS textbook of bariatric surgery. The development of this book reflects the commitment of the ASMBS leadership's goal of providing the most up-to-date education for our members.

Designed to be the *most* inclusive textbook on the topic of bariatric surgery and integrated health services to date, this textbook comprises two volumes. The first volume is devoted to the science and practices of bariatric surgery and is divided into five sections detailing basic considerations, including bariatric surgery's history and evolution, the pathophysiology of obesity, mechanisms of action, primary operations and management of complications, revision of primary bariatric surgery for failure of weight loss, the role of metabolic surgery, and specific considerations such as the role of endoscopy in bariatric surgery and coding and reimbursement. The second volume focuses on the medical, psychological, and nutritional management of the bariatric patients.

Each chapter in this book was written by a world-renowned expert in their field. A comprehensive text that adheres to the highest standards is a major undertaking, and we, the editors, are grateful and indebted to every author who has devoted time and effort to research the most important evidence-based information and report it in a concise and easy-to-read chapter. We believe that this *ASMBS Textbook of Bariatric Surgery* is the leading source of scientific information for surgeons, physicians, residents, students, and integrated health members today and for years to come.

Orange, CA, USA	Ninh T. Nguyen, MD
Scottsdale, AZ, USA	Robin Blackstone, MD
Standford, CA, USA	John Morton, MD
Dalton, GA, USA	Jaime Ponce, MD
University Park, FL, USA	Raul Rosenthal, MD
Falls Church, VA, USA	Jeanne Blankenship, RD
Philadelphia, PA, USA	David B. Sarwer, PhD
Danville, PA, USA	Christopher Still, DO

Contents

Part I Psychosocial

1. **Psychosocial Characteristics of Bariatric Surgery Candidates** 3
   David B. Sarwer, Kelly C. Allison, Brooke A. Bailer,
   and Lucy F. Faulconbridge

2. **Psychopathology and Bariatric Surgery** 11
   James E. Mitchell and Martina de Zwaan

3. **Quality of Life** 19
   David B. Sarwer, Chanelle T. Bishop-Gilyard, and Ray Carvajal

4. **Eating Disorders and Eating Behavior Pre- and Post-bariatric Surgery** 25
   Martina de Zwaan and James E. Mitchell

5. **Introduction to Psychological Consultations for Bariatric Surgery Patients** 33
   Katherine L. Applegate and Kelli E. Friedman

6. **Psychosocial Issues After Bariatric Surgery** 43
   Leslie J. Heinberg and Megan E. Lavery

7. **Technology to Assess and Intervene on Weight-Related Behaviors with Bariatric Surgery Patients** 55
   J. Graham Thomas and Dale S. Bond

8. **Psychosocial Issues in Adolescent Bariatric Surgery** 65
   Meg H. Zeller and Jennifer Reiter-Purtill

Part II Nutrition

9. **Perioperative Nutrition Assessment of the Bariatric Surgery Patient** 77
   Laura Lewis Frank

10. **Nutrition Education and Counseling of the Bariatric Surgery Patient** 91
    Toni Piechota

11. **Macronutrient Recommendations: Protein, Carbohydrate, and Fat** 101
    Mary Demarest Litchford

12. **Identification, Assessment, and Treatment of Vitamin and Mineral Deficiencies After Bariatric Surgery** 111
    Margaret M. Furtado

13. **Managing Common Nutrition Problems After Bariatric Surgery** 119
    Claire M. LeBrun

14 Nutrition Care Across the Weight Loss Surgery Process 129
Julie M. Parrott and J. Scott Parrott

Part III Obesity Medicine

15 Lifestyle Modification for the Treatment of Obesity 147
David B. Sarwer, Meghan L. Butryn, Evan Forman,
and Lauren E. Bradley

16 Pharmacotherapy Management of Obesity 157
Amanda G. Powell and Caroline Apovian

17 Medical Preparation for Bariatric Surgery 165
Peter N. Benotti and Gregory Dalencourt

**18 The Perioperative and Postoperative Medical Management
of the Bariatric Surgery Patient** 175
Christopher Still, Nadia Boulghassoul-Pietrzykowska,
and Jennifer Franceschelli

19 The Importance of a Multidisciplinary Team Approach 185
Tracy Martinez

**20 Genomic and Clinical Predictors Associated with Long-Term Success
After Bariatric Surgery** 195
Glenn S. Gerhard and G. Craig Wood

21 Medical Approach to a Patient with Postoperative Weight Regain 205
Robert F. Kushner and Kirsten Webb

**22 The Role of Physical Activity in Optimizing Bariatric
Surgery Outcomes** 217
Dale S. Bond and Wendy C. King

Index 231

Contributors

Kelly C. Allison, PhD Department of Psychiatry, Perelman School of Medicine at the University of Pennsylvania, Philadelphia, PA, USA

Caroline Apovian, MD, FACP, FACN Department of Medicine, Boston University School of Medicine, Boston, MA, USA

Nutrition and Support Service, Boston Medical Center, Boston, MA, USA

Katherine L. Applegate, PhD Department of Psychiatry, Duke Center for Metabolic and Weight Loss Surgery, Duke University Health System, Durham, NC, USA

Brooke A. Bailer, PhD Department of Psychiatry, Center for Weight and Eating Disorders, Perelman School of Medicine at the University of Pennsylvania, Philadelphia, PA, USA

Peter N. Benotti, MD, FACS Obesity Institute, Geisinger Medical Center, Danville, PA, USA

Chanelle T. Bishop-Gilyard, PsyD, MS Department of Psychiatry, Center for Weight and Eating Disorders, The University of Pennsylvania, Philadelphia, PA, USA

Jeanne Blankenship, MS, RD, CLE Policy Initiatives and Advocacy, American Dietetic Association, Falls Church, VA, USA

Dale S. Bond, PhD Department of Psychiatry and Human Behavior, The Weight Control and Diabetes Research Center, Brown Alpert Medical School, The Miriam Hospital, Providence, RI, USA

Nadia Boulghassoul-Pietrzykowska, MD, FACP Center for Medical Weight Management, Nutrition, Fitness and Lifestyle, Weight & Life MD, Ewing, NJ, USA

Lauren E. Bradley, MS Department of Psychology, Drexel University, Philadelphia, PA, USA

Meghan L. Butryn, PhD Department of Psychology, Drexel University, Philadelphia, PA, USA

Ray Carvajal, PsyD Department of Psychiatry, Center for Weight and Eating Disorders, Perelman School of Medicine at the University of Pennsylvania, Philadelphia, PA, USA

Perelman School of Medicine at the University of Pennsylvania, Philadelphia, PA, USA

Gregory Dalencourt, MD Faxton St. Luke's Healthcare, William A. Graber, MD, PC Weight Loss Surgery, New Hartford, NY, USA

Martina de Zwaan, MD Department of Psychosomatic Medicine and Psychotherapy, Hannover Medical School, Hanover, Lower Saxony, Germany

Lucy F. Faulconbridge, PhD Department of Psychiatry, Center for Weight and Eating Disorders, Perelman School of Medicine at the University of Pennsylvania, Philadelphia, PA, USA

Evan Forman, PhD Department of Psychology, Drexel University, Philadelphia, PA, USA

Jennifer Franceschelli, DO Department of GI and Nutrition, Geisinger Obesity Institute, Geisinger Medical Center, Danville, PA, USA

Laura Lewis Frank, PhD, MPH, RD, CD Coordinated Program in Dietetics, Program in Nutrition & Exercise Physiology (NEP), MultiCare Health System, College of Pharmacy, Washington State University, Tacoma, WA, USA

Frank Nutrition & Exercise Consulting, LLC, Gig Harbor, WA, USA

Kelli E. Friedman, PhD Department of Psychiatry, Duke Center for Metabolic and Weight Loss Surgery, Duke University Health System, Durham, NC, USA

Margaret M. Furtado, MS, RD, LDN, RYT Department of Bariatric Surgery, University of Maryland Medical Center, Baltimore, MD, USA

Glenn S. Gerhard, MD Institute for Personalized Medicine, Pennsylvania State University, College of Medicine, Hershey, PA, USA

Leslie J. Heinberg, PhD Behavioral Services, Bariatric and Metabolic Institute, Cleveland, OH, USA

Department of Medicine, Cleveland Clinic Lerner College of Medicine, Cleveland, OH, USA

Wendy C. King, PhD Department of Epidemiology, University of Pittsburgh, Pittsburgh, PA, USA

Robert F. Kushner, MD Division of General Medicine, Department of Medicine, Northwestern University Feinberg School of Medicine, Chicago, IL, USA

Megan E. Lavery, PsyD Cleveland Clinic Foundation, Cleveland, OH, USA

Claire M. LeBrun, MPH, RD, LD Department of Surgery, George Washington Medical Faculty Associates, Washington, DC, USA

Mary Demarest Litchford, PhD, RD, LDN Case Software & Books, Greensboro, NC, USA

Tracy Martinez, RN, BSN, CBN Wittgrove Bariatric Center, La Jolla, La Jolla, CA, USA

James E. Mitchell, MD Neuropsychiatric Research Institute, University of North Dakota School of Medicine and Health Sciences, Fargo, ND, USA

Julie M. Parrott, MS, RD, CPT Central Jersey Bariatrics, Freehold, NJ, USA

J. Scott Parrott, PhD Department of Interdisciplinary Studies, SHRP, Newark, NJ, USA

Department of Quantitative Methods, School of Public Health, University of Medicine and Dentistry of NJ, Newark, NJ, USA

Toni Piechota, MS, MPH, RD Department of Food and Nutrition, University of California, Davis, Sacramento, CA, USA

Amanda G. Powell, MD Department of Endocrinology, Diabetes, Nutrition and Weight Management, Boston Medical Center, Boston, MA, USA

Jennifer Reiter-Purtill, PhD Department of Behavioral Medicine and Clinical Psychology, Cincinnati Children's Hospital Medical Center, Cincinnati, OH, USA

David B. Sarwer, PhD Department of Psychiatry, Director of Clinical Services Center for Weight and Eating Disorders, Perelman School of Medicine at the University of Pennsylvania, Philadelphia, PA, USA

Christopher Still, DO, FACN, FACP Department of GI and Nutrition, Geisinger Obesity Institute, Geisinger Medical Center, Danville, PA, USA

J. Graham Thomas, PhD Weight Control and Diabetes Research Center, The Miriam Hospital, The Warren Alpert Medical School of Brown University, Providence, RI, USA

Kirsten Webb, MSN, CNP, CDE Center for Lifestyle Medicine, Northwestern Medical Faculty Foundation, Chicago, IL, USA

G. Craig Wood, MS Geisinger Health System, Geisinger Obesity Institute, Danville, PA, USA

Meg H. Zeller, PhD Department of Behavioral Medicine and Clinical Psychology, Cincinnati Children's Hospital Medical Center, University of Cincinnati College of Medicine, Cincinnati, OH, USA

Part I
Psychosocial

Psychosocial Characteristics of Bariatric Surgery Candidates

David B. Sarwer, Kelly C. Allison, Brooke A. Bailer, and Lucy F. Faulconbridge

Chapter Objectives

At the end of this chapter, the reader will be able to identify the most relevant psychosocial characteristics of individuals who present for bariatric surgery. The reader will also understand how these characteristics may be related to postoperative outcomes, both in terms of weight loss and psychosocial adaptation to the significant changes in weight and health that occur after bariatric surgery.

Psychosocial Characteristics of Bariatric Surgery Candidates

Motivations for and Expectations About Bariatric Surgery

For most individuals who present for bariatric surgery, improvements in weight-related comorbidities, as well as increased life expectancy, are among the primary motivations for surgery. At the same time, concerns about physical appearance and body image also influence the decision to seek surgery. Appropriate candidates for surgery often are

D.B. Sarwer, PhD (✉)
Department of Psychiatry, Director of Clinical Services Center for Weight and Eating Disorders, Perelman School of Medicine at the University of Pennsylvania, Philadelphia, PA, USA
e-mail: dsarwer@mail.med.upenn.edu

K.C. Allison, PhD
Department of Psychiatry, Perelman School of Medicine at the University of Pennsylvania, 3535 Market St., Suite 3028, Philadelphia, PA 19104-3309, USA
e-mail: kca@mail.med.upenn.edu

B.A. Bailer, PhD • L.F. Faulconbridge, PhD
Department of Psychiatry, Center for Weight and Eating Disorders, Perelman School of Medicine at the University of Pennsylvania, 3535 Market Street, Suite 3021, Philadelphia, PA 19104, USA
e-mail: bbailer@mail.med.upenn.edu; lucyhf@mail.med.upenn.edu

able to articulate these "internal" motivations for surgery. In contrast, those who are "externally" motivated for surgery, and interested in surgery for some secondary gain such as saving a troubled marriage, may be less appropriate candidates for surgery, as the procedure and subsequent weight loss may not have the desired effect on those external influences.

Individuals who present for all forms of weight loss treatment, including bariatric surgery, typically have unrealistic expectations regarding the amount of weight they will lose. For example, individuals with obesity who are being treated with lifestyle modification have reported "goal" weight losses of 33 % of their initial body weight, when in reality losses of 7–10 % of initial weight are typical [1]. Candidates for bariatric surgery have reported that they expect to lose 40–50 % of their initial body weight, which is much greater than the 25–30 % of weight typically achieved with the most common surgical procedures and for the majority of patients. Clinically, these unrealistic expectations were thought to put individuals at risk for weight regain. However, studies have suggested that they are not associated with any negative weight-related or psychosocial consequences [2].

Candidates for surgery likely have expectations about the impact of surgery on other areas of their lives, including quality of life, body image, and sexual relationships. This literature is reviewed in detail in Chap. 3.

Knowledge of Bariatric Surgery

Well known by most professionals who work in the area of bariatric surgery, less than 2 % of Americans who meet the recommended criteria for bariatric surgery undergo surgery each year. The reasons for this are both multiple and complex. Insurance coverage is likely a major barrier; lack of knowledge about the safety and efficacy of procedures also contributes to this disparity. While some physicians are knowledgeable about bariatric surgery and have favorable impressions about surgery as a treatment for obesity as well as type 2 diabetes, this is not universal [3]. At the same time, many patients who are eligible for bariatric surgery display a lack of knowledge about the safety and efficacy of surgery, the impact of the procedures on weight-related health problems, or the need to make significant, lifelong dietary and behavioral changes in order to experience an optimal postoperative outcome. This lack of knowledge underscores the important role of preoperative preparation and education during the initial consultation with the surgeon, consultations with the dietitian and mental health professional, and attendance in preoperative support groups [4]. These consultations are discussed in detail in several chapters throughout this volume.

Weight and Dieting Histories

Many members of the bariatric team—surgeon, nurse, dietitian, and/or mental health professional—may inquire about patients' weight and dieting histories. This includes assessing the age of onset of obesity and the history of obesity in family members. Candidates for surgery typically have an earlier age of onset of obesity and stronger family history of the disorder than do persons with less severe obesity [5]. This history may be a phenotypical expression of a genetic predisposition to obesity.

The majority of candidates for bariatric surgery has made multiple efforts to lose weight and can be described as "dieting veterans." Patients reported an average of 4.7 ± 2.9 previous weight loss efforts in which they lost at least 10 lb [6]. Self-directed diets and commercial programs were the most common weight loss approaches, although many report using pharmacological methods as well. While these experiences may not have been entirely successful, they have provided many patients with a foundation of knowledge regarding nutrition and healthy eating. Those without such a history often lack this knowledge and can benefit from additional dietary counseling, preoperative medical weight management, and attendance in the program's support group.

Intellectual Functioning

The discussion of the intellectual functioning of bariatric surgery patients has been a "hot-button" issue ever since an insurance company in Tennessee attempted to enact a policy that would require intelligence (IQ) testing of all patients prior to surgery. The recommendation was not based upon any available evidence and likely was a by-product of the pejorative attitudes and stigmatization that obese individuals often experience (as detailed later). Encouragingly, public outcry prevented the implementation of the policy.

Nevertheless, individuals across the spectrum of intelligence levels present for bariatric surgery, just as they do for other forms of medical and surgical treatment. Impairments in intellectual functioning, either from organic mental retardation or acquired brain injury, are not, by themselves, contraindications to surgery. If the patient can understand and adhere to the behavioral requirements of surgery and is in an environment where those behavioral changes could be supported, then surgery will likely improve their physical and mental quality of life. These situations often require some modification from the standard operating procedures, such as the delivery of instructional information in multiple domains, often repeatedly, as well as active involvement from other members of the patient's support system.

Interestingly, a number of recent studies have suggested that individuals with obesity, and in particular those with extreme obesity who are presenting for bariatric surgery, show some deficits in cognitive functioning. For example, obese individuals show deficits in memory, executive functioning (i.e., working memory, mental flexibility), motor speed, and complex attention [7]. These deficits could impact comprehension as well as retention of information presented to patients as part of the preoperative consultation process. Encouragingly, other studies have shown that there are improvements in these areas within the first year after surgery [8]. At present, the specific factors that contribute to these deficits, as well as the mechanisms of their improvements, are not well understood.

Self-Esteem

Self-esteem is a central psychological construct for many individuals. It can be strongly influenced by quality of life and body image, as discussed in detail in Chap. 3.

Excess body weight, and likely extreme obesity in particular, has the potential to detrimentally impact self-esteem. Some candidates for bariatric surgery struggle to recognize and appreciate their talents and abilities because of their body weight. However, this is not universal; others with extreme obesity may be comfortable with their work and home life, but maintaining a lower body weight has been the one area where they have not been successful. Obesity may be more likely to impact the self-esteem of women, likely given our society's overemphasis on thinness as the criterion for physical beauty.

Personality Characteristics

Interest in the personalities of individuals with extreme obesity and who present for bariatric surgery predates the current obesity crisis in the Western world as well as the renaissance of bariatric surgery seen this century. In many of the early studies, the Minnesota Multiphasic Personality Inventory (MMPI) was used to investigate the personality characteristics of bariatric patients. As reviewed in detail elsewhere, these studies concluded that a large minority to small majority of patients presented for surgery with significant psychopathology or character disorders [9]. It is not clear, however, whether these rates are higher than rates of these disorders in the general population, as most of these studies did not include appropriate comparison or control groups of individuals not presenting for surgery.

However, the relationship between specific MMPI profiles or characteristics and postoperative outcomes is still largely unknown. Likely as a result, personality testing of this kind is not widely used as part of the preoperative psychological evaluation at present (see Chap. 5).

Symptoms of Depression

Several studies have shown both cross-sectional and longitudinal relationships between excess body weight and depression. Persons with extreme obesity—body mass index (BMI) ≥40 kg/m^2—for example, are almost five times more likely to have experienced an episode of major depression in the past month as compared to average-weight individuals [10]. Our research team, and others, have found that extremely obese women seeking bariatric surgery scored significantly higher on the Beck Depression Inventory II (13.2 versus 8.1) than moderately obese women seeking lifestyle modification [11].

This relationship between excess weight and depression is consistently stronger for women than for men. Obese women were more likely to experience a major depressive episode in the past year as compared to average-weight women [12]. In contrast, obesity in men was associated with significantly reduced risks of depression as compared to men of average weight, suggesting a protective effect of excess weight. The factors that make obese women more vulnerable to depression than men are not yet well established, but likely moderators include physiological differences in hormones and fat metabolism, as well as society's strong emphasis on a lean physical appearance in women but not men.

Between 25 and 30 % of candidates for bariatric surgery report clinically significant symptoms of depression at the time of surgery. The reasons for this are not well understood but could include the experience of weight-related prejudice and discrimination, the presence of physical pain or other impairments in quality of life, repeated failed attempts to sustain weight loss, or the occurrence of disordered eating.

The remaining 70–75 % of surgery candidates report minimal to mild symptoms of depression that generally are not of clinical concern [11]. Those who score in the moderate to severe range of depression require further examination and are asked about their sleep, concentration, cognition, vocational and social functioning, as well as the presence of suicidal ideation during preoperative psychological assessment. Many of these patients are already under psychiatric or psychotherapeutic care [13]. In these cases, permission to contact practitioners is requested to obtain their assessment of the patient's psychiatric status and whether they support the individual's decision to have surgery.

Mental Health Treatment

A number of studies have investigated the use of mental health treatment among persons who present for bariatric surgery. Between 16 and 40 % of patients report ongoing mental health treatment at the time of surgery [14]. Up to 50 % have reported a history of psychiatric treatment. Both of these rates are higher than the rate in the general population.

The most common form of treatment appears to be the use of antidepressant medications. For a number of reasons, primary care physicians appear to be the medical providers typically prescribing and managing these medications. Presently, little is known about how these medications interact with the different surgical procedures [15]. Dramatic changes in absorption of medications may potentially occur due to a reduction in gastrointestinal surface area and other changes. Rapid changes in body weight and fat mass may also affect the efficacy and tolerability of antidepressant medications. To date, there has been little guidance on the management of these medications peri- or postoperatively.

Eating and Activity Habits

Eating and physical activity habits are behaviors that require attention from the entire bariatric surgery team both before and again after surgery. Registered dietitians often evaluate these domains and make recommendations to patients, although in some programs, including our own, the mental health professional also assesses these behaviors as part of the preoperative psychological consultation.

Studies have found that patients typically consume approximately 2,400 kcal/day prior to surgery [16, 17]. This is more than the total daily caloric intake recommended by the US Department of Agriculture, and continued consumption of this amount of calories and over a period of years has likely been a significant contributing factor to the development and maintenance of extreme obesity. However, patients report a large range of caloric intake; some may be consuming 3,000–4,000 kcal/day and report daily consumption of food from fast food and takeout restaurants. In contrast, others who present for bariatric surgery may already be consuming a recommended calorie goal from a nutritionist, doctor, or commercial program in an effort to control their weight and other comorbidities.

Beyond total calories, it is important to assess the number and types of meals and snacks consumed daily. After surgery, patients are expected to follow a strict meal and beverage schedule that is often very different from their preoperative routines. Breakfast skipping is a common presentation, with a small minority of patients reporting not eating a full meal until dinner. In one study that included a sample of 147 patients seeking bariatric surgery, 59 % reported morning anorexia more than half of the time, and 17 % reported that they delayed their first meal until noon or later [18]. Fasting for extended periods of time increases the risk of loss of control eating and binge episodes, and loss of control eating has been emerging as a predictor of weight regain postoperatively [19]. Breakfast skipping and daytime fasting could also represent a shift in the circadian pattern of eating consistent with night eating syndrome [20]. Persons experiencing nocturnal ingestions (waking from sleep to eat) preoperatively may continue to experience them after surgery and, as such, would be an important behavior to modify.

Patients have also reported that certain eating behaviors have contributed significantly to their weight gain. Fabricatore and colleagues [21] examined the 20 eating behaviors contained in the Weight and Lifestyle Inventory (WALI) [22] and generated five factors that summarized problematic eating influences. These factors included (1) eating in response to negative affect, (2) eating in response to positive affect and social cues, (3) general overeating and impaired appetite regulation, (4) overeating at early meals, and (5) snacking. Surgery patients with mild to severe (as opposed to minimal) depressive symptoms reported a significantly greater influence of negative affect on their eating. Additionally, the 27 % of the sample meeting criteria for binge eating disorder scored higher on every factor as compared to those without disorder. Snacking or "grazing" after surgery also seems to represent a risk for attenuated weight loss and weight regain. Thus, raising awareness with patients about the impact of these eating behaviors on their past weight history, and their likely influence on weight loss and retention postoperatively, is an important part of the preoperative evaluation and education process.

Family Support

The decision to seek bariatric surgery is a significant one, not only for the patient but for his or her family members. Intuitively, the satisfaction with and quality of those relationships could impact postoperative outcomes, although this issue has received little empirical study. In rare cases, family members may be opposed to surgery or may try to sabotage patients' weight loss efforts. For these reasons, family relationships are typically discussed during the preoperative psychological evaluation. Surgery candidates who report they are dissatisfied with their marriages (or other intimate relationships) are informed that surgery and weight loss are unlikely to resolve these problems.

Childhood Maltreatment

In the general population, approximately one third of women and 8 % of men report a history of childhood sexual abuse [23]. Similar percentages of adults report a history of physical abuse, although estimates of the rates for both experiences vary depending upon study methodology. Both sexual and physical abuse are believed to be risk factors for the development of obesity. The experience of childhood maltreatment has been associated with a 1.4–1.6-fold increased risk of a BMI >35 kg/m^2 [24]. The rate of childhood maltreatment may be even greater among those with extreme obesity, with studies suggesting that up to 32 % of candidates for bariatric surgery reported a history of sexual abuse and 29 % a history of physical abuse [25, 26]. Almost 70 % reported a history of childhood maltreatment, including emotional neglect, imprisonment of a parent, substance abuse in the home, or other unfortunate experiences.

Encouragingly, at least two studies have suggested that a history of childhood sexual abuse is not associated with the magnitude of weight loss after bariatric surgery [27, 28]. However, patients with a history of sexual abuse may experience some "emotional turbulence" as they go through the period of rapid weight loss and experience significant changes in their physical appearance and body image. This distress and discomfort may interfere with dietary adherence and, in some cases, may indirectly lead some individuals to return to maladaptive eating behaviors and food choices as they use eating as a coping mechanism. For these reasons, we routinely ask patients about a history of childhood maltreatment during their preoperative evaluation and counsel them about how these issues hold the potential to remerge postoperatively.

Stigma and Discrimination

Weight-related stigmatization or overt discrimination of obese individuals is believed to be a common, if not pervasive, experience. Intuitively, these experiences may contribute to the psychosocial distress seen in persons with obesity. Bias against persons with obesity has been found in social, educational, occupational, and even medical settings [29]. Somewhat surprisingly, weight-related stigma and discrimination have received relatively little attention in the bariatric surgery literature. A history of weight-based teasing, which is probably the most ubiquitous form of stigma, has been found to be associated with greater levels of depression, body image dissatisfaction, and poorer self-esteem in bariatric surgery patients [30]. However, at least two studies have suggested that the rate of the most overt forms of stigma and bias against those with extreme obesity who present for bariatric surgery may not be as common as intuitively thought [31, 32]. In general, these individuals reported very little weight-related stigma, with the most common form of stigma being experienced "several times" in participants' lives. Nevertheless, the occurrence of stigmatization is associated with poorer weight-related quality of life and greater symptoms of depression. Thus, the experience of stigma and discrimination hold the potential to have detrimental psychosocial effects.

Timing of Surgery

While not a psychosocial characteristic, consideration of the timing of surgery in relation to other circumstances in a patient's life is considered to be an important part of the preoperative evaluation process. Ideally, patients have chosen to pursue surgery at a time that is relatively free of significant life stressors such as a change in employment, living situations, or romantic relationships. Ideally, the patient should have 3–4 weeks of time set aside to undergo the operation, recover from it physically, and begin to adapt to the postoperative dietary and behavioral changes required of surgery. In cases in which candidates report extremely stressful life events, it may be useful to recommend that they delay surgery until the stressors have resolved.

Psychological Characteristics and Postoperative Outcomes

Patients who undergo bariatric surgery have been found to experience, on average, significant reductions in symptoms of depression, anxiety, and binge eating disorder and significant improvements in quality of life [33]. An important question, however, is the relationship between preoperative psychological characteristics and postoperative outcomes. At present, the relationship between preoperative psychological status and postoperative outcomes is unclear [34, 35]. Some studies have suggested that preoperative psychopathology and eating behavior are associated with suboptimal weight loss; others have suggested that preoperative psychopathology may not be associated with smaller weight losses but may be associated with untoward psychosocial outcomes. Unfortunately, the complex relationship between obesity, personality characteristics, and psychopathology and a number of methodological issues within this literature make drawing definitive conclusions difficult at this time. It may be that psychiatric symptoms that are largely attributable to weight, such as impaired quality of life, may be associated with more positive outcomes, whereas those symptoms representative of psychiatric illness, that is, independent of obesity, are associated with less positive outcomes.

Most mental health professionals who work in the area have likely been asked, either by surgeon colleagues, other medical professionals, laypersons, or patients themselves, "Can you predict postoperative outcome based upon the preoperative evaluation?" While one of the axioms of mental health is "past behavior typically predicts future behavior," there is currently no appropriate level of evidence that allows us to conclude, with any degree of certainty, that specific preoperative personality characteristics or traits can be used to predict postoperative outcomes, either in terms of weight loss or psychosocial adaptation.

Conclusion

This chapter has reviewed the more general psychosocial characteristics seen in men and women who present for bariatric surgery. Many patients share commonalities with regard to their motivations for surgery, personality characteristics, common eating and activity behavior patterns, and expectations of postoperative outcomes. Others vary tremendously with regard to their developmental history, family relationships, and other life experiences. Nevertheless, stories in the mass media will often make reference to the "obese personality" suggesting that there is a cluster of psychosocial characteristics shared by individuals with obesity. The reality is that the worldwide spread of the obesity problem has confirmed what many have argued for years—there is no such thing as an "obese personality" and that the disease is the end result of countless genetic, physiological, psychosocial, and environmental variables that interact and impact most individuals in a heterogeneous manner. This may be particularly true when individuals who suffer from extreme obesity and present for bariatric surgery are considered.

This conclusion, however, does not mean that there is no value in trying to understand the psychosocial characteristics of individuals who present for bariatric surgery and, most importantly, how these variables may be related to postoperative outcomes, both in terms of weight loss and psychosocial adaptation to the significant changes in weight and health that occur after bariatric surgery. Nor does this conclusion suggest that there is no value in or need for the preoperative psychological evaluation prior to bariatric surgery as discussed in Chap. 5. Research on psychosocial characteristics of patients has played an important role in the development and refinement of those preoperative evaluations over the past decade. This research, as well as those evaluations, will continue to play an important role in attempting to identify the psychological and behavioral variables that may lead to suboptimal postoperative outcomes. Furthermore, mental health professionals play and likely will continue to play an important role in the continued development of bariatric surgery, both in terms of continued advances in quality and also as part of the argument for greater access to bariatric surgery for more individuals in the future.

Question and Answer Section

Questions

1. Obesity is more likely to impact the self-esteem of:
   A. Men
   B. Women
   C. Men and women equally
2. If a bariatric surgery candidate has a history of depression, what is the most likely outcome after the patient has surgery?
   A. The patient will lose a significant amount of weight and will no longer be depressed.
   B. The patient will lose a significant amount of weight but will still suffer from depression.
   C. There is no way to predict the postoperative outcome based on the preoperative psychological assessment.

Answers

1. **B**. Given society's overemphasis on thinness as the criterion for beauty, the self-esteem of women is more likely to be affected by obesity than for men.
2. **C**. Psychosocial variables may be related to postoperative outcomes; however, there is no level of evidence allowing mental health professionals to conclude that specific preoperative personality characteristics or traits can be used to predict postoperative outcomes, either in terms of weight loss or psychosocial adaptation.

Acknowledgments Completion of this article supported, in part, by grants:
NIH Grant HL109235
NIDDK Grant 1RC1DK086132
University of Pennsylvania Diabetes Research Center Grant 2P30DK019525-36
NIH Grant R01-DK072452
NIH Grant NCT00721838

Disclosures Dr. Sarwer has received consulting compensation from Allergan, BAROnova, EnteroMedics, and Ethicon Endo-Surgery, which are manufacturers of products for obesity. None of these entities provided financial support for his work on this manuscript.

References

1. Foster GD, Wadden TA, Vogt R, Brewer G. What is a reasonable weight loss? Patients' expectations and evaluations of obesity treatment outcomes. J Consult Clin Psychol. 1997;65(1):79–85.
2. Fabricatore AN, Wadden TA, Womble LG, Sarwer DB, Berkowitz RI, Foster GD, et al. The role of patients' expectations and goals in the behavioral and pharmacological treatment of obesity. Int J Obes (Lond). 2007;31(11):1739–45.
3. Sarwer DB, Ritter S, Wadden TA, Spitzer JC, Vetter ML, Moore RH. Physicians' attitudes about referring their type 2 diabetes patients for bariatric surgery. Surg Obes Relat Dis. 2012 (in press).
4. Wadden TA, Sarwer DB. Behavioral assessment of candidates for bariatric surgery: a patient-oriented approach. Obes Res. 2006;14 Suppl 2:53S–62.
5. Crerand CE, Wadden TA, Sarwer DB, Fabricatore AN, Kuehnel RH, Gibbons LM, et al. A comparison of weight histories in women with class III vs. class I-II obesity. Surg Obes Relat Dis. 2006;2(2):165–70.
6. Gibbons LM, Sarwer DB, Crerand CE, Fabricatore AN, Kuehnel RH, Lipschutz PE, et al. Previous weight loss experiences of bariatric surgery candidates: how much have patients dieted prior to surgery? Surg Obes Relat Dis. 2006;2(2):159–64.
7. Sellbom KS, Gunstad J. Cognitive function and decline in obesity. J Alzheimers Dis. 2012;30:S89–95.
8. Gunstad J, Strain G, Devlin MJ, Wing R, Cohen RA, Paul RH, et al. Improved memory function 12 weeks after bariatric surgery. Surg Obes Relat Dis. 2011;7(4):465–72.
9. Sarwer DB, Wadden TA, Fabricatore AN. Psychosocial and behavioral aspects of bariatric surgery. Obes Res. 2005;13(4):639–48.
10. Onyike CU, Crum RM, Lee HB, Lyketsos CG, Eaton WW. Is obesity associated with major depression? Results from the third national health and nutrition examination survey. Am J Epidemiol. 2003;158(12):1139–47.
11. Wadden TA, Butryn ML, Sarwer DB, Fabricatore AN, Crerand CE, Lipschutz PE, et al. Comparison of psychosocial status in treatment-seeking women with class III vs. class I-II obesity. Surg Obes Relat Dis. 2006;2(2):138–45.
12. Carpenter KM, Hasin DS, Allison DB, Faith MS. Relationships between obesity and DSM-IV major depressive disorder, suicide ideation, and suicide attempts: results from a general population study. Am J Public Health. 2000;90(2):251–7.
13. Pawlow LA, O'Neil PM, White MA, Byrne TK. Findings and outcomes of psychological evaluations of gastric bypass applicants. Surg Obes Relat Dis. 2005;1(6):523–7; discussion 528–9.
14. Sarwer DB, Cohn N, Gibbons LM, Magee L, Crerand CE, Raper SE, Rosato EF, Williams NN, Wadden TA. Psychiatric diagnoses and psychiatric treatment among bariatric surgery candidates. Obes Surg. 2004;14:1148–56.
15. Sarwer DB, Faulconbridge LF, Steffen KJ, Roerig JL, Mitchell JE. Managing patients after surgery: changes in drug prescription, body weight can affect psychotropic prescribing. Curr Psychiatry. 2010;10(1):3–9.
16. Sarwer DB, Wadden TA, Moore RH, Baker AW, Gibbons LM, Raper SE, et al. Preoperative eating behavior, postoperative dietary adherence, and weight loss after gastric bypass surgery. Surg Obes Relat Dis. 2008;4(5):640–6.
17. Sjostrum CD, Lindroos AK, Peltonen M, Torgerson J, Bouchard C, Carlsson B, et al. Lifestyle, diabetes, and cardiovascular risk factors 10 years after bariatric surgery. N Engl J Med. 2004;351(26):2683–93.

18. Allison KC, Engel SG, Crosby RD, de Zwaan M, O'Reardon JP, Wonderlich SA, et al. Evaluation of diagnostic criteria for night eating syndrome using item response theory analysis. Eat Behav. 2008;9(4):398–407.
19. de Zwann M, Mitchell JE, Howell LM, Monson N, Swan-Kremeier L, Crosby RJ, et al. Characteristics of morbidly obese patients before gastric bypass surgery. Compr Psychiatry. 2003;44(5):428–34.
20. Allison KC, Lundgren JD, O'Reardon JP, Geliebter A, Gluck ME, Vinai P, et al. Proposed diagnostic criteria for night eating syndrome. Int J Eat Disord. 2010;43:241–7.
21. Fabricatore AN, Wadden TA, Sarwer DB, Kuehnel RH, Lipschutz PE, et al. Self-reported eating behaviors of extremely obese persons seeking bariatric surgery: a factor analytic approach. Obesity. 2006;14(Suppl):83S–9.
22. Wadden TA, Foster GD. Weight and Lifestyle Inventory (WALI). Surg Obes Relat Dis. 2006;2(2):180–99.
23. Gustafson TB, Sarwer DB. Childhood sexual abuse and obesity. Obes Rev. 2004;5(3):129–35.
24. Felitti VJ, Anda RF, Nordenberg D, Williamson DF, Spitz AM, Edwards V, et al. Relationship of childhood abuse and household dysfunction to many of the leading causes of death in adults. The Adverse Childhood Experiences (ACE) Study. Am J Prev Med. 1998;14(4):245–58.
25. Grilo CM, Masheb RM, Brody M, Toth C, Burke-Martindale CH, Rothschild BS. Childhood maltreatment in extremely obese male and female bariatric surgery candidates. Obes Res. 2005;13(1):123–30.
26. Gustafson TB, Gibbons LM, Sarwer DB, Crerand CE, Fabricatore AN, Wadden TA, et al. History of sexual abuse among bariatric surgery candidates. Surg Obes Relat Dis. 2006;2(3):369–74; discussion 375–6.
27. Buser A, Dymek-Valentine M, Hilburger J, Alverdy J. Outcome following gastric bypass surgery: impact of past sexual abuse. Obes Surg. 2004;14(2):170–4.
28. Larsen JK, Geenen R. Childhood sexual abuse is not associated with a poor outcome after gastric banding for severe obesity. Obes Surg. 2005;15(4):534–7.
29. Puhl RM, Heuer CA. The stigma of obesity: a review and update. Obesity. 2009;17(5):941–64.
30. Petry NM, Barry D, Pietrzak RH, Wagner JA. Overweight and obesity are associated with psychiatric disorders: results from the national epidemiologic survey on alcohol and related conditions. Psychosom Med. 2008;70(3):288–97.
31. Friedman KE, Ashmore JA, Applegate KL. Recent experiences of weight-based stigmatization in a weight loss surgery population: psychological and behavioral correlates. Obesity. 2008;16 Suppl 2:S69–74.
32. Sarwer DB, Fabricatore AN, Eisenberg MH, Sywulak LA, Wadden TA. Self-reported stigmatization among candidates for bariatric surgery. Obesity. 2008;16 Suppl 2:S75–9.
33. Wadden TA, Sarwer DB, Fabricatore AN, Jones L, Stack R, Williams NS. Psychosocial and behavioral status of patients undergoing bariatric surgery: what to expect before and after surgery. Med Clin North Am. 2007;91(3):451–69, xi–xii.
34. Herpertz S, Kielmann R, Wolf AM, Hebebrand J, Senf W. Do psychosocial variables predict weight loss or mental health after obesity surgery? A systematic review. Obes Res. 2004;12(10):1554–69.
35. van Hout GC, Verschure SK, van Heck GL. Psychosocial predictors of success following bariatric surgery. Obes Surg. 2005;15(4):552–60.

Psychopathology and Bariatric Surgery

James E. Mitchell and Martina de Zwaan

Chapter Objectives

1. To present an overview of various types of psychopathology frequently seen in candidates for bariatric surgery
2. To discuss the implications of psychopathology on postoperative outcomes
3. To review the elements that should be included in the presurgical psychosocial evaluation

Introduction

It is now well established that high rates of psychopathology are seen in bariatric surgery candidates [1–3]. However, in considering this observation, several factors need to be considered. First, candidates for bariatric surgery are, by definition, severely obese. This raises the interesting question as to the relationship between psychopathology and obesity in general. Can obesity be considered a psychiatric disorder, particularly in those with severe obesity [4]? However, if this notion is rejected as a global conclusion, a second question is whether or not a subgroup (or subgroups) of patients with obesity develop the disorder as a reflection of underlying psychopathology. A third proposition would be that the comorbidity between psychopathology and obesity may be attributable to other variables that are not necessarily causal but mediate or moderate the interaction. Those three propositions are not mutually exclusive, and there is evidence to support each among certain subgroups of persons with obesity.

In this chapter, we will first briefly review the relationship between obesity and psychopathology, particularly among the severely obese who constitute the group of potential candidates for bariatric surgery. We will then turn to rates of psychiatric disorders and psychological symptoms, such as anxiety and depression, in presurgical pre-bariatric surgery populations, and examine the prevalence of such problems (either their continuation or emergence) after surgery. Third, we will briefly focus on the issue of the assessment of psychopathology prior to bariatric surgery and how this is best accomplished. Fourth, we will discuss what forms of psychopathology might serve as useful exclusion criteria for the procedure, as well as criteria that might dictate the need for special monitoring or intervention prior to or following surgery. Lastly, we will discuss the impact of psychopathology on the outcome of bariatric surgery particularly as it relates to amount of weight loss and the risk of substantial weight regain. Admittedly, the literature in some of these areas is modest at best. However, we will review the data that are available.

Of note, in this chapter we will use the term "psychopathology" rather broadly to incorporate not only specific psychiatric disorders but also symptoms of a psychological nature, such as depression, anxiety, and eating pathology that have been linked to psychiatric disorders, which may impact both on the risk of obesity and bariatric surgery outcome.

Obesity and Psychopathology

The question as to whether or not obesity may constitute a form of psychopathology has been widely debated in the literature for an extended period of time. It remains a focus of considerable interest, particularly given the current plan to revise the psychiatric nomenclature in the fifth edition of the Diagnostic and Statistical Manual of Mental Disorders (DSM-5), to be published shortly [4]. It has been widely recognized for some time that populations of patients with

J.E. Mitchell, MD (✉)
Neuropsychiatric Research Institute, University of North Dakota School of Medicine and Health Sciences, 1208th St. South, Fargo, ND 58102, USA
e-mail: mitcelle@medicine.nodak.edu

M. de Zwaan, MD
Department of Psychosomatic Medicine and Psychotherapy, Hannover Medical School, Carl-Neuberg-Strasse 1, Hannover, Lower Saxony 30625, Germany
e-mail: deZwaan.Martina@mh-hanover.de

obesity tend to have higher than expected prevalence rates of a variety of psychiatric disorders, including in particular affective (mood) disorders, anxiety disorders, and eating disorders—in particular binge eating disorder (BED) [5]— and that these rates in general tend to increase in prevalence with an increasing severity of the obesity. Also of note, a meta-analysis suggested that this is a bidirectional relationship, with obese individuals being at increased risk for developing depression, and that there also is an increased risk of developing obesity in those with depression [6]. However, in general most authors have concluded that not all forms of obesity are caused by psychopathology and that clearly many obese individuals function quite well, free of any significant psychiatric symptoms or disorders. Nevertheless, most, if not all, encounter significant problems with stigma and discrimination, depending on various factors including the culture in which they live.

The relationship, however, between the high comorbidity levels of obesity and psychopathology is nonetheless well established and consistently found, and the veracity of this conclusion has been widely accepted by experts in both psychopathology and obesity. For example, in the National Epidemiological Survey on Alcohol and Related Conditions (NESARC) [2], obese and extremely obese individuals were more likely than those at a normal body weight to be depressed, with high rates of mood disorders, anxiety disorders, alcohol use disorders, and personality disorders. These results are similar to those obtained in the National Comorbidity Replication Survey (NCS-R) [7].

The exact nature of these relationships remains controversial. One possibility that has emerged increasingly in recent years is the idea that individuals with obesity may have a form of addictive disorder similar to other addictive disorders, such as alcohol or drug abuse, whereas in contradistinction to these other forms of abuse, the abused substance is food. As has been well documented in this literature, there are similarities between obesity and addictive disorders, including craving for the desired substance (drug or highly palatable food), a sense of loss of control when using, repeated attempts to control use, use despite clear adverse consequences, and the dedication of much time in obtaining and using the substance [8–10]. Also some neurobiological data as well seem to support that common pathways are involved in both groups of disorders, particularly data related to the endogenous dopamine neurotransmitter system in the central nervous system (CNS) and its role in appetitive and reenforcing behaviors. However, the addiction model also is widely criticized [8–10]. Shortcomings of the addiction model include, most importantly, the observation that appetite and food ingestion are necessary for human survival, while the use or abuse of drugs is not. Nonetheless, the literature in this area continues to develop, and the nature of this relationship will continue to fuel both debate and research going forward.

Another variable linking obesity and psychopathology is a literature indicating that disordered eating, particularly binge eating—wherein subjects engage in overeating characterized by a sense of loss of control—may also be linked to the development of obesity, particularly more severe forms of obesity [4]. Actually, aberrant eating pre- and postbariatric surgery is of considerable importance in predicting outcome after bariatric surgery. This is discussed below and reviewed in depth in Chap. 4.

Another issue of relevance to this association between obesity and psychopathology is the use of psychotropic medication. Many of the available psychotropic agents that are used commonly for depression and anxiety may result in significant weight gain, while the number of such medications associated with weight loss or that are weight neutral is small. Given that the prescription medication most commonly taken by candidates for bariatric surgery are antidepressants, and given the high rates of psychopathology in this population (particularly rates of anxiety disorders and major depression), the use of these medications and other forms of mental health treatment is a central role of the preoperative psychological evaluation (see Chap. 5). Also, as discussed below, certain bariatric surgery procedures may impact on the pharmacokinetics of medications including antidepressant drugs.

Psychopathology Prior to Bariatric Surgery

As previously mentioned, it must be remembered that the stigmatization of and discrimination against the obese must be considered in evaluating psychopathology in severely obese patients who present for bariatric surgery. The data are consistent in showing significantly higher than expected rates of DSM-IV Axis I disorders (such as major depression and anxiety disorders) in bariatric surgery candidates. However, a problem in evaluating this literature concerns the nature of the assessments that have been utilized. Many times, rates of psychopathology have been based on patient self-report rather than structured clinical interviews, the accepted "gold standard" for assessing for the presence of psychopathology. Also, in some studies, the prevalence rates are based on assessments that have been conducted in the context of the psychological assessment often required to evaluate candidates for the appropriateness for bariatric surgery. Patients may bias their reports in such situations in an attempt to minimize a history of psychiatric problems in hopes of obtaining the surgery. Also, the concordance between routine clinical interviews and structured interviews using diagnostic criteria, which are seldom used in routine clinical practice, is not particularly high across all psychiatric disorders [11].

To date, six studies have been published or presented detailing rates of psychopathology in bariatric surgery candidates

Table 2.1 Lifetime psychiatric diagnoses

Authors/year	Rosenberger et al. 2006 [3]	Kalarchian et al. 2007 [15]	Mauri et al. 2008 [12]	Mühlhans et al. 2009 [5]	Jones-Corneille et al. 2010 [14]	Mitchell et al. (in submission)
Sample size	174	288	282	146	105	199
Axis I diagnosis						
Psychiatric disorder	36.8 %	66.3 %	37.6 %	72.6 %	50.5 %	68.6 %
Affective disorder		45.5 %	22.0 %	54.8 %	35.2 %	44.2 %
Anxiety disorder	15.5 %	37.5 %	18.1 %	21.2 %	24.8 %	31.7 %
Substance use disorder	5.2 %	32.6 %	1.1 %	15.1 %	28.8 %	35.7 %
Alcohol abuse or dependence	4.0 %	30.9 %	0.7 %	11.0 %	10.5 %	33.2 %
Eating disorder	13.8 %	NA	NA	50.0 %	NA	26.6 %
Binge eating disorder	4.6 %	27.1 %	11.1 %	NA	NA	13.1 %
Bulimia nervosa	0.0 %	3.5 %	1.8 %	6.8 %	NA	2.5 %
EDNOS[a]	9.2 %	NA	NA	NA	NA	13.1 %

[a]Eating disorders not otherwise specified

Table 2.2 Current psychiatric diagnoses

Authors/year	Rosenberger et al. 2006 [3]	Kalarchian et al. 2007 [15]	Mauri et al. 2008 [12]	Mühlhans et al. 2009 [5]	Jones-Corneille et al. 2010 [14]	Mitchell et al. (in submission)
Sample size	174	288	282	146	105	199
Axis I diagnosis						
Psychiatric disorder	24.1 %	37.8 %	20.9 %	55.5 %	29.5 %	33.7 %
Affective disorder	10.9 %	15.6 %	6.4 %	31.5 %	14.3 %	11.6 %
Anxiety disorder	11.5 %	24.0 %	12.4 %	15.1 %	16.2 %	18.1 %
Substance use disorder	0.6 %	1.7 %[a]	NA	1.4 %	0.9 %	1.0 %
Alcohol abuse or dependence	0.6 %	0.7 %[a]	NA	0.7 %	NA	0.5 %
Eating disorder	10.3 %	NA	NA	37.7 %	NA	NA
Binge eating disorder	3.4 %	16.0 %	6.7 %	23.3 %	41.9 %	10.1 %
Bulimia nervosa	0.0 %	0.3 %	0.4 %	0.0 %	NA	1.0 %
EDNOS[a]	6.9 %	NA	NA	14.4 %	NA	NA

[a]Eating disorder not otherwise specified

and using structured diagnostic instruments [3, 5, 12–15]. These data are summarized in Tables 2.1 and 2.2. The first, published by Rosenberger et al. in 2006, found lifetime prevalence rates of 22 % for affective disorders and 16 % for anxiety disorders [3]. Mauri and colleagues in 2008 reported lifetime prevalence rates of affective disorders of 22 % and lifetime prevalence rates for any Axis I psychiatric disorder of 38 % [12]. Jones-Corneille and colleagues reported lifetime rates of any psychiatric disorder of 50.5 % [14].

Three of the studies, by Kalarchian et al. [15], Mühlhans et al. [5], and Mitchell et al. [13], used structured diagnostic psychiatric interviews separate from the routine evaluation process, and patients in these series were told that the results would not be shared with the surgical team under most circumstances (unless some particularly dangerous problem was reported such as active suicidal ideation). The results of all of these studies, including the latter three, included sample sizes that have varied considerably, with the number of subjects ranging from 105 to 288. Despite the similarity in methodologies, lifetime prevalence rates of psychiatric disorders still have varied widely, from a low of 36.8 % to a high of 72.6 %. Rates of any affective disorder (22–54.8 %), any anxiety disorder (15.5–37.5 %), and any substance use disorder (1.1–35.7 %) also varied. Relative to current psychiatric diagnoses, as shown in Table 2.1, there also has been considerable variability. Therefore, our best data on the prevalence of such problems have provided highly variable results, probably attributable to some extent to demographic and other differences between the populations studied.

Given the previous discussion about a possible association between obesity and substance use disorders, as well as obesity and eating problems such as binge eating disorder, it is particularly interesting to focus on the data in Tables 2.1 and 2.2 for these conditions. Several of these studies—including two of the three studies where the interviews were done independent of the routine psychological evaluation—found very high rates for a lifetime risk of alcohol abuse and dependence, although rates of such problems at the time of assessment were consistently low. Whether this reflects a desire to withhold information that patients fear might jeopardize their consideration for surgery, or reflect true prevalence rates, is unknown. The rate of binge eating disorder, both current and lifetime history, also was substantial.

Two recent reports of the relationship between preoperative psychopathology and postoperative outcomes are of great interest. Kalarchian and colleagues [16] reported that those with an Axis I disorder prior to surgery, in particular mood and anxiety disorders, experienced smaller weight loss 6 months after surgery. Further reports from this cohort, which continues to be followed, will provide interesting, important data. De Zwaan and colleagues recently reported similar findings, focusing on presurgical depression and long-term outcome [17].

Postsurgery Psychiatric Status

Relative to the impact of bariatric surgery on psychiatric disorders, much of the available literature suggests that rates of psychopathology for many, but not all, patients tend to improve postoperatively and at least in the first few years [18, 19]. Although the data in this regard are inconsistent, and longitudinal data that would be of particular importance are lacking, the available reports do suggest that, in general, improvement in psychopathology is to some extent mitigated over time with the reemergence or development of psychopathology distal to the procedures. Whether this reflects dissatisfaction with the outcome of the procedures over time or eventual weight gain after reaching weight nadir is not clear, but a number of variables clearly might impact on this outcome. Predicting which patients may experience a recrudescence of previously remitted psychopathology will be a critically important contribution to this body of research.

Another variable of considerable interest is the observation that the mortality from suicide may actually increase after bariatric surgery [20, 21]. The reasons for this are unclear, although the available reports suggest that suicide tends to occur in the 1–4-year span after bariatric surgery. Most of the data reported thus far has been cross-sectional, and very little is known about specific factors that may predict an increased risk for the actual occurrence of suicide, which remains a relatively rare event in this population. However, the literature here does suggest a variety of hypothetical reasons why the suicide rate may be increased. One is the persistence or reoccurrence of medical comorbidities after bariatric surgery, which may result in patient disappointment with their outcome. Also the disinhibition and impulsivity secondary to changes in alcohol absorption may be involved, as may the cognitive impairment associated with hypoglycemia, at least on a theoretical basis. Also patients will have a marked diminution in their serum cholesterol level, and in epidemiological studies hypocholesterolemia has been linked to increased risk in suicide, although it is unusual for patients to actually become hypocholesterolemic following these procedures. There is also a variety of changes in various peptidergic systems after bariatric surgery, including ghrelin and glucagon-like peptide-1 (GLP-1). These peptides appear to have active central effects as well, including on cognitive functioning. There has been a particular interest in GLP-1, and it is conceivable that changes in the peptidergic regulation systems are involved in the suicide risk. Of particular interest have been psychosocial issues, including lack of improvement in quality of life in a subgroup of patients, continued or recurrent physical mobility restrictions, continued low self-esteem, as well as continued recurrence of sexual dysfunction and romantic relationship difficulties.

Psychiatric Assessment of Bariatric Candidates

A detailed discussion of the psychiatric assessment of candidates for bariatric surgery can be found in Chap. 5. However, a brief overview is provided here. Most bariatric surgery programs routinely utilize, and many third-party payers require, psychosocial evaluation prior to surgery [22]. While one purpose of such interviews clearly is to examine for evidence of psychopathology, in particular to identify any contraindications to surgery (which is rare), it is important for the evaluator to realize that most patients present for surgery to address their obesity and weight-related health problems and not their psychological functioning. With this in mind, the interview and its results can be useful to the team in not only ruling out contraindications but also in designing a treatment plan that both addresses potential problems and also recognizes the patient's strengths and supports.

While these evaluations can and should include a psychoeducational component, much of the focus is on establishing the prevalence of psychopathology, both current and prior. In particular, there is a need for strong emphasis to establish whether or not the patients may have a form of psychopathology that may increase their risk, or the liability, for not being able to be compliant with proper aftercare. In some cases, such problems may dictate the need for intervention prior to surgery. This is particularly true of patients with severe depression or untreated anxiety problems, as well as for those with active substance abuse or dependency problems.

Patients with a history of trauma, physical or sexual, may be at increased risk for psychopathology but also for problems with coping postoperatively. Thus, these areas should be assessed. It is also important to obtain a detailed history of current and prior mental health treatment including psychotropic medications used.

As part of the assessment, it is important to examine the patient's social support system. Are there people in their environment that can be helpful to the patient as she transitions to her new life? Are there current sources of conflict that should be addressed? What are the current major life stressors and what are the patient's coping skills?

Structured interviews and self-report measures are often used in these evaluations [22, 23]; however, the use of these measures is limited by both time and cost. At minimum, strong consideration should be given in utilizing a well-validated measure of mood and depression such as the Beck Depression Inventory (BDI) or the Patient Health Questionnaire (PHQ). The cutdown, annoyed, guilty, eye-opener (CAGE) questionnaire can be useful in terms of evaluating substance abuse. Another self-report instrument to consider is the Questionnaire of Eating and Weight Patterns (QEWP), which was specifically designed to assess problems with binge eating and includes the criteria for binge eating disorder. When it is permitted, a more detailed and at times more expensive arsenal should be considered, perhaps including the use of Millon Clinical Multi-axial Inventory-3, which has established norms in bariatric surgery populations, and a measure of quality of life, such as the Impact of Weight on Quality of Life-Lite, which is the most widely used obesity-specific quality of life measure. When possible, the use of structured diagnostic interviews such as the Structured Clinical Interview for DSM-IV and the Eating Disorders Examination can be considered, although these are time-consuming and require the use of trained interview personnel. However, the data obtained using such instruments can be extremely useful, and both measures have well-established validity and reliability.

Psychopharmacology Before and After Bariatric Surgery

As mentioned previously, given the high rates of psychopathology in candidates for bariatric surgery and the fact that these problems may persist after surgery, it is clear that psychotropic medications will commonly be used in these patients and will need to be used on an ongoing basis among a subgroup of these patients. The most frequently used medications are the antidepressant drugs. Although many medications that they receive presurgery, including antidiabetic, antihypertensive, and antilipidemic agents, may be discontinued following the procedure as medical comorbidities normalize or improve, antidepressant medication use typically continues. This raises interesting questions concerning the pharmacokinetics of these drugs. In this discussion, we will assume that Roux-en-Y gastric bypass is our model in discussing these pharmacokinetic changes.

Although the amount of data here are limited, the available literature suggests that there are abnormalities, at least in the short term, in the absorption of various psychopharmacological agents after Roux-en-Y gastric bypass. This is not surprising, given that the duodenum is essentially excluded from the alimentary flow and that many of these drugs are absorbed primarily in the duodenum. The drug studies thus far have primarily focused on serotonin reuptake inhibitors. However, other psychotropic agents may be involved as well. Available reports suggest that serotonin reuptake inhibitors may be malabsorbed by at least 50 % during acute administration. There is also a limited amount of data suggesting that over time, this may be compensated for to some extent. The reasons for this are unclear and may relate to adaptive changes in the bowel. For example, we know that certain medications can be absorbed more distally after bariatric surgery. This may be true of antidepressant drugs. There also may be changes in the hypertrophy of villi over time, as well as adaptations in the cytochrome P450 enzyme distributions, and the distribution of transport proteins involved in drug absorption. Given these changes, it is important for clinicians to carefully consider monitoring psychotropic blood levels, particularly antidepressant levels, following surgery and perhaps every 6 months for a period of several years after the procedure. This would be particularly important in patients where there is a concern about a return of depressive symptoms or some other form of psychopathology.

Psychosocial Interventions

Psychosocial interventions can be used either preoperatively or postoperatively. However, the amount of research that has been done in this area is quite small, and therefore many of the reports that have appeared, while clinically informative, are not supported by a great deal of data.

In terms of preparing patients for bariatric surgery, the focus can be on encouraging preoperative weight loss, which has been shown to have benefits in terms of risks associated with the procedure itself, as well as preparing patients for the changes that will be necessitated after surgery. Generally, lifestyle interventions can also be useful, including education about obesity, the process of weight loss, the necessity for implementing a reduced calorie nutritionally balanced eating plan, the physical activity changes that will be necessary, and the self-monitoring that will be required as well. Postoperative programs have also been advocated, and there is some evidence that attendance in support group meeting or other aftercare services may result in increased weight loss and improved quality of life, as well as better overall compliance with other postsurgical recommendations. Postoperative interventions can be conducted in either group or individual formats. These sessions can use established counseling techniques that have been shown to be helpful in long-term weight maintenance. It is important to identify specific problems that develop, such as dietary difficulties, problems with instituting a better plan of exercise, and relationship issues. Also it is useful to focus on coping stress management techniques. Specific eating problems may emerge after bariatric surgery, which are reviewed in Chap. 4. Those include binge eating or "loss of control" eating, grazing, and night eating.

Conclusion

It is now widely recognized that high rates of psychopathology are seen among those with extreme obesity and who present for bariatric surgery, although the nature of this relationship and its directionality remain unclear. It has also been suggested that certain subtypes of obesity should be regarded as an addiction to food—an idea supported by some empirical animal work and phenomenological observations, but still remains controversial. Also, certain forms of psychopathology, in particular binge eating disorder, may impact on outcome, given the aberrant eating patterns involved.

While it is reassuring that some cases of psychopathology remit after surgery, others do not or may later reoccur. There also appears to be an increased risk of suicide after bariatric surgery, perhaps attributable to a variety of reasons, and evidence of malabsorption of certain medications, in particular antidepressants postsurgery, which may impact on the rates of psychopathology. There is also a growing interest in developing psychosocial interventions to improve weight loss and other outcomes after surgery, although this field is still in its infancy.

Question and Answer Section

Questions

1. Possible contributors to depression pre-bariatric surgery include all of the following except:
   A. High rates of depression among the obese in general
   B. Social stigma and discrimination
   C. Mobility problems
   D. Low serum cortisol
2. Premorbid depression among bariatric surgery candidates may be associated with:
   A. Improved weight loss after surgery
   B. Impaired weight loss after surgery
   C. Change in distribution of weight loss on body compartments after surgery
   D. Increased perioperative complication rate

Answers

1. **D.** The first three are all probably important contributors. The obese, however, generally have elevated cortisol serum levels.
2. **B.** Depression generally has been associated with less weight loss, not more, and at least theoretically with increased rates of suicide. There are no firm data on differential weight loss across body compartments according to depression.

Acknowledgments Completion of this article was supported, in part, by National Institutes of Health (NIH) grants:
NIH RO1 DK84979
NIH RO3 AA19573
NIH UO1 DK66471

References

1. Herpertz S, Burgmer R, Stang A, de Zwaan M, Wolf AM, Chen-Stute A, Hulisz T, Jöcket KH, Senf W. Prevalence of mental disorders in normal-weight and obese individuals with and without weight loss treatment in a German urban population. J Psychosom Res. 2006;61:95–103.
2. Petry NM, Barry D, Pietrzak RH, Wagner JA. Overweight and obesity are associated with psychiatric disorders: results from the National Epidemiologic Survey on Alcohol and Related Conditions. Psychosom Med. 2008;70:288–97.
3. Rosenberger PH, Henderson KE, Grilo CM. Psychiatric disorder comorbidity and association with eating disorders in bariatric surgery patients: a cross-sectional study using structured interview-based diagnosis. J Clin Psychiatry. 2006;67:1080–5.
4. Marcus MD, Wildes JE. Obesity: is it a mental disorder? Int J Eat Disord. 2009;42:739–53.
5. Mühlhans B, Horbach T, de Zwaan M. Psychiatric disorders in bariatric surgery candidates: a review of the literature and results of a German pre-bariatric surgery sample. Gen Hosp Psychiatry. 2009;31:414–21.
6. Luppino FS, de Wit LM, Bouvy PF, Stijnen T, Cuijpers P, Penninx BW, Zitman FG. Overweight, obesity and depression: a systematic review and meta-analysis of longitudinal studies. Arch Gen Psychiatry. 2010;67:220–9.
7. Simon GE, Von Korff M, Saunders K, Miglioretti DL, Crane PK, van Belle G, et al. Association between obesity and psychiatric disorders in the US adult population. Arch Gen Psychiatry. 2006;63:824–30.
8. Ziauddeen H, Farooqi IS, Fletcher PC. Obesity and the brain: how convincing is the addiction model? Nat Rev Neurosci. 2012;13:279–86.
9. Allen PJ, Batra P, Geiger BM, Wommack T, Gilhooly C, Pothos EN. Rationale and consequences of reclassifying obesity as an addictive disorder: neurobiology, food environment and social policy perspectives. Physiol Behav. 2012;107:126–37.
10. Avena NM, Gold JA, Kroll C, Gold MS. Further developments in the neurobiology of food and addiction: update on the state of the science. Nutrition. 2012;28:341–3.
11. Mitchell JE, Steffen KJ, de Zwaan M, Ertelt TW, Marino JM, Müller A. Congruence between clinical and research-based psychiatric assessment in bariatric surgical candidates. Surg Obes Relat Dis. 2010;6:628–34.
12. Mauri M, Rucci P, Calderone A, Santini F, Oppo A, Romano A, et al. Axis I and II disorders and quality of life in bariatric surgery candidates. J Clin Psychiatry. 2008;69:295–301.
13. Mitchell JE, Selzer F, Kalarchian MA, Devlin MJ, Strain G, Elder KA, et al. Psychopathology prior to surgery in the Longitudinal Assessment of Bariatric Surgery-3 (LABS-3) Psychosocial Study. Paper presented at The ASMBS meeting, 6/10, Las Vegas.
14. Jones-Corneille J, Wadden TA, Sarwer DB, Faulconbridge LF, Fabricatore AN, Stack RM, et al. Axis I psychopathology in bariatric surgery candidates with and without binge eating disorder: results of structured clinical interviews. Obes Surg. 2010. doi:10.1007/s11695-010-0322-9.
15. Kalarchian MA, Marcus MD, Levine MD, Courcoulas AO, Pilkonis PA, Ringham RM, et al. Psychiatric disorders among bariatric surgery candidates: relationship to obesity and functional health status. Am J Psychiatry. 2007;164:328–34.

16. Kalarchian MA, Marcus MD, Levine MD, Soulakova JN, Courcoulas AO, Wisinski MS. Relationship of psychiatric disorders to 6-month outcomes after gastric bypass. Surg Obes Relat Dis. 2008;4:544–9.
17. de Zwaan M, Enderle J, Wagner S, Mühlhans B, Ditzen B, Gefeller O, et al. Anxiety and depression in bariatric surgery patients: a prospective, follow-up study using structured clinical interviews. J Affect Disord. 2011;133:61–8.
18. Herpertz S, Kielmann R, Wolf AM, Langkafel M, Senf W, Hebebrand J. Does obesity surgery improve psychosocial functioning? A systematic review. Int J Obes Relat Metab Disord. 2003;27:1300–14.
19. Herpertz S, Kielmann R, Wolf AM, Hebebrand J, Senf W. Do psychosocial variables predict weight loss or mental health after obesity surgery? A systematic review. Obes Rev. 2004;12:1554–69.
20. Adams TD, Gress RE, Smith SC, Halverson RC, Simper SC, Rosamond WD, et al. Long-term mortality after gastric bypass surgery. N Engl J Med. 2007;357:753–61.
21. Tindle HA, Omalu B, Courcoulas A, Marcus M, Hammers J, Kuller LH. Risk of suicide after long-term follow-up from bariatric surgery. Am J Med. 2010;123:1036–42.
22. Sogg S. The clinical interview. In: Mitchell JE, de Zwaan M, editors. Psychosocial assessment and treatment of bariatric surgery patients. New York: Routledge; 2012. p. 15–35.
23. Peterson CB, Berg KC, Mitchell JE. Structured interviews and self-report measures. In: Mitchell JE, de Zwaan M, editors. Psychosocial assessment and treatment of bariatric surgery patients. New York: Routledge; 2012. p. 37–60.

Quality of Life

David B. Sarwer, Chanelle T. Bishop-Gilyard, and Ray Carvajal

Chapter Objectives

1. To characterize the impairments in health- and weight-related quality of life in persons with extreme obesity
2. To review the literature on changes in health- and weight-related quality of life in persons who undergo bariatric surgery
3. To discuss the relationship between other aspects of quality of life, such as body image and sexuality, and bariatric surgery

Introduction

The psychological construct of "quality of life" has long been of interest to mental health professionals. Over the past two decades, there has been a growing interest in quality of life because of its relationship to health and chronic disease. A now sizable body of research has investigated the relationship of quality of life to specific health conditions, including obesity and its comorbidities (most frequently type 2 diabetes, hypertension, and osteoarthritis). Other studies have investigated changes in quality of life that occur with weight loss, both the modest weight losses seen with lifestyle modification interventions and the more sizable weight losses seen with bariatric surgery.

Quality of life is a multidimensional construct. It includes a number of elements—the most common of which, when applied to obesity, are health-related and weight-related quality of life. At the same time, the psychological construct of body image is thought to be an important part of quality of life for many individuals. Finally, another important aspect of quality of life for many is sexuality.

Health-Related and Weight-Related Quality of Life

Obesity has been associated with impairments in quality of life in countless studies. Many of these investigations have focused on the relationship between excess body weight and health-related quality of life (HRQOL). HRQOL refers to the burden of suffering and the limitations in physical, vocational, and social functioning associated with illness [1]. HRQOL may be assessed by paper-and-pencil measures, the most common of which is the Medical Outcomes Survey Short-Form 36 (SF-36) [2]. The SF-36 is a standardized self-report measure that assesses eight separate domains of HRQOL including physical functioning, role functioning related to physical and emotional problems, social functioning, bodily pain, general mental health, vitality, and perception of general health. These subscales can be further grouped together to calculate physical health and mental health composite scores.

Numerous studies have shown a correlation between body mass index (BMI) and the degree of impairment in most of the subscales of the SF-36 [3, 4]. More specifically, the degree of obesity is commonly associated with increased physical limitations, bodily pain, and fatigue. The strain of excess weight can impede even the most basic physical func-

D.B. Sarwer, PhD (✉)
Department of Psychiatry, Director of Clinical Services Center for Weight and Eating Disorders, Perelman School of Medicine at the University of Pennsylvania, Philadelphia, PA, USA
e-mail: dsarwer@mail.med.upenn.edu

C.T. Bishop-Gilyard, PsyD, MS
Department of Psychiatry, Center for Weight and Eating Disorders, The University of Pennsylvania, Philadelphia, PA, USA

Perelman School of Medicine at the University of Pennsylvania, Philadelphia, PA, USA
e-mail: chaneltb@mail.med.upenn.edu

R. Carvajal, PsyD
Department of Psychiatry, Center for Weight and Eating Disorders, Perelman School of Medicine at the University of Pennsylvania, 3535 Market St., Suite 3031, Philadelphia, PA 19104, USA
e-mail: carvajar@mail.med.upenn.edu

tions and personal care tasks, including walking, climbing stairs, bathing, toileting, and dressing for some individuals. Impairments in HRQOL also may account for increased symptoms of depression, especially among individuals with extreme obesity. Approximately three-quarters of candidates for bariatric surgery report minimal to mild symptoms of depression as assessed by the Beck Depression Inventory-II [5]. Individuals with extreme obesity are approximately five times more likely to have experienced a major depressive episode in the past year as compared to those of average weight [6]. In addition, the risk of attempted suicide has been found to increase as BMI exceeds 40 kg/m^2 [7]. The increased risk of depression and suicide among persons with extreme obesity may be attributable, in part, to their severe impairment in HRQOL. These difficulties are among the most distressing aspects of extreme obesity and may be among the strongest motivators for seeking bariatric surgery.

There also are a number of disease-specific measures of quality of life that can assess the effects of a single illness, such as obesity. Two of the most commonly used measures in the obesity literature are the Impact of Weight on Quality of Life (IWQOL) scale [8] and its more commonly used short form, the IWQOL-Lite [9]. The IWQOL consists of 74 items designed to assess the effects of weight on eight domains of quality of life, including health, social/interpersonal functioning, work, mobility, self-esteem, sexual life, activities of daily living, and comfort with food. The IWQOL-Lite version contains 31 items and, in addition to a total score, provides sub-scores in physical functioning, self-esteem, sexual life, public distress, and work. This version has been used in number of recent studies of bariatric surgery patients and has demonstrated that impairments in weight-related quality of life are strongly associated with BMI [10, 11].

Improvements in Quality of Life After Bariatric Surgery

Numerous studies have suggested that individuals report improvements in psychosocial functioning with weight reduction [12]. Perhaps the most consistent finding in this area is the association between weight loss (particularly surgically induced weight loss) and quality of life. Following bariatric surgery, individuals report statistically and clinically significant improvements in both health- and weight-related quality of life [13–16]. Many of these improvements occur in the first few months after surgery and during the period of rapid weight loss. For example, in a recent study, bariatric surgery patients reported significant improvements in almost all domains of the SF-36 as early as 20 weeks after surgery and after a weight loss of approximately 25 % of their initial body weight [16]. The Swedish Obese Subjects study similarly reported peak improvements in quality of life within the first few postoperative years [17]. In several of these studies, the magnitude of improvement has been impressively large and with patients, in some studies, reporting a postoperative quality of life comparable to individuals in the general population and who likely never experienced the physical and emotional toll of extreme obesity.

In contrast, at least two studies suggest that improvements in HRQOL postoperatively may be restricted to specific domains. Although patients experienced normal levels of psychological and social quality of life 1–3 years following surgery, one study [18] found that patients' physical functioning, general health, and vitality remained below population norms. Likewise, using the SF-36, Horchner and colleagues' results indicated that only general health perceptions, bodily pain, and mental health significantly improved 2 years postoperatively [19]. Thus, these two studies contrast the broad improvements in HRQOL found in most other research. Horchner and colleagues postulate that more general measures of HRQOL, such as the SF-36, may be inadequate measures of HRQOL in persons with extreme obesity [19]. Supporting this hypothesis, a review of 34 randomized control trials concluded that obesity-specific measures are more likely to demonstrate increases in HRQOL following weight loss than generic measures [20].

Improvements in quality of life appear to be well maintained for the first few postoperative years and are superior to improvements experienced by individuals who lose weight with lifestyle modification or pharmacotherapy. Nevertheless, individuals who experience improvements in physical discomfort and quality of life are likely to be able to engage in more physical activity (see Chap. 3) as well as experience improvements in work-related activities and occupational functioning. Two reviews have concluded that patients report improvements in job status, performance, and satisfaction postoperatively [21, 22]. These findings, coupled with recent research that has shown improvements in some domains of cognitive functioning following substantial weight loss (see Chap. 15), suggest that surgically induced weight loss (along with its concurrent improvements in areas such as sleep quality) may have a significant impact on both work performance and work-related quality of life that was underappreciated by both patients and providers a decade ago.

Improvements in weight-related quality of life also have been documented, with studies using these instruments showing essentially similar patterns of results to those investigations that focused on HRQOL. For example, Kolotkin and colleagues found that gastric bypass patients reported significant improvements in weight-related quality of life domains as compared to individuals with obesity who did not undergo surgery [23]. Sarwer and colleagues also found significant improvements in weight-related quality of life following gastric bypass [16]. Like HRQOL, patients reported statistically significant improvements in weight-related quality of life as early as 20 weeks after surgery and significantly improved (compared to preoperative levels) into the second postoperative year. These improvements were correlated with the postoperative weight loss.

In summary, it appears that health- and weight-related quality of life improves following weight loss. When individuals with extreme obesity and those who present for and undergo bariatric surgery are considered, the relationship appears to be somewhat more complex. While many areas of HRQOL appear to improve with the larger weight losses seen with bariatric surgery, other domains appear to be less likely to change. This may be a function of some of the physical limitations that some individuals may continue to experience even following a substantial weight loss. In contrast, studies that have assessed weight-related quality of life have almost uniformly found significant and sustained improvements following bariatric surgery.

Other Domains of Quality of Life

Body Image

The psychological construct of "body image" has been of interest to scholars for much of the past century. While a definition of body image may seem intuitive, the nature of the construct makes articulation of a specific, user-friendly definition more difficult. One of the most concise definitions suggests that body image consists of perceptions, thoughts, and feelings associated with the body and bodily experience [24]. While this definition describes the multidimensional nature of the construct, it does not highlight body image behaviors, such as motivations for changing one's appearance through weight loss. Recently, Cash and Smolak have described body image as "the psychological experience of embodiment" [25]. This description conveys a sense of importance of the role of body image in larger psychological constructs like quality of life.

Theoretical development and empirical research on body image has grown exponentially in the past two decades. This scholarship has solidified body image as an important area of quality of life and psychosocial functioning. A great deal of the previous work on body image has been focused on the weight and shape concerns of individuals with eating disorders. As research into the worldwide obesity problem matured in the 1990s, the body image concerns of overweight and obese individuals garnered more attention [26]. Body image concerns can be both global and specific. A number of studies have suggested that body image dissatisfaction is associated with degree of excess body weight (e.g., Sarwer et al. [27]; Sarwer et al. [28]; Latner [29]). However, the strength of this relationship is modest. This finding is consistent with theories of body image, which have suggested that there may be little relationship between what one thinks about the body and the objective reality of one's appearance [25].

At the same time, many individuals report some specific concerns with their appearance. For example, in a sample of 79 obese women, almost half (47 %) reported that they were most dissatisfied with their waist and abdomen, whereas only 10 % reported dissatisfaction with their overall body [27]. Forty-two percent of average weight women also indicated that they were most dissatisfied with their waist and abdomen, suggesting that dissatisfaction with the waistline may be independent of actual body weight. In general and not surprisingly, women are typically far more dissatisfied with their body image than men [30]. Differences also exist across ethnic groups. African-American women, as compared to Caucasian women, typically report less body image dissatisfaction [28]. Interestingly, however, Cox and colleagues found body image to be a partial mediator between BMI and weight-specific quality of life among black women [31]. Among other ethnic groups, body image dissatisfaction appears to be related to the degree of acculturation into more Westernized lifestyles [32].

Regardless of ethnicity or acculturation, some degree of body image dissatisfaction appears to be "normative" in Western society and likely results from society's pervasive emphasis on thinness as the ideal. This dissatisfaction is believed to motivate a number of appearance-enhancing behaviors, including both surgical and nonsurgical weight loss treatment. A small number of individuals, however, report an excessive degree of dissatisfaction with their weight and shape, which may negatively impact behavior and, in some cases, may be a symptom of more significant psychological distress that goes beyond the "norm." For example, a significantly greater percentage of women with obesity, as compared to women without obesity, reported, on more than half of the days of the month, camouflaging their obesity with clothing, changing their posture or body movements, avoiding looking at their bodies, and becoming upset when thinking about their appearance [27]. Similarly, a greater percentage of women with obesity also reported moderate to extreme embarrassment in social situations, such as work or parties, because of their weight [27]. Other studies have found a relationship between decreased body image satisfaction, low self-esteem, and increased self-reported depressive symptoms in obese women [27, 33, 34].

Numerous studies have reported that weight loss after bariatric surgery is associated with marked improvements in body image [4, 8, 9, 12, 26, 35]. A recent study examining changes in quality of life and body image in patients who underwent gastric bypass surgery found significant improvements in body image within the first 2 years of surgery [10]. This study also reported a relationship between percent weight loss and improvements in body image quality of life (as assessed by the Body Image Quality of Life Inventory), but not on scores on the Body Shape Questionnaire (BSQ). Though one might expect agreement between these two measures, the results may indicate that larger weight losses are associated with improvements in quality of life domains, but not with general weight and shape concerns (as measured on the BSQ).

These results also may help to explain anecdotal reports that some patients express dissatisfaction with their bodies after losing massive weight through surgery. This dissatisfaction typically is attributed to excess, loose skin of the abdomen, thighs, and arms [26, 36]. In 2012, approximately 55,000 Americans underwent plastic surgical procedures following a massive weight loss typically associated with bariatric surgery [37]. The most common of these procedures is breast reduction surgery, although plastic surgeons can perform procedures on most areas of the body to improve their appearance following weight reduction. Although little research has examined the influence of these body-contouring procedures on the bariatric patient specifically, a more general body of literature suggests that plastic surgery patients experience significant improvements in their body image postoperatively [36, 38]. Unfortunately, these procedures are rarely covered by third-party payers and, as a result, can become cost prohibitive for many individuals.

Sexual Function

Recently, two reviews have detailed the relationship between obesity and sexual functioning [39, 40]. Both concluded that obesity appears to have a detrimental impact on sexual functioning. Problems in functioning appear to be more common in women than men. Women struggling with obesity often report reductions in sexual desire as well as difficulty with other aspects of the sexual response cycle. While some of these difficulties may be attributed to psychosocial causes, such as body image dissatisfaction, others may be attributed to weight-related comorbidities, such as type 2 diabetes or hypertension. These conditions, and their treatments, can profoundly impact sexual functioning in women and men. Both conditions likely account for the majority of cases of erectile dysfunction, the most common sexual dysfunction in men.

Problems in sexual functioning are highly prevalent in the general population and are associated with both impaired mood and lower quality of life [41]. The relationship between obesity and sexual functioning is complex, and a comprehensive discussion requires consideration of reproductive hormones and weight-related comorbidities [40]. The discussion here will focus more specifically on the relationship between quality of life and other psychosocial factors, and marital and sexual relationships.

Quality of life, body image, and sexual functioning are intricately related constructs [42]. Intuitively, it is easy to imagine how an individual with obesity, dissatisfied with his or her body image, would be reluctant to engage in sexual behavior. Similarly, physical limitations associated with extreme obesity may make sexual activity unpleasant, difficult, painful, or even impossible. Nevertheless, it is important to realize that sexual dysfunction, while often characterized as a condition of an individual, occurs in the context of a relationship. That is, other problems or issues in a romantic relationship can contribute to the development and maintenance of a sexual dysfunction, just as the presence of dysfunctional sexual behavior can negatively impact the quality of a romantic relationship.

There likely are other psychosocial contributors to the relationship between obesity and impaired sexual functioning. Depression, for example, also may contribute to sexual dysfunction. As detailed in Chaps. 1 and 2, increased symptoms of depression, as well as formal diagnoses of depression, are related to BMI. Independent of obesity, there is a strong relationship between depression and sexual dysfunction in men as well as women, although, as will be discussed later, body weight, mood, and sexual function are intertwined for some individuals [43–45].

A relatively modest body of research has looked at changes in sexual functioning following weight reduction [39, 40]. Most of these studies have been conducted on individuals with a weight-related comorbidity. Men with hypertension, and who lost weight through a lifestyle modification program, experienced significant improvements in both self-report and physiologic measures of sexual function as compared to men treated with a beta-blocker (propranolol) or central alpha agonist (clonidine) [46]. Other studies with hypertensive patients have similarly shown improvements in sexual function following weight reduction or increased physical activity [47]. Men with obesity, but free of major weight-related comorbidities, have been able to lose approximately 15 kg of weight in a behavioral modification program and experience significant improvements in erectile functioning [48].

Only a small number of studies that have looked at changes in sexual functioning in persons who undergo bariatric surgery have been published to date. Ninety-seven men who underwent gastric bypass reported improvements in all domains of sexual functioning within the first few postoperative years [49]. The amount of weight loss was associated with the degree of improvement in sexual functioning. In a study of women who underwent bariatric surgery, female sexual dysfunction (diagnosed before surgery) resolved in 68 % of women, and women reported statistically significant improvements in sexual functioning after surgery in all areas [50, 51].

Conclusions

A sizable body of research confirms the intuitive thought of most professionals who work in the area of bariatric surgery—extreme obesity is associated with substantial and significant impairments in quality of life. Excessive body weight can limit physical functioning and also contributes to numerous comorbidities that can further erode health and quality of life. At the same time, the psychosocial burden of extreme obesity cannot be underestimated. These relationships underscore the necessity of seeing quality of life as multidimensional, an umbrella-like term that encompasses both health-related and weight-related quality of life.

At the same time, body image and sexual functioning are central aspects of quality of life for many individuals. Not surprisingly, those affected with extreme obesity report heightened levels of body image dissatisfaction. They also report impairments in sexual functioning. The potential mechanisms for these impairments in sexual functioning can be hard to pinpoint. Some impairments in sexual behavior may be the result of body image dissatisfaction, while others may be the result of obesity-related comorbidities, like type 2 diabetes and hypertension, and their treatments.

Encouragingly, studies have suggested that even a modest weight loss is associated with improvement in quality of life, as well as body image and sexual functioning. The magnitude of these improvements often appears to be associated with the size of the weight loss. Many studies have documented the improvements in health- and weight-related quality of life that occur after bariatric surgery. At present, fewer studies have documented changes in body image and sexual functioning after the larger weight losses seen with surgery. However, these studies suggest that these important areas of quality of life also improve following bariatric surgery.

Question and Answer Section

Questions

1. Extreme obesity is associated with all of the following, except:
   A. Health-related quality of life
   B. Weight-related quality of life
   C. Body image dissatisfaction
   D. Sexual orientation
2. In contrast to other areas of quality of life, relatively few studies have demonstrated a relationship between the massive weight loss seen with bariatric surgery and:
   A. Weight-related quality of life
   B. Body image
   C. Marital satisfaction
   D. Sexual functioning

Answers

1. **D**. Extreme obesity is associated with sexual dysfunction, not sexual orientation.
2. **C**. Relatively few studies have shown that marital satisfaction improves following bariatric surgery. Well-developed bodies of research have shown that bariatric surgery is associated with improvements in weight-related quality of life, body image, and sexual functioning.

Conflict of Interest Statement Dr. Sarwer discloses that he currently receives grant support from:

The American Society of Metabolic and Bariatric Surgery ("Improvements in Reproductive Status Following Bariatric Surgery")

National Institutes of Health (RC1-DK086132 "Lifestyle Modification Versus Bariatric Surgery for Type 2 Diabetes"; R01-DK072452-01 "Changes in Sexual Function Following Bariatric Surgery"; and R01-DK080738 "Dietary Intake and Eating Behavior in Adolescents Who Undergo Bariatric Surgery")

He discloses that he is a consultant with Allergan, BariMD, BaroNova, EnteroMedics, and Ethicon Endo-Surgery and Galderma. These relationships have had no influence on the material in this paper.

References

1. Wadden TA, Phelan S. Assessment of quality of life in obese individuals. Obes Res. 2002;10S:50S–7.
2. Ware JE, Snow KK, Kosinski M, Gandek B. SF-36 Health survey: manual and interpretation guide. Boston: The Health Institute; 1993.
3. Fontaine KR, Barofsky I. Obesity and health-related quality of life. Obes Rev. 2001;2:173–82.
4. Kolotkin RL, Meter K, Williams GR. Quality of life and obesity. Obes Rev. 2001;2:219–29.
5. Sarwer DB, Faulconbridge LF, Mitchell JE, Steffen KJ, Roerig JL. The management of mood disorders with anti-depressant medications after bariatric surgery. Curr Psychiatr. (in press).
6. Onyike CU, Crum RM, Lee HB, Lyketsos CG, Eaton WW. Is obesity associated with major depression? Results from the Third National Health and Nutrition Examination Survey. Am J Epidemiol. 2003;158(12):1139–47.
7. Dong C, Li W-D, Li D, Price RA. Extreme obesity is associated with attempted suicides: results from a family study. Int J Obes. 2006;30:388–90.
8. Kolotkin RL, Head S, Hamilton M, Tse CK. Assessing the impact of weight on quality of life. Obes Res. 1995;3:49–56.
9. Kolotkin RL, Crosby RD, Kosloski KD, Williams GR. Development of a brief measure to assess quality of life in obesity. Obes Res. 2001;9:102–11.
10. Boan J, Kolotkin RL, Westman EC, McMahon RL, Grant JP. Binge eating, quality of life and physical activity improve after Roux-en-Y gastric bypass for morbid obesity. Obes Surg. 2004;14(3):341–8.
11. Dymek MP, Le Grange D, Neven K, Alverdy J. Quality of life after gastric bypass surgery: a cross-sectional study. Obes Res. 2002;10:1135–42.
12. Sarwer DB, Wadden TA, Fabricatore AN. Psychosocial and behavioral aspects of bariatric surgery. Obes Res. 2005;13:639–48.
13. Pilone V, Mozzi E, Schettino AM, Furbetta F, Di Maro A, Giardiello C, Italian Group for Lap-Band, et al. Improvement in health-related quality of life in first year after laparoscopic adjustable gastric banding. Surg Obes Relat Dis. 2012;8(3):260–8.

14. Lier HO, Biringer E, Hove O, Stubhaug B, Tangen T. Quality of life among patients undergoing bariatric surgery: associations with mental health- a 1 year follow-up study of bariatric surgery patients. Health Qual Life Outcomes. 2011;9:79.
15. Kolotkin RL, Crosby RD, Gress RE, Hunt SC, Adams TD. Two-year changes in health-related quality of life in gastric bypass patients compared with severely obese controls. Surg Obes Relat Dis. 2009;5:250–6.
16. Sarwer DB, Wadden TA, Moore RH, Eisenberg MH, Raper SE, Williams NN. Changes in quality of life and body image after gastric bypass surgery. Surg Obes Relat Dis. 2010;6(6):608–14.
17. Sjöström L, Lindroos AK, Peltonen M, Torgerson J, Bouchard C, Carlsson B, et al. Lifestyle, diabetes, and cardiovascular risk factors 10 years after bariatric surgery. N Engl J Med. 2004;351(26):2683–93.
18. Schok M, Greenen R, van Antwerpen T, de Wit P, Brand N, van Ramshorst B. Quality of life after laparoscopic adjustable gastric banding for severe obesity: postoperative and retrospective preoperative evaluations. Obes Surg. 2000;10(6):502–8.
19. Horchner R, Tuinebreijer W, Kelder H. Quality-of-life assessment of morbidly obese patients who have undergone a lap-band operation: 2 year follow-up study. Is the MOS SF-36 a useful instrument to measure quality of life in morbidly obese patients? Obes Surg. 2001;11(2):212–8.
20. Maciejewski ML, Patrick DL, Williamson DF. A structured review of randomized controlled trials of weight loss showed little improvement in health-related quality of life. J Clin Epidemiol. 2005;58(6):568–78.
21. Bocchieri LE, Meana M, Fisher BL. A review of psychosocial outcomes of surgery for morbid obesity. J Psychosom Res. 2002;52:155–65.
22. Herpertz S, Kielmann R, Wolf AM, Langkafel M, Senf W, Hebebrand J. Does obesity surgery improve psychosocial functioning? A systematic review. Int J Obes Relat Metab Disord. 2003;27(11):1300–14.
23. Kolotkin RL, Davidson LE, Crosby RD, Hunt SC, Adams TD. Six-year changes in health-related quality of life in gastric bypass patients versus obese comparison groups. Surg Obes Relat Dis. 2012;8:625–33.
24. Cash TF, Pruzinsky T, editors. Body images: development, deviance, and change. New York: The Guilford Press; 1990.
25. Cash TF, Smolak L, editors. Body image handbook: a handbook of science, practice and prevention. 2nd ed. New York: The Guilford Press; 2011.
26. Sarwer DB, Thompson JK, Cash TF. Body image and obesity in adulthood. Psychiatr Clin N Am. 2005;28(1):68–87.
27. Sarwer DB, Wadden TA, Foster GD. Assessment of body image dissatisfaction in obese women: specificity, severity, and clinical significance. J Consult Clin Psychol. 1998;66(4):651–4.
28. Sarwer DB, Dilks RJ, Spitzer JC. Weight loss and changes in body image. In: Cash TF, Smolak L, editors. Body image: a handbook of science, practice and prevention. 2nd ed. New York: The Guilford Press; 2011. p. 369–93.
29. Latner JD. Body weight and body image in adults. In: Cash TF, editor. Encyclopedia of body image and human appearance. New York: Elsevier; 2012. p. 264–9.
30. Schwartz MB, Brownell KD. Obesity and body image. Body Image. 2004;1:43–56.
31. Cox TL, Ard JD, Beasley TM, Fernandez JR, Howard VJ, Affuso O. Body image as a mediator of the relationship between body mass index and weight-related quality of life in black women. J Womens Health. 2011;20(10):1573–8.
32. Soh NL, Touyz SW, Surgenor LJ. Eating and body image disturbances across cultures: a review. Eur Eat Disord Rev. 2006;14:54–65.
33. Foster GD, Wadden TA, Vogt RA. Body image in obese women before, during, and after weight loss treatment. Health Psychol. 1997;16(3):226–9.
34. Grilo CM, Wilfley DE, Brownell KD, Rodin J. Teasing, body image, and self-esteem in a clinical sample of obese women. Addict Behav. 1994;19(4):443–50.
35. Fabricatore AN, Wadden TA, Sarwer DB, Faith MS. Health-related quality of life and symptoms of depression in extremely obese persons seeking bariatric surgery. Obes Surg. 2005;15:304–9.
36. Sarwer DB, Didie ER, Gibbons LM. Cosmetic surgery of the body. In: Sarwer DB, Pruzinsky T, Cash TF, Goldwyn RM, Persing JA, Whitaker LA, editors. Psychological aspects of reconstructive and cosmetic plastic surgery: clinical, empirical, and ethical perspectives. Philadelphia: Lippincott Williams & Wilkins; 2006. p. 251–66.
37. American Society of Plastic Surgeons. American Society of Plastic Surgeons 2011 plastic surgery statistics report. Arlington Heights: ASPS; 2012.
38. Sarwer DB, Wadden TA, Pertschuk MJ, Whitaker LA. The psychology of cosmetic surgery: a review and reconceptualization. Clin Psychol Rev. 1998;18:1–22.
39. Kolotkin RL, Zunker C, Ostbye T. Sexual functioning and obesity: a review. Obesity (Silver Spring). 2012;20(12):2325–33. doi:10.1038/oby.2012.104. Epub 2012 Apr 23.
40. Sarwer DB, Lavery M, Spitzer JC. A review of the relationships between extreme obesity, quality of life, and sexual function. Obes Surg. 2012;22(4):668–76.
41. Laumann EO, Paik A, Rosen RC. Sexual dysfunction in the United States: prevalence and predictors. JAMA. 1999;281:537–44.
42. Widerman M. Body image and sexual functioning. In: Cash TF, editor. Encyclopedia of body image and human appearance. New York: Elsevier; 2012. p. 148–52.
43. Rizvi SJ, Kennedy SH, Ravindran LN, Giacobbe P, Eisfeld BS, Mancini D, et al. The relationship between testosterone and sexual function in depressed and healthy men. J Sex Med. 2010;7(2):816–25.
44. McCabe M, Althof SE, Assalian P, Chevret-Measson M, Leiblum SR, Simonelli C. Psychological and interpersonal dimensions of sexual function and dysfunction. J Sex Med. 2010;7(1):4279–36.
45. Clayton AH. Sexual dysfunction related to depression and antidepressant medications. Curr Womens Health Rep. 2010;2(3):182–7.
46. Kostis JB, Rosen RC, Brondolo E, Taska L, Smith DE, Wilson AC. Superiority of nonpharmacological therapy compared to propranolol and placebo in men with mild hypertension: a randomized, prospective trial. Am Heart J. 1992;123:466–74.
47. Rosen RC, Kostis JB, Brondolo E. Nondrug treatment approaches for hypertension. Clin Geriatr Med. 1989;5:791–803.
48. Esposito K, Giugliano F, Di Palo C, Giugliano G, Marfella R, D'Andrea F, et al. Effect of lifestyle changes on erectile dysfunction in obese men: a randomized controlled trial. JAMA. 2004;291(24):2978–84.
49. Dallal RM, Chernoff A, O'Leary MP, Smith JA, Braverman JD, Quebbemann BB. Sexual dysfunction is common in the morbidly obese male and improves after gastric bypass surgery. J Am Coll Surg. 2008;207(6):859–64.
50. Bond DS, Vithiananthan S, Leahey TM, Thomas JG, Sax HC, Pohl D, et al. Prevalence and degree of sexual dysfunction in a sample of women seeking bariatric surgery. Surg Obes Relat Dis. 2009;5(6):698–704. Epub 2009 Jul 24.
51. Bond DS, Wing RR, Vithiananthan S, Sax HC, Roye GD, Ryder BA, et al. Significant resolution of female sexual dysfunction after bariatric surgery. Surg Obes Relat Dis. 2011;7(1):1–7. Epub 2010 Jun 4.

Eating Disorders and Eating Behavior Pre- and Post-bariatric Surgery

Martina de Zwaan and James E. Mitchell

Chapter Objectives

1. To present an overview of various types of eating pathology prior to bariatric surgery
2. To present the course of eating pathology after bariatric surgery
3. To discuss the implications of eating pathology for bariatric surgery outcome

Introduction

For the past three decades, research has examined bariatric surgery patients and sought to determine the prevalence of eating pathology and eating-related problems both before and after surgery. This chapter will describe and discuss eating disorders and eating problems in both pre- and post-bariatric surgery patients. The assessment of eating disorders has been recommended as a routine part of preoperative evaluation of candidates for bariatric surgery.

Eating Pathology Prior to Bariatric Surgery

The current literature suggests that individuals with extreme obesity who seek bariatric surgery are likely to exhibit eating pathology such as binge eating, night eating, emotional eating, sweet eating, or grazing. Even though one might assume that all persons with severe obesity will have some kind of pathological eating behavior or problematic eating styles, studies on the prevalence of formal eating disorders do not support this clinical impression.

Binge Eating

Binge eating disorder (BED) has been included in the and Statistical Manual of Mental Disorders (DSM-5). BED is defined by recurrent binge eating episodes that occur, in contrast with those in bulimia nervosa (BN), in the absence of inappropriate weight control behaviors (e.g., purging). A series of characteristics are associated with binge eating, such as rapid consumption of food, eating until uncomfortably full, and marked distress regarding the behavior. For a BED diagnosis, binge eating episodes must have occurred at least once a week over a time period of 3 months. The loss of control item distinguishes those with binge eating from patients who eat very large amounts of food at a meal because they believe that they are genuinely hungry for excessive portion sizes. Binge eating frequently serves an affect regulation function. BED is the most prevalent eating disorder affecting 2–5 % in the general population. Bulimia nervosa, which involves binge eating and the engagement of inappropriate compensatory behaviors such as self-induced vomiting, overuse of laxatives, or excessive exercise, occurs less frequently in both the general population and among candidates for bariatric surgery [1].

The median frequency of current binge eating disorder (BED) in bariatric surgery candidates is approximately 20 %, which is definitely higher than can be expected in the general population [2, 3]. The prevalence rates of BED in the different studies vary widely (from 2 % to 50 %) depending on the time of assessment (prospectively or retrospectively) and on the instruments used to assess its presence. Overall, BED does appear to be a substantial problem in many patients who will be undergoing bariatric surgery. In addition, it must be

M. de Zwaan, MD (✉)
Department of Psychosomatic Medicine and Psychotherapy, Hannover Medical School, Carl-Neuberg-Strasse 1, Hanover, Lower Saxony 30625, Germany
e-mail: deZwaan.Martina@mh-hannover.de

J.E. Mitchell, MD
Neuropsychiatric Research Institute, University of North Dakota School of Medicine and Health Sciences, 1208th St. South, Fargo, ND 58102, USA
e-mail: mitchell@medicine.nodak.edu

remembered that some patients may minimize their eating problems prior to surgery out of concern that the bariatric team will find the behavior particularly problematic and recommend against proceeding with surgery.

Earlier studies assessed binge eating or BED using self-report instruments or diagnosed BED retrospectively. Both approaches have significant limitations. More recent studies applied more sophisticated methodology, e.g., the Eating Disorder Examination Interview (EDE), which is considered the reference standard for the assessment of aberrant eating behaviors. The EDE assesses the core features of all formal eating disorders and allows the calculation of four subscale scores: dietary restraint, eating concerns, weight concerns, and shape concerns. The dietary restraint subscale pertains to conscious efforts to limit food intake for shape and weight reasons. The three other subscales reflect dysfunctional attitudes regarding eating and overvalued ideas regarding weight and shape. However, the interview is lengthy and probably is not feasible for routine clinical practice. There is a questionnaire version (EDE-Q) available. Alternatively, the Eating Inventory (EI) can be applied to assess the degree of cognitive restraint, the tendency to lose control over food intake (disinhibition), and physical and psychological sensations of hunger.

Not surprisingly, binge eating is associated with increased eating-related and general psychopathology. Bariatric surgery candidates with BED have been shown to exhibit higher rates of depression, anxiety, and alcohol abuse. They have higher scores on ratings assessing disinhibition of eating and perceived hunger as well as greater dissatisfaction with weight and shape compared to bariatric surgery candidates without BED. Finally, BED appears to have a pronounced impact on important dimensions of health-related quality of life that exceeds the impact of obesity per se. This is important to consider since there is evidence that patients with more than two mental disorders might have a less favorable bariatric surgery outcome compared to patients with one or no psychiatric diagnoses [4].

A number of research groups have studied whether binge eating and full syndromal BED might represent a relative contraindication, or predict a poorer outcome, in persons who undergo different bariatric procedures. The results with regard to binge eating and binge eating disorder (BED) as predictors for postsurgery weight loss are somewhat mixed. While some studies have found that preoperative binge eating predicts poorer weight loss, other studies have suggested that binge eating is not associated with smaller weight losses (e.g., White et al. [5], de Zwaan et al. [6], Wadden et al. [7], Livhits et al. [8]) (Table 4.1). This appears to be true for short- and medium-term follow-up durations as well as for long-term follow-ups of up to 5–6 years [4, 9].

In summary, there is a lack of conclusive evidence that binge eating behavior that is present presurgery is a strong predictor for attenuated weight loss or weight regain after surgery independent of the kind of surgical procedure applied. As a result, there currently is a lack of consensus as to how to manage these patients. Psychological interventions for bariatric surgery patients, including some that address binge eating, have been described. There is some evidence that responders to brief preoperative treatment for binge eating behavior might have better short-term postsurgical weight loss outcomes [10]; however, controlled trials are needed. More importantly, patients should be monitored for recurrence of disordered eating patterns after the operation.

Night Eating

The night eating syndrome (NES) is characterized by morning anorexia, evening hyperphagia, and sleep difficulty and more recently by recurrent awakenings from sleep to eat (nocturnal eating [11]). These core symptoms must be accompanied by an awareness of the behaviors such that the patient does not have amnesia for the event and there must also be some impairment associated with the behavior. In contrast to binge eating disorder (BED), NES lacks the defining characteristics of a binge. NES is listed as a Feeding and Eating Disorder Not Elsewhere Classified in the DSM-5. A number of studies have reported relatively high rates of NES in bariatric surgery patients ranging between 8 and 26 %. In addition, NES appears to be associated with higher rates of depression and lower self-esteem (see de Zwaan [12]).

Grazing

Another eating behavior that is frequently considered in bariatric patients is "grazing." While the term is commonly used in both clinical practice and the scientific literature, it is ill defined. There is a clear overlap with the terms "nibbling," "picking," or "frequent snacking throughout the day." The term "grazing" has been used to describe "eating smaller quantities of food continuously throughout the day with accompanying feelings of loss of control" [13]. It also has been described as "permanent eating." The lack of valid and reliable instruments to diagnose grazing remains problematic, but there is evidence that 30–60 % of surgery candidates report the behavior [3]. Nevertheless, in clinical practice, it may be difficult to differentiate between "grazing" or "permanent eating" and individuals who are following the recommendation of the bariatric program to eat five to six smaller meals on a regular schedule and throughout the day (see Chap. 13).

Table 4.1 Influence of binge eating behavior pre- and postsurgery on weight loss/regain postsurgery

Authors	Sample size (completer)	Surgical procedure	Duration of follow-up	Assessment instruments	Pre-BE/BED/EE/grazing predicts weight loss/regain	Post-BE/BED/LOC eating correlates with weight loss/regain
Rowston et al. (1992)	16	BPD, Gazet	2 years	BITE, clinical interview	–	Yes
Pekkarinen et al. (1994)	27	VBG	5.4 years	BES, BITE	–	Yes
Busetto et al. (1996)	80	GBP	12 months	Clinical interview	No	–
Hsu et al. (1996)	24	VBG	3.5 years	EDE	No	Yes
Hsu et al. (1997)	27	GBP	21 months	EDE	Yes	–
Powers et al. (1999)	72	Restriction	5.5 years	EDQ, BES, EAT	No	–
Dymek et al. (2001)	32	GBP	6 months	QEWP, EI, BES	Yes	–
Mitchell et al. (2001)	78	GBP	14 years	M-FED, QEWP	–	Yes
Busetto et al. (2002)	260	Banding	3 years	Clinical interview	No	–
Kalarchian et al. (2002)	99	GBP	2–7 years	EDE-Q, EI	–	Yes
Sabbioni et al. (2002)	82	VBG	2 years	1 question clinical interview	No	–
Guisado and Vaz (2003)	140	VBG	18 months	BES, EI	–	Yes
Boan et al. (2004)	40	GBP	6 months	EI, BES	No	–
Green et al. (2004)	65	GBP	6 months	SCID, QEWP	Yes	–
Larsen et al. (2006)	157	Banding	>2 years	BES, EDE, DEBQ	–	Yes
Burgmer et al. (2005)	118	Banding	>1 year	EI, SIAB	No	–
Busetto et al. (2005) [17]	379	Banding	5 years	Clinical interview	No	–
Malone and Alger-Mayer (2004)	109	GBP	1 year	BES	No	–
Kinzl et al. (2006) [4]	140	Banding	30–84 months	Clinical interview	No	–
Bocchieri-Ricciardi et al. (2006)	72	GBP	18 months	QEWP	No	–
White et al. (2006)	139	GBP	1 year	EDE-Q	No	–
Sallet et al. (2007)	216	GBP	2 years	Clinical interview	Yes	–
Scholtz et al. (2007)	29	Banding	5 years	EDE-I	–	Yes
Kalarchian et al. (2008)	207	GBP	6 months		No	–
Colles et al. (2008) [15]	129	Banding	1 year	QEWP clinical interview	No	Yes
Fujiko et al. (2008)	118	GBP	2 years	1 question self-report	No	–
Toussi et al. (2009) [20]	67	GBP	2 years	Clinical interview	Yes	–
Alger-Mayer et al. (2009) [9]	20	GBP	6 years	BES	No	–
Gorin and Raftopoulos (2009) [19]	196	GBP	6 months	Clinical interview	No	–
White et al. (2010) [5]	361	GBP	1 and 2 years	EDE, LOC eating	No	Yes
de Zwaan et al. (2010) [6]	59	GBP	2 years	EDE-I (BSV)	No	Yes
Kofman et al. (2010) [16]	497	GBP	3–10 years (4.2 years)	Modified QEWP Internet survey	–	Yes
Crowley et al. (2011)	48	GBP	6 months	IBES	Yes	–
Wadden et al. (2011) [7]	95	GBP, banding	1 year	QEWP, EDE-I	No	No
Legenbauer et al. (2011)	151	Banding	1 and 4 years	SIAB	No	–
De Man Lapidoth et al. (2011)	173	–	3 years	–	No	No
Crowley et al. (2011)	48	GBP	6 months	IBES	Yes	–
Wood and Ogden (2012)	49	Banding	3–6 months	Questionnaires	No	No
Brunault et al. (2012)	34	Sleeve	1 year	BITE	Yes	–

BES Binge Eating Scale, *BITE* Bulimic Inventory Test, Edinburgh, *DEBQ* Dutch Eating Behavior Questionnaire, *EAT* Eating Attitude Test, *EDE* (Q or I) (BSV) Eating Disorder Examination (Questionnaire or Interview) (Bariatric Surgery Version), *EI* Eating Inventory, *EDI* Eating Disorder Inventory, *EDQ* Eating Disorder Questionnaire, *IBES* Inventory of Binge Eating Situations (number of triggers for binge eating), *QEWP* Questionnaire on Eating and Weight Patterns, *SIAB* Structured Interview for Anorexia and Bulimia, *banding* gastric banding, *BE* binge eating, *BED* binge eating disorder, *BPD Gazet* biliopancreatic diversion with partial gastrectomy, *EE* emotional eating, *GBP* gastric bypass, *LOC eating* loss of control eating, *restriction* restrictive type surgery, *sleeve* sleeve gastrectomy, *VBG* vertical banded gastroplasty

Sweet Eating

Another behavior of clinical and research interest has been the eating of sweets. As with grazing, there are no validated diagnostic instruments to specifically assess the consumption of sweets, although the percentage of calories from sweets can be determined through 24 food recalls. Sweet eating is usually defined as "overeating of high-caloric sweet foods." It has been suggested that high-sugar foods, such as chocolate, can be potent reinforcers and be used, by some individuals, as a coping strategy for emotional distress. Engagement in this behavior for a period of years, and even short of the volume necessary to meet diagnostic criteria for BED, likely contributes to the development of obesity.

Summary

Binge eating, grazing, sweet eating, and night eating appear to be common in bariatric surgery candidates. According to the evidence so far, bariatric surgery candidates with a comorbid BED have significantly higher rates of lifetime psychiatric comorbidity compared to obese patients without BED. A recent review, however, concludes that neither preoperative binge eating nor other preoperative maladaptive eating behaviors such as grazing, sweet eating, and night eating are predictive of postoperative weight loss [8].

Eating Pathology After Bariatric Surgery

Outcome research after bariatric surgery traditionally focuses more on change in weight and somatic comorbidity while underemphasizing, if not disregarding, the role of eating behavior. Initially after surgery, patients do not have much interest in food, and they usually experience less hunger, less preoccupation with food, and are focused on eating the "right things." At approximately 18 months after surgery, they often experience a weight plateau. Caloric intake begins to increase and most patients experience some weight regain. Adherence to the reduced portion sizes is believed to be a significant challenge for many patients over time, and patients may try to "push their limits" with regard to food quantities but also with regard to high-fat and high-sugar content food.

Bariatric surgery itself leads to major changes in eating patterns; the different procedures are believed to have considerable and differential effects on eating patterns. Patients need to relearn to eat and drink in the first weeks and months after surgery. It is inherently difficult to distinguish between "normal" and "abnormal" eating postoperatively, since most eating behavior will be different from the eating behavior of the general population. Patients are instructed to restrict their portion sizes and food varieties while increasing their meal frequency. They need to reduce the speed of eating and the size of their bites and sips, and they need to extensively chew their food before swallowing. They need to learn new cues for satiety in order to avoid overeating. The modified anatomy of the upper gastrointestinal tract might even promote the development of new eating pathology. In addition, medical complications (such as vomiting) and specialized diets may mimic eating disordered behaviors. Other symptoms following surgery, such as "plugging" (defined as food getting stuck in the small opening of the pouch with epigastric discomfort), "dumping," constipation, nausea, or excessive salivation may lead patients to engage in restrictive or compensatory behaviors in an effort to deal with the difficulties they encounter with food intake. In considering whether or not these behaviors are pathological, one must consider the motivation behind them and understand if they are driven by excessive concerns about shape or weight or if they are merely a way of accommodating the considerable changes in the digestive tract that result from the surgery.

Since there is no commonly agreed categorization of postoperative pathological eating behavior, our group developed a Bariatric Surgery Version of the EDE (EDE-BSV, available upon request). The EDE-BSV allows a fine-grained analysis of eating behavior after bariatric surgery taking into account the altered anatomical situation of the upper gastrointestinal tract. The EDE-BSV contains several additional probes in order to differentiate compensatory behaviors for shape or weight reasons from behaviors due to surgery: "Did you vomit because of plugging or dumping?" "Have you had thoughts about how vomiting might influence your weight or shape?" "Would you be concerned if you vomited less but ate the same?" "Do you sometimes eat certain foods even though you know that there is a high likelihood that this will result in nausea and/or vomiting?" In addition, probes to characterize adverse physical effects of bariatric surgery related to eating were added (e.g., for plugging and dumping). All symptoms are rated in terms of presence and monthly frequency during the last 6 months prior to the interview (Fig. 4.1).

Binge Eating and the Loss of Control of Eating

Most studies have demonstrated that, in the short-term, bariatric surgery has a pronounced positive effect on binge eating and associated psychopathology. Eating unusually (objectively) large amounts of food in a single sitting is physically not possible, likely due to the small size of the gastric pouch and the small outlet that restricts the volume of ingestible food. In addition, overeating after surgery is often followed by vomiting or regurgitation of food. Thus, bariatric surgery seems to be able to "cure" binge eating, at least for a period of time. However, there is evidence that as postoperative time increases, patients are able to consume larger quantities of food [14]. Even though BED prevalence will be greatly diminished, feelings of loss of control (LOC)

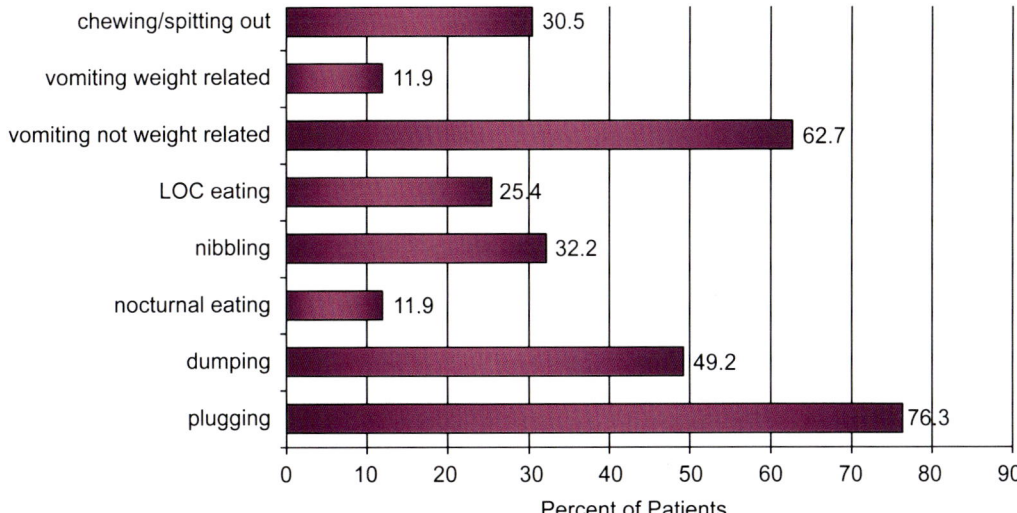

Fig. 4.1 Nonnormative eating behavior 2 years after gastric bypass (n=59, after de Zwaan et al. [6]). *LOC eating* loss of control eating (eating a subjectively large amount of food with a feeling of loss of control), *plugging* food getting stuck in the small opening of the pouch, *nocturnal eating* an episode of eating after the subject has been to sleep

can still persist since the dynamics responsible for binge eating, such as emotional distress, may remain.

Consequently, researchers have focused more on the "sense of loss of control" rather than objective overeating as the essential diagnostic criterion for problematic eating behavior postsurgery. LOC eating seems to be an important indicator of eating problems postoperatively. In most studies, the number of patients with LOC eating decreases after surgery; however, many patients report the reemergence of LOC eating postoperatively with increasing rates as postoperative time increases [5, 15]. The prevalence rates of LOC eating have been found to increase to up to 50 % of patients 3 or more years postoperatively [16]. LOC eating after surgery is significantly more common in participants with preoperative binge eating (disorder) and is associated with more postoperative vomiting as well as with more pathological scores on measures of eating-related and general psychopathology.

Most studies that have investigated this association reported that LOC eating following surgery seems to be a negative prognostic indicator for weight loss. However, the amount of weight loss is usually still clinically significant—superior to what likely would have been experienced with more conservative weight loss efforts–and with greater improvements in obesity-related comorbidities. At the same time, there is some evidence that abnormal eating behavior postsurgery might lead to increased complication rates, readmissions, and nonadherence with postoperative dietary and physical activity recommendations [17–19].

These findings suggest that periodic monitoring of eating behavior could be useful in patients postsurgery, especially if the weight loss is suboptimal [7]. LOC eating appears to be a marker not only for weight outcomes but also for more global psychopathology. These patients might potentially benefit from psychotherapeutic interventions teaching them new approaches to the management of negative emotions and stress to ensure weight maintenance or continued losses as well as to improve associated psychopathology in the years following surgery. Whether such interventions should be targeted prior to surgery or following surgery is unclear. So far, there have been no systematic trials of preventative interventions. Most importantly there is evidence that patients with binge eating may be more likely to miss appointments after surgery, and thus targeted efforts should be made to have these patients attend postoperative visits [20].

Vomiting

Following bariatric surgery procedures with a restrictive component, patients report an increased occurrence of involuntary vomiting, especially during the first few postoperative weeks. Vomiting usually occurs when patients eat too much in relation to their pouch size or when food gets stuck in the small opening of the pouch ("plugging"), which is a painful experience. Others self-induce vomiting as a response to fullness and epigastric discomfort. Patients usually use their fingers to self-induce vomiting. Some may drink water and others just need to bend over the toilet to facilitate vomiting. Others drink meat tenderizer to decrease the discomfort. Postoperative vomiting is distressing to some patients and surprisingly well tolerated by others.

There seems to be a subgroup of patients after bariatric surgery who use vomiting as an additional method to regulate weight (Fig. 4.1). When the patients reach their weight plateau, they frequently develop an intense fear of weight regain, which given their previous history of weight loss and regain is understandable. It is difficult to establish the extent to which the patients accept vomiting in order not to regain weight or to lose more weight. Even if the vomiting occurs spontaneously, some patients might welcome the effect that they believe this might have on their weight or shape. Some patients might even intentionally overeat knowing that it might result in spontaneous vomiting, which some patients believe will help to prevent weight gain.

Chewing and Spitting Out Food

A significant number of patients start chewing and spitting out food postoperatively. This behavior is usually not accompanied by distress and mostly serves to avoid plugging. It is either planned (e.g., to get a taste of red meat, which they usually avoid because it easily gets stuck) or unplanned (e.g., "the one bite too much that would make me vomit").

Formal Eating Disorders

A number of case reports and case series have described the development of syndromes closely resembling BN and anorexia nervosa (AN) following bariatric surgery [2]. AN is characterized by an intense fear of gaining weight or becoming fat, leading to restriction of energy intake and to significantly low body weight. In these cases, patients eat less than they would be able to and develop anorexic and bulimic beliefs and, in some cases, eventually full-blown AN or BN. Patients might meet all criteria for BN except for "ingestion of a large amount of food" because this is simply not possible. Others might meet all criteria for AN, except for the weight criterion because it takes many months or even years before formerly obese patients reach a low body weight. While some may not meet the weight criteria early on, others may do so over time. One explanation for the development of an eating disorder might be that individuals with a psychological vulnerability might become preoccupied with food and weight loss. They may report an intense fear of regaining weight or fail to be satisfied when reaching a reasonable postoperative weight.

However, the prevalence of BN and AN after bariatric surgery is unknown. Health-care professionals who encounter these individuals might develop a negative attitude toward obesity surgery. They need to be cautioned that this appears to occur only in a small minority of patients who are most likely not representative of bariatric surgery patients in general.

Night Eating

After surgery, night eating is usually observed less frequently than before surgery. There is also some evidence that the reoccurrence of night eating may contribute to weight regain. The phenomenon of night eating after bariatric surgery has not been adequately studied, particularly as to how it might relate to inadequate intake during the day.

Grazing

Similar to before surgery, few data are available on postoperative grazing behavior. Some may consider this behavior as adaptive eating style promoting weight maintenance. Postoperative grazing appears to be common with up to 30 % reporting permanent eating postsurgery, and this behavior has been shown to be negatively correlated with weight loss and positively correlated with weight regain [15, 16]. Grazing might result in a total daily caloric intake that will exceed optimal postoperative consumption. There is no means to reliably differentiate LOC eating and grazing postoperatively. Saunders suggested that postoperative grazing may fulfill a similar function as binge eating [13]. Overall, a sense of loss of control, regardless of how the behavior is labeled, appears to be the core symptom of maladaptive eating behaviors, given that the consumption of small amounts of food continuously over extended periods is still possible following bariatric surgery.

Sweet Eating

Overeating on high-caloric sweet foods is possible after purely restrictive surgery but not after bypass surgery where dumping occurs after ingestion of sweet foods. However, dumping is no longer considered universal and also appears to decrease in frequency for some over time, suggesting some intestinal adaptation that then allows for more sweet eating without dumping. It has been postulated that "sweet eaters" might benefit more from gastric bypass since they would consciously avoid eating sweets for fear of developing dumping syndrome but will do poorly after other procedures. However, there is evidence that sweet eating behavior is not predictive of weight outcome after restrictive surgical procedures (see de Zwaan [12]). In addition, there is evidence that gastric banding might alter postoperative eating behavior with a shift toward soft, high-calorie foods also in patients who did not report sweet eating tendencies preoperatively.

Consequently, there is no contemporary evidence that sweet eating behavior should be used as a preoperative selection criterion for bariatric surgery. The applied definitions of "sweet eaters" remain arbitrary, and as Lindroos et al. [21] pointed out, 62 % of all women included in the SOS study (including normal-weight control subjects) consumed more than 15 % of their calories from sweet foods, with non-sweet eaters being a minority in normal-weight subjects.

Conclusion

Binge eating behavior is common in bariatric surgery candidates and generally improves after surgery. The relationship between preoperative binge eating and weight loss or weight regain does not appear to be very strong [8]. During the first postoperative phase, patients are rapidly losing weight and receive a substantial amount of positive reinforcement. However, research suggests that preoperative binge eating may place patients at higher risk for the reemergence of disordered eating postoperatively, which is associated with poorer weight loss and greater weight regain in the long term. Usually, maladaptive eating after bariatric surgery typically represents a continuation or recurrence of preoperative eating patterns. It must be kept in mind, however, that also patients who redevelop abnormal eating behaviors still show a satisfactory weight loss—even though smaller compared with patients without eating problems. Consequently, BED prior to surgery is not a contraindication for the procedure. However, the identification and treatment of postoperative eating problems might improve long-term weight outcome in these patients. Detection of postoperative problems requires regular postoperative follow-up clinic visits; however, there is evidence that general compliance is lower after surgery when compared to before surgery, especially in patients with psychological problems [20] and motivating patients to participate in such treatments is often a challenge.

Question and Answer Section

Questions

1. The contraindications to gastric bypass surgery include:
   A. Binge eating
   B. Grazing
   C. Sweet eating
   D. None of the above
2. In general, binge eating:
   A. Improves after bariatric surgery
   B. Remains unchanged after bariatric surgery
   C. Worsens after bariatric surgery
   D. Increases the mortality associated with bariatric surgery.

Answers

1. **D.** All of these behaviors should be assessed, but none are absolute contraindications.
2. **A.** Binge eating may change into loss of control eating after surgery but generally improves. There is no evidence for D.

References

1. Sarwer DB, Dilks RJ, West Smith L. Dietary intake and eating behavior after bariatric surgery: threats to weight loss maintenance and strategies for success. Surg Obes Relat Dis. 2011;7:644–51.
2. Marino JM, Ertelt TW, Lancaster K, Steffen K, Peterson L, de Zwaan M, Mitchell JE. The emergence of eating pathology after bariatric surgery: a rare outcome with important clinical implications. Int J Eat Disord. 2012;45:179–84.
3. Engel SG, Mitchell JE, de Zwaan M, Steffen KJ. Eating disorders and eating problems pre- and post bariatric surgery. In: Mitchell JE, de Zwaan M, editors. Psychosocial assessment and treatment of bariatric surgery patients. New York: Routledge; 2010.
4. Kinzl JF, Schrattenecker M, Traweger C, Mattesich M, Fiala M, Biebl W. Psychosocial predictors of weight loss after bariatric surgery. Obes Surg. 2006;16:1609–14.
5. White MA, Kalarchian MA, Masheb RM, et al. Loss of control over eating predicts outcome in bariatric surgery patients: a prospective 24-month follow-up study. J Clin Psychiatry. 2010;71:175–84.
6. de Zwaan M, Hilbert A, Swan-Kremeier L, Simonich H, Lancaster K, Howell LM, Monson T, Crosby RD, Mitchell JE. Comprehensive interview assessment of eating behavior 18–35 months after gastric bypass surgery for morbid obesity. Surg Obes Relat Dis. 2010;6:79–87.
7. Wadden TA, Faulconbridge LF, Jones-Corneille LR, Sarwer DB, Fabricatore AN, Thomas G, Wilson GT, Alexander MG, Pulcini ME, Webb VL, Williams NN. Binge eating disorder and the outcome of bariatric surgery at one year: a prospective, observational study. Obesity. 2011;19:1220–8.
8. Livhits M, Mercado C, Yermilov I, Parikh JA, Dutson E, Mehran A, Ko CY, Gibbons MM. Preoperative predictors of weight loss following bariatric surgery: systematic review. Obes Surg. 2012;22:70–89.
9. Alger-Mayer S, Rosati C, Polimeni JM, Malone M. Preoperative binge eating status and gastric bypass surgery: a long-term outcome study. Obes Surg. 2009;19:139–45.
10. Ashton K, Heinberg L, Windover A, Merrell J. Positive response to binge eating intervention enhances postoperative weight loss. Surg Obes Relat Dis. 2011;7:315–20.
11. Allison KC, Lundgren JD, O'Reardon JP, Geliebter A, Gluck ME, Vinai P, Mitchell JE, Schenck CH, Howell MJ, Crow SJ, Engel SG, Latzer Y, Tzischinsky O, Mahowald MW, Stunkard AJ. Proposed diagnostic criteria for night eating syndrome. Int J Eat Disord. 2010;43:241–7.
12. de Zwaan M. Weight and eating changes after bariatric surgery. In: Mitchell JE, de Zwaan M, editors. Bariatric surgery: a guide for mental health professionals. New York: Brunner-Routledge; 2005. p. 77–100.
13. Saunders R. "Grazing": a high-risk behavior. Obes Surg. 2004;14:98–102.
14. Sarwer DB, Wadden TA, Moore RH, Baker AW, Gibbons LM, Raper SE, Williams NN. Preoperative eating behavior, postoperative dietary adherence and weight loss following gastric bypass surgery. Surg Obes Relat Dis. 2008;5:640–6.
15. Colles SL, Dixon JB, O'Brien PE. Loss of control is central to psychological disturbance associated with binge eating disorder. Obesity. 2008;16:608–14.
16. Kofman MD, Lent MR, Swencionis C. Maladaptive eating patterns, quality of life, and weight outcomes following gastric bypass: results of an internet survey. Obesity. 2010;18:1938–43.
17. Busetto L, Segato G, De Luca M, De Marchi F, Foletto M, Vianello M, Valeri M, Favretti F, Enzi G. Weight loss and postoperative complications in morbidly obese patients with binge eating disorder treated by laparoscopic adjustable gastric banding. Obes Surg. 2005;15:195–201.

18. Wölnerhanssen BK, Peters T, Kern B, Schötzau A, Ackermann C, von Flüe M, Peterli R. Predictors of outcome in treatment of morbid obesity by laparoscopic adjustable gastric banding: results of a prospective study of 380 patients. Surg Obes Relat Dis. 2008;4:500–6.
19. Gorin AA, Raftopoulos I. Effect of mood and eating disorders on the short-term outcome of laparoscopic Roux-en-Y gastric bypass. Obes Surg. 2009;19:1685–90.
20. Toussi R, Fujioka K, Coleman KJ. Pre- and postsurgery behavioral compliance, patient health, and postbariatric surgical weight loss. Obesity. 2009;17:996–1002.
21. Lindroos AK, Lissner L, Sjostrom L. Weight change in relation to intake of sugar and sweet foods before and after weight reducing gastric surgery. Int J Obes Relat Metab Disord. 1996;20:634–43.

Introduction to Psychological Consultations for Bariatric Surgery Patients

Katherine L. Applegate and Kelli E. Friedman

Chapter Objectives

Readers of this chapter will be able to:
1. Understand the common assessment formats used by behavioral health clinicians to conduct preoperative psychological consultations.
2. List and describe many specific domains relevant for psychological consultations with bariatric surgery patients.
3. Discuss the use of psychometric instruments as a way to improve the standardization and thoroughness of psychological consultations for bariatric surgery.

Introduction

The psychological consultation became a recommended component of the preoperative assessment process for bariatric surgery candidates after the 1991 National Institutes of Health (NIH) Consensus Panel emphasized the relevance of multidisciplinary evaluations [1]. When conducted by a behavioral health provider with expertise in obesity and bariatric surgery, the psychological consultation can function less as a requirement to qualify for surgery and more as an opportunity for patients to receive guidance on behavioral and psychosocial preparation for surgery. In this way, an effective psychological consultation goes well beyond a traditional diagnostic assessment and includes several topics specific to bariatric surgery [2, 3]. A primary objective of the psychological consultation is to develop a behavioral treatment plan with specific recommendations to enhance the perioperative course and effectiveness of bariatric surgery for each individual patient. The consultation also can assist the surgical practice as a whole by minimizing untreated psychopathology, recommending additional educational activities for selected patients, or providing targeted behavioral interventions (e.g., smoking cessation, improved medication adherence) prior to surgery to improve patient safety and potential success of surgery.

Because the psychological consultation for surgery goes well beyond a general diagnostic assessment, domains specifically relevant to bariatric surgery need to be assessed. This in-depth information is most commonly gathered through a semi-structured interview, which may be augmented with psychometric measures of various psychological domains [4]. This chapter will review the basic tenants of the preoperative psychological evaluation. Common assessment areas, including dieting history, psychopathology, eating pathology, substance use, knowledge about bariatric surgery, and psychosocial stressors will also be discussed. This is followed by a review of common psychometric instruments used with this population, treatment planning options, and clinician training issues.

Clinical Assessment Strategies

There are numerous topics included in the pre-bariatric surgery psychological consultation beyond those issues commonly covered during a general psychiatric evaluation. Interestingly, although psychosocial consultations are currently required by the vast majority of third-party payers in the United States and by over 80 % of surgical programs [5], a specific, standardized method of conducting pre-bariatric surgery psychological consultations has not yet emerged. One reason that a standardized format has not yet been developed may be the lack of an empirically supported consensus on the behavioral and psychosocial factors that impact or predict surgical outcome [6, 7]. As a result, the format for these consultations varies across practitioners.

K.L. Applegate, PhD (✉) • K.E. Friedman, PhD
Department of Psychiatry, Duke Center for Metabolic and Weight Loss Surgery, Duke University Health System, Durham, NC 27704, USA
e-mail: katherine.applegate@duke.edu; kelli.friedman@duke.edu

The vast majority of behavioral health clinicians conducting pre-bariatric surgery psychological consultations include a clinical interview as part of their protocol [4]. Wadden and Sarwer [7] proposed that the Weight and Lifestyle Inventory (WALI) [8] could be employed as a presurgical assessment tool. This pencil and paper measure is completed by the patient prior to the clinical interview and assesses the patient's weight history, weight-loss goals, substance use, eating patterns, physical activity, social support, psychological factors, recent psychosocial stressors, and medical history. In this "patient-oriented approach," the clinician incorporates the results of the WALI into the pre-bariatric surgery consultation. The information gathered, along with the patient's knowledge level about surgery and plans for the perioperative period, can then be used to develop a treatment plan for each patient.

The Boston Interview for Bariatric Surgery is another semi-structured interview that was originally published in 2004 and updated in 2008 [6]. It is based on empirical data and specifically tailored to pre-bariatric surgery psychological evaluations. This measure covers many topics including the patient's weight history and weight-loss goals, substance use, eating habits, physical activity, family issues, recent psychosocial stressors, medical history (patient's knowledge and understanding, adherence), surgery knowledge, relationships and social support, and psychiatric functioning. This empirically based interview has modules that can be administered by other members of the treatment team (if available) to shorten the interview.

Both Wadden and Sarwer [7] and Sogg and Mori [6] suggest trying to put the patient at ease before starting the actual psychological consultation. Although this may seem intuitive, quite often bariatric surgery patients have not had contact with mental health providers and may be particularly concerned about the outcome of the assessment (e.g., questioning if they will they be "approved" for surgery). As Wadden and Sarwer [7] emphasize, the purpose of the consultation is not to "psychoanalyze" patients, but rather to help patients in their decision-making process about surgery and to prepare for upcoming behavioral changes. In addition, by taking time to put patients at ease, behavioral health providers are building rapport with patients that may extend their professional relationship to postoperative support if needed. Clinicians can normalize patients' anxiety and structure questions to put them more at ease with the topics. For example, when assessing adherence it is often useful to acknowledge that people sometimes struggle with this issue (e.g., "How often do you miss doses of your medication?" versus "Do you miss doses of your medication?").

During the consultation, patients may try to present themselves in a favorable light to "qualify" for surgery. In a well-designed study comparing the results of presurgical psychological interviews with a research-based psychiatric assessment (separate from the clinical evaluation), there was only moderate congruence—the agreement rate was lower than expected [9]. In another study, a substantial percentage of patients' validity scales of the Minnesota Multiphasic Personality Inventory-2 (MMPI-2) suggested that they had invalid profiles, which necessitated retesting with new instructions for openness in response to the questions [10]. In both clinical interviews and personality testing, minimization of symptoms can interfere with the clinician's ability to develop an accurate conceptualization of the patient's psychosocial issues and may complicate these assessments.

After completing the assessment, the behavioral health provider develops an individualized treatment plan that often is communicated to the referring surgical team as well as the patient. The results of the assessment and the resulting treatment plan frequently are requested by the patient's insurance company as well. In general, however, most patients are unconditionally recommended for surgery at the time of their initial consultation [4, 11–13]. Several studies have reported that 64–86 % of patients are "approved" for surgery after their first consultation. A small percentage of patients are deemed inappropriate for surgery (~3–4 %). Deferral/delay rates in published studies range from a low of 8 % to a high of 31 % [11–13]. Although there are not standardized reasons for delaying a patient's surgery, there do seem to be common themes among providers, including untreated or undertreated psychiatric disorders, significant life stressors, and poor educational preparation for bariatric surgery [4, 11, 13]. A referral for additional psychiatric treatment seems to be the most common reason for delay [11, 13].

Friedman and colleagues [11] investigated patients' responses to being given a psychological treatment plan that included a delay for additional assessment or treatment. Of the 837 patients that were evaluated in their study, 68 (8 %) were given activities to complete before proceeding to surgery. Of the patients delayed for treatment, 56 % were adherent with their treatment plan and subsequently underwent bariatric surgery, and 44 % were not adherent with the treatment plan and were not offered surgery. Those factors that predicted being nonadherent were male gender, a more complicated treatment plan (e.g., starting therapy and consulting about psychotropic medication), and higher hostility scores.

Recently, Heinberg et al. [14] described the Cleveland Clinic Behavioral Rating System (CCBRS), which proposes a continuous rating scale methodology for pre-bariatric surgery psychological consultations in place of the more commonly used categorical systems noted previously (i.e., pass, delay, deny). In this system, trained clinicians rate patients on a 5-point scale (poor, guarded, fair, good, excellent) across eight domains culled from the empirical literature. The eight domains include:

1. Consent (ability to consent, cognitive impairment)
2. Expectations (e.g., knowledge of surgery, weight-loss goals, relationship changes)
3. Social support (specifically addressing support for bariatric surgery)

4. Mental health (e.g., psychiatric conditions and history, past treatment)
5. Chemical abuse/dependence (past and current substance use habits)
6. Eating behaviors
7. Adherence (past dieting history outcomes, medical regimen adherence, likelihood of program adherence)
8. Coping and stressors (coping styles, stress management)

The rating system concludes with an overall impression score as well as the individual scores from each of the eight domains. Investigating the results of the CCBRS in 389 patients, summary scores were correlated with unemployment, lower levels of education, higher body mass index (BMI), current tobacco use, and current psychotropic medication use [14]. This CCBRS appears to be a brief, internally consistent, reliable strategy for determining patients' suitability for bariatric surgery [14].

In a recent study, the CCBRS was used to identify possible psychological factors that may influence patients' failure to complete the preoperative assessment process [15]. The most common explanations for not reaching surgery were withdrawal from the program and incomplete program requirements. Those patients who did not complete their requirements for surgery were more likely to be enrolled in outpatient behavioral health treatment, to be on psychotropic medication, and to have met criteria for current or past alcohol abuse or dependence when compared to those who had failed to reach surgery for other reasons.

Bariatric-Specific Areas of Assessment

The American Society for Metabolic and Weight Loss Surgery (ASMBS) released recommendations for the pre-bariatric surgery psychological consultation in 2004 [16]. This document is fairly general and was created to provide an overview of important aspects of the presurgical psychosocial assessment. The recommendations are divided into broad content categories including behavioral, cognitive/emotional, developmental, current life situations, and motivation/expectations for surgery. ASMBS is currently working on a new set of clinical guidelines for behavioral health providers conducting pre-bariatric surgery psychological consultations; however, the release date has yet to be announced. The ASMBS, along with other groups of researchers, recommend the assessment of the following areas.

Dieting/Weight History

If the multidisciplinary team includes a registered dietician (RD), the bulk of the dieting history can be gathered and summarized by this professional. Subsequently, the relevant points from the RD assessment can be incorporated into the patient's behavioral treatment plan as needed. If this resource is not available, the behavioral health provider can review the degree to which patients have used behavioral diets in the past, their adherence to the diet (i.e., pounds lost, length of diet), and behavioral lessons learned from past diets that may be relevant after bariatric surgery. Also, obtaining and reviewing the patient's lifelong weight history may provide information about triggers for past weight gain (e.g., emotional eating, medication side effects, inactivity, life transitions) that can be discussed during the evaluation [3].

Physical Activity Level

Activity level and potential/perceived barriers to activity can be assessed during the consultation. Patients with obesity may present with a variety of physical activity levels depending on their general medical health, mobility, joint health, familiarity with structured exercise, and motivational level. Many patients can benefit from suggestions about modified exercises they could perform, information about low-intensity/short-duration options for exercise, and activity options for patients with chronic joint pain (e.g., water aerobics, chair exercises, stationary bicycling). The heightened motivation that patients often feel when they present for bariatric surgery can be directed into encouragement of increased physical activity in the weeks before surgery. Patients can be reminded that, in addition to weight loss, health and fitness are also goals of increased physical activity, as well as better chances of long-term success with their weight-loss maintenance, as discussed in Chap. 22. Patients may need encouragement to initiate physical activity plans prior to surgery, rather than waiting until after their procedure. Problem solving through perceived obstacles and motivational enhancement can be useful to patients at the assessment stage [16].

Eating Pathology

While many bariatric surgery patients report poor or unstructured eating habits during the preoperative psychological consultation, only a portion of these individuals will meet criteria for an eating disorder (also see Chap. 4). Grazing and emotionally triggered eating are two common forms of eating patterns noted in this population. Grazing is commonly defined as constant or continuous eating that may be the result of habit, low appetite awareness, compulsion, or negative affect regulation [16]. To reduce grazing, patients can be instructed in stimulus control, meal planning, and appetite awareness principles. Emotional eating can function as a coping skill to manage negative affective states such as anxiety, sadness, loneliness, or anger [2, 3]. If emotionally triggered eating patterns are present, patients can be educated about the importance of developing alternative coping strategies before surgery since these behaviors will not be available to them after their procedures. Also, there is a concern that if grazing and emotional eating return after the initial postoperative period, patients may be at risk for weight regain [3].

Bariatric surgery patients are commonly screened for both binge eating disorder (BED) and night eating syndrome (NES) during the pre-bariatric surgery consultations. BED is the most common eating disorder documented among bariatric surgery patients, with prevalence estimates ranging from 2 to 57.5 % depending on the assessment methodology used [2]. Research investigating the effect of BED on patients' outcome after bariatric surgery has been inconsistent, though there is preliminary evidence that binge eating improves during the first 6–18 months after bariatric surgery [17]. Thus, delaying surgery for preoperative treatment of BED is rarely recommended and likely only takes place when patients have extreme cases of BED [2]. Instead, patients can be educated about the possibility that binge eating may return in the years after bariatric surgery and that the symptoms may require behavioral intervention at that point to minimize the risk of postoperative weight regain. Importantly, patients with BED are still likely to achieve significantly more weight loss with bariatric surgery than with any nonsurgical weight-loss intervention available [3].

Patients may acknowledge other types of eating disorders during the psychological consultation, including NES. The syndrome has four primary characteristics: morning anorexia, hyperphagia in the evening, nighttime awakenings, and night eating [18, 19]. Rates of NES vary widely depending on the assessment method used. Clinical interview data suggests that nearly 9 % of bariatric surgery patients report aspects of NES. At present, there is no evidence linking NES to postoperative outcome; a referral for the behavioral treatment of this condition is not typically given prior to surgery [2]. Although the presence of self-induced vomiting among preoperative bariatric surgery patients is rare, recurrent postoperative vomiting (whether self-induced or spontaneous) can be potentially dangerous (e.g., dehydration, abdominal pain). As such, patients who acknowledge self-induced vomiting preoperatively may warrant treatment before proceeding with surgery to reduce the potential for postoperative complications [7, 11].

Psychopathology and Treatment History

The prevalence rates of psychopathology among bariatric surgery patients, as well as the relevance of these disorders to postoperative weight-loss outcome, have long been of interest to surgeons and mental health professionals who work with persons with extreme obesity. The literature in this area is reviewed in detail in Chap. 2. Kalarchian and colleagues [20] conducted clinical assessments of candidates administered independently of the psychological screening process for bariatric surgery with the expectation that patients would be more forthcoming about their symptoms in this context. At the time of screening, 38 % of candidates met criteria for at least one Axis I disorder, which includes diagnoses such as mood and anxiety disorders. This rate increased to 66 % when considering the lifetime history of having at least one of these disorders. They also reported that 28.5 % of their sample met criteria for a personality disorder. The authors suggest that the rates of psychopathology may be higher among bariatric surgery patients, compared to community samples, because of the treatment-seeking nature of the group, the severity of obesity among bariatric surgery patients, and the associated medical comorbidities linked to obesity [20].

Given these findings, information on past and current psychological functioning/symptoms, use of psychotropic medication, outpatient and inpatient mental health treatment, and previous psychological testing (e.g., neuropsychological reports, psychiatric disability claims) can be helpful in understanding the nature and severity of any existing psychopathology. How recently the patient was in treatment, the length, and the patient's adherence to treatment can shed light on the psychological issues as well. When evaluating a patient's suitability for bariatric surgery, lifetime or current psychopathology, even severe psychopathology, does not necessarily prevent a patient from proceeding with surgery [2, 3]. Instead, a goal of the pre-bariatric surgery psychological consultation should be to assess if existing psychopathology is as well managed as possible during the perioperative period with the intent of limiting the risk of treatment nonadherence, to reduce symptom interference with weight-loss efforts (e.g., low motivation impacting physical activity level), and to verify that patients have the cognitive capacity to give informed consent for surgery. Thus, the behavioral health provider is assisting the surgical team in managing severe mental illness for as many patients as possible. This strategy allows more patients the opportunity to take advantage of the potential benefits of bariatric surgery [21].

A substantial percentage of patients seeking bariatric surgery report taking one or more psychotropic medications at the time of their psychological consultation [11, 12, 14]. This rate of psychotropic medication usage is approximately six times higher than the general population [2]. The long-term effectiveness of these medications on weight-loss outcome and psychological symptom management, as well as the pharmacokinetics of psychotropic medication in general after bariatric surgery, is unclear at the present time. However, some common practices have emerged to assist in the potential absorption of these medications [2]. For example, patients are often transitioned from sustained-release to instant-release formulations of their psychotropic medications. Some programs direct patients to crush their medications (especially post-Roux-en-Y gastric bypass [RYGB]) in an effort, at least in theory, to promote absorption. Patients on these medications should be carefully monitored for changes in their psychiatric symptoms after surgery and by a health care provider familiar with bariatric surgery.

Substance Use Habits

Use of nicotine, alcohol, narcotic pain medication, and illicit drugs are commonly assessed in the psychological consultation [16]. A discussion of patients' current and past substance use is important not only to assess for substance abuse or dependence, but also to facilitate a review of postoperative recommendations regarding substance use. Patients can be educated about how their substance use may need to be modified in an effort to reduce perioperative risks (e.g., dehydrating effects of caffeine, risk of ulcers and blood clots from nicotine, liver complications from alcohol use).

Alcohol use after bariatric surgery has received significant attention in the popular press and more recently in the scientific literature; thus, patients may have questions about risk of addiction after surgery. Although a significant percentage of bariatric surgery patients (32.6 %) meet criteria for a lifetime history of substance abuse disorder, only a small percentage (1.7 %) of patients meet criteria for a substance use disorder at the time of their psychological consultation [20]. Behavioral health providers can discuss with patients the function that substance use has played in the past (i.e., to manage sleep difficulties, chronic pain, or negative affect) and work to generate lower-risk behaviors that can replace substance use postoperatively. Those patients who acknowledge current substance abuse and dependence are commonly referred for treatment prior to proceeding with bariatric surgery [2, 4, 5, 11, 22].

Knowledge About Bariatric Surgery

The importance of preoperative patient education and informed consent for this elective surgery cannot be overstated. Bariatric surgery requires lifelong behavioral changes for optimal outcome and for a reduction in the risk of medical complications (e.g., dehydration, dumping syndrome, vitamin deficiencies). During the consultation, patients can be asked to explain bariatric surgery procedures and to describe known risks or possible complications. This allows the behavioral health clinician to assess the amount of information the patient has already gathered about the desired bariatric surgery and the accuracy of that information [7, 16]. Patients can be asked to describe the postoperative dietary and lifestyle recommendations for thoroughness and accuracy. Most patients are generally familiar with this information from speaking with other patients, postings on the Internet, or speaking with a medical provider. Those who have significant gaps in their understanding of surgery can be further assessed for motivation, reading comprehension, literacy, cognitive capacity, or seriousness about proceeding with surgery. Some patients may indicate that they have assigned the responsibility of learning the perioperative educational information to a support person; however, it is vital that patients with the capacity to review and process this information themselves do so. Overall, the clinical team should have a reasonable expectation that each patient will be adherent with the postoperative dietary regimen as evidenced by active participation in the preoperative education process.

Adherence with Medical/Psychological Treatment

A critical goal during the consultation is to gather information about the patient's adherence to past medical and/or psychological treatment to develop an estimation of the likelihood of their future adherence to the post-bariatric surgery regimen. Adherence information can be gathered from the patient based on their medication habits, frequency of missed medication doses, adherence with treatment recommendations, self-discontinuation of medication, and dropping out of past treatment programs. If a patient has diabetes or a similar chronic illness, the patient's health behaviors relevant to that condition can be reviewed (e.g., testing frequency for blood glucose levels, HbA1c levels, etc.). Any opportunity to speak with other treating providers or to review medical records also can be a source of information about past treatment adherence. If an adherence issue is present, suggestions for improving the behavior going forward can be provided to the patient (e.g., establishing behavioral reminders for medication), as well as education about how dietary/vitamin adherence will be essential for long-term safety and success.

Social Support

The availability of emotional, functional, and informational support should be assessed as these resources can be beneficial to patients and to the surgical practice. Specifically, patients can be asked about the type and quality of their current primary social relationships (i.e., romantic partners, parents, children, friends, coworkers, other bariatric surgery patients) and how these individuals may react to the common changes that occur after surgery [14, 16]. An understanding of the nature and stability of their current relationships is useful, as well as any acute medical or psychiatric issues in their partner, the presence of domestic violence, financial stressors, an impending marital separation, caregiving responsibilities, etc. Patients sometimes are reluctant to tell other people about their decision to have bariatric surgery and may benefit from guidance on how to recruit positive social support. In addition, patients can be encouraged to involve their existing support people in educational seminars, medical and RD appointments, nutritional classes, and support group meetings.

Psychosocial Stressors/Recent Life Events

Major life events can distract patients from the intense lifestyle modifications required perioperatively. As such, a review of ongoing or anticipated psychosocial stressors is relevant for the appropriate timing of bariatric surgery. Patients can work with the surgical team to plan their procedures for a relatively low-stress time period if possible (e.g., summer break for teachers). Since it is recommended that patients allow several weeks to focus on surgery [7], a postponement after a recent marital separation, significant/acute health problem of a family member, or the death of a loved one may be recommended.

Legal Issues

A brief review of past or current litigation, arrests, or pending legal issues is useful for treatment planning purposes [16]. These circumstances may interfere with the patient's ability to be present for postoperative medical care and to control access to appropriate dietary options (e.g., incarceration). The timing of bariatric surgery may need to be postponed until such cases are resolved and the patient's availability for standard postoperative care can be better assured.

Psychometric Measures

The use of psychometric measures during pre-bariatric surgery psychological consultations varies widely [4]. Some behavioral health providers use none, while others include an extensive battery of measures that include symptom inventories or personality assessments. Perhaps no standardized protocol has yet emerged because only a few measures have been validated for use with bariatric surgery patients and none have been shown to reliably predict postsurgical weight loss or psychosocial outcomes [3]. Nonetheless, measures of eating pathology, mood disorders, substance use disorders, and personality inventories are commonly incorporated into the psychological consultations [4]. Survey results indicate that about 69 % of clinicians use at least one symptom inventory or screening instrument. More specifically, nearly 52 % of clinicians use scales that assess depressive symptoms, 36 % use inventories of disordered eating, 42 % use objective personality tests, and 33 % use tools to assess cognitive impairment. Only about 3 % of clinicians report using projective personality tests [4]. Certainly, the cost of the assessment instruments, the necessary clinician training and their previous familiarity with the instruments, and the time associated with administering and scoring the measures have an impact on which measures are selected [23]. The following are several commonly used measures (for a comprehensive review of specific measures used with bariatric surgery patients, see Peterson et al. [23]):

Beck Depression Inventory

The Beck Depression Inventories (BDI and BDI-II) are the most frequently used measures of depressive symptoms among behavioral health providers conducting pre-bariatric surgery psychological consultations [4]. The BDI-II is a 21-item self-report questionnaire that assesses depressive symptomatology for the previous 2 weeks on a 4-point scale and includes items on mood, suicidal ideation, somatic changes, and cognitive symptoms with higher scores indicating more symptomatology [24]. The reliability and validity of this measure have been well documented among various patient populations, and patients with class III obesity have been shown to have significantly higher BDI-II scores than their less obese counterparts [25]. The association with severe obesity may result from the number of somatic items included in the BDI (concerns with physical health, fatigue) that may be related to obesity rather than depression. This is particularly problematic given that untreated or undertreated depression may delay bariatric surgery [10]. Thus, if using the inventories, the clinician should investigate item level information rather than simply the total score [26]. Both the Hamilton Rating Scale for Depression (Ham-D) and the Patient Health Questionnaire (PHQ-9) also can be used to assess depressive symptoms. The Ham-D is administered by a health care professional and surveys the type and magnitude of depressive symptoms [27]. The PHQ-9 is a quickly scored self-report screening instrument for measuring the severity of depression [28]. Because these two measures have less focus on the somatic features of depression, they may more accurately assess mood among bariatric surgery patients.

Questionnaire for Eating and Weight Patterns-Revised

Questionnaire for Eating and Weight Patterns-Revised (QEWP-R) is a self-administered measure that assesses for the presence of binge episodes, the frequency of such episodes, rapid eating, eating past feeling full, eating when not hungry, disgust after overeating, and other eating experiences [29]. This scale also assesses for purgative behaviors including: self-induced vomiting; fasting; excessive exercising; and abuse of laxatives, diuretics, and diet pills. Although the QEWP-R may be a useful screening measure for BED, this instrument is not intended as a diagnostic tool as the agreement between the QEWP-R and structured clinical interviews is only moderate.

The estimates of BED among bariatric surgery patients vary widely, related at least in part to the assessment method used (e.g., self-report questionnaire vs. clinical interview) [18]. Patients may over- or underreport disordered eating behavior on the QEWP-R, and the concepts of binge volume and loss of control may be difficult for people to answer reliably without additional prompting from a well-trained clinician. Overall, the discrepancies between interview and questionnaire data on the prevalence rates of BED suggest that a clinical interview is necessary to assign a valid diagnosis of BED [18].

Symptoms Checklist-90-R

The Symptoms Checklist-90-R (SCL-90-R) is a 90-item self-report questionnaire designed to assess a broad range of psychiatric symptoms [30]. There are nine primary dimensions: somatization, obsessive–compulsive, interpersonal sensitivity, depression, anxiety, anger–hostility, phobic anxiety, paranoid ideation, and psychoticism (social isolation). In addition, three global indices measure overall psychological distress: Global Severity Index, Positive Symptom Index, and Positive Symptom Distress Index. Normative data are now available for weight-loss surgery patients on this instrument showing good internal consistency and validity ratings when used as a screening instrument during assessments [31].

Minnesota Multiphasic Personality Inventory-2

Minnesota Multiphasic Personality Inventory-2 (MMPI-2) is a 567 true/false questionnaire that includes validity and clinical scales that tap a wide range of personality and psychopathology domains [32]. Though the scale is lengthy to complete, has a copyright fee, and requires training to learn the scoring procedure, Walfish and colleagues [10, 33] have highlighted the benefit of including a psychometric measure with a validity scale because patients may have motivation to minimize their symptoms on the inventory. Those who engage in impression management in this way may require special instructions or repeated administrations before producing valid profiles. New research on the use of the restructured form of this instrument (MMPI-2-RF) is underway, investigating its psychometric properties among bariatric surgery patients.

Treatment Planning

In 2008, the American Association of Clinical Endocrinologists, The Obesity Society, and the American Society for Metabolic and Bariatric Surgery (AACE/TOS/ASMBS) published bariatric guidelines that included a section on psychiatric factors to be considered in the assessment and selection process [34]. They recommended a psychosocial–behavioral evaluation, which assesses environmental, familial, and behavioral factors for all patients before bariatric surgery. Those patients with a known or suspected psychiatric illness would be referred on to a formal mental health evaluation before surgery. Overall, these guidelines highlight the importance of determining a patient's ability to incorporate the necessary nutritional and behavioral changes associated with bariatric surgery. These guidelines are being updated and the updated version is scheduled for publication in 2013.

Greenberg et al. [2] published an update on evidence-based guidelines for pre-bariatric surgery behavioral treatment plans covering a variety of areas including psychopathology, disordered eating patterns, and substance abuse. Nevertheless, surgical programs and behavioral health providers vary in the use of these guidelines in treatment recommendations and planning. Regardless, certain issues are generally considered to be contraindications for surgery, including current substance abuse, active psychosis, purgative behaviors (specifically self-induced vomiting), untreated or undertreated psychopathology, and documented medical nonadherence [4, 11].

If patients present with a clinical issue that may impact their suitability for bariatric surgery, a brief behavioral intervention may be indicated. Recently, Heinberg and colleagues published examples of such interventions for alcohol abuse and binge eating [22, 35]. According to their alcohol protocol, patients are initially categorized into high, medium, and low risk for alcohol misuse after surgery. Patients who are actively abusing substances are referred for substance abuse treatment and nonsurgical weight-loss intervention for 1 year. Those patients with a history of substance abuse, a strong family history of substance abuse, evidence of drug-seeking behavior, or patterns of frequent social drinking are referred to a 90-min relapse prevention/psychoeducational group prior to surgery. During this session, patients are educated about the increased intoxicating effects of alcohol after surgery, the risk for prolonged intoxication, the high caloric value of alcohol, the risk of liver problems, and the disinhibiting effects of alcohol on food intake. The authors encourage additional research to examine the efficacy of such preoperative educational programs on reducing alcohol abuse after bariatric surgery. The binge eating protocol consists of a brief 4-session preoperative cognitive behavioral group intervention [35]. Those patients who responded positively to this intervention lost a significantly greater percent of their excess weight (%EWL) at 6 and 12 months than those who did not respond. Overall, these problem-specific cognitive behavioral interventions for bariatric surgery patients show great promise in improving readiness and suitability for bariatric surgery.

The decision to defer an eligible patient's bariatric surgery for psychosocial reasons should be made with great care because these treatment plans can generate frustration, disappointment, and anger among patients, who then may not return to the program. Thus, potential psychosocial concerns must be considered in the context of the likely medical and functional benefits of moving forward with surgery. Pawlow and colleagues [12] reported that they deferred 15.8 % of their patients based on the results of the psychological consultation and that only 10 % of those delayed patients went on to have bariatric surgery within 27 months of the deferral. Friedman and colleagues [11] reported greater success with transitioning delayed patients through a behavioral treatment plan to surgery; 56 % of their deferred patients ultimately went on to have surgery. Several factors were noted as strategies to increase the chances of moving patients toward surgery, including (1) a tracking system to manage patients currently completing a behavioral treatment plan, (2) detailed written instructions for patients about the steps they need to take, and (3) case management to assess each patient's progress with the set goals [12].

While the majority of patients are cleared for surgery at the time of their initial evaluation, some have argued that requiring all patients to undergo a psychological evaluation before bariatric surgery is a manifestation of weight-related bias and represents just another "obstacle" for patients. However, while most non-bariatric surgical patients are not required to see a mental health provider prior to approval for their procedures, some forms of surgery are greatly affected by, and greatly affect, psychological and behavioral factors. Thus, a psychological consultation seems warranted in this context [6]. As more empirical data emerge on predictors of long-term bariatric surgery success, there will likely be a clearer picture on the most relevant psychological and behavioral factors to address preoperatively. Until that time, the pre-bariatric surgery psychological consultation can be conceptualized as an educational opportunity for patients, a time to review behavioral preparations, and a chance to discuss potential obstacles to weight-loss success [5–7].

Clinician Preparation

As noted previously, there is a good degree of variability regarding the nature of the preoperative psychological evaluation. While some programs have doctoral-level health psychologists who specialize in eating disorders and obesity on staff within the surgical clinic, other centers may refer their patients to community-based providers who may have less experience with bariatric surgery. To better understand the potential issues associated with developing a credential for bariatric behavioral health providers, West-Smith and Sogg [36] conducted a survey of the members of ASMBS. Of the respondents, 95 % believed that specialty knowledge in bariatric surgery was important and 87 % indicated that prior clinical experience was central to performing these consultations.

Content knowledge and clinical experience for clinicians enhances the quality of the psychosocial consultation for patients and likely improves the resulting behavioral treatment plan. Inexperienced clinicians may defer a patient for surgery unnecessarily or clear a patient for surgery before a relevant clinical issue can be addressed. These treatment decisions ultimately can have a significant impact on the overall quality of the patient's medical care and, as with any medical intervention planning, should be undertaken only by qualified professionals and based on empirical information when available.

Conclusion

The pre-bariatric surgery psychological consultation serves many purposes including enhancing behavioral preparation for surgery, educating patients about psychosocial aspects of the bariatric surgery experience, and building rapport for future clinical support as needed. Although the consultation may be viewed as merely another requirement in getting patients to surgery, when done well, the session can benefit both the patient and the surgical team.

The use of empirical literature and sound clinical judgment to inform and justify clinical decision making is critical for the appropriate preoperative treatment planning of bariatric surgery candidates. There is a high bar when deferring or denying a patient for medically indicated surgical care for psychosocial reasons. If at all possible, the behavioral health provider and the surgical team can develop a plan to minimize the potential impact of the identified psychosocial issues on the patient's perioperative experience. The focus of the pre-bariatric surgery psychological consultation remains on assisting patients to better prepare for bariatric surgery through multidisciplinary treatment planning, rather than on preventing complex patients from progressing to surgery.

Question and Answer Section

Questions

1. All of the following may require a behavioral treatment plan prior to proceeding with bariatric surgery EXCEPT:
   A. A suicide attempt within the past 30 days with subsequent psychiatric hospitalization
   B. Active alcohol dependence and refusal to seek treatment
   C. Binge eating disorder
   D. Florid psychosis resulting from medication nonadherence in a patient with paranoid schizophrenia
2. Which of the following is NOT a common psychometric measure used by behavioral health providers working with bariatric surgery patients?
   A. The Beck Depression Inventory-II
   B. Rorschach Projective Technique
   C. Minnesota Multiphasic Personality Inventory-II
   D. Questionnaire on Eating and Weight Patterns-Revised
3. If a patient is diagnosed with alcohol dependence during the pre-bariatric surgery psychological consultation, a typical recommendation by the behavioral health provider would be:
   A. Proceed with surgery and reduce alcohol intake for the first 3 months.
   B. Patient should never have bariatric surgery because of their substance abuse.
   C. Proceed with surgery and request a medical staff member to prescribe Antabuse.
   D. Refer the patient for long-term substance abuse treatment.

Answers

1. **C**. Binge eating disorder is not generally considered a behavioral contraindication for bariatric surgery [2].
2. **B**. The Rorschach Projective Technique is used by less than 1 % of behavioral health providers working with bariatric surgery patients [4].
3. **D**. One of the most common psychosocial reasons to defer a patient for bariatric surgery is substance abuse/dependence. A recent paper suggests that patients with alcohol dependence attend substance abuse treatment and pass drug screens for at least 1 year prior to bariatric surgery [22].

References

1. NIH Consensus Development Conference Panel. Gastrointestinal surgery for severe obesity. Ann Intern Med. 1991;115:956–61.
2. Greenberg I, Sogg S, Perna FM. Behavioral and psychological care in weight loss surgery: best practice update. Obesity. 2009;17:880–4.
3. Sogg S, Mori DL. Psychosocial evaluation for bariatric surgery: the Boston interview and opportunities for intervention. Obes Surg. 2009;19:369–77.
4. Fabricatore AN, Crerand CE, Wadden TA, Sarwer DB, Krasucki JL. How do mental health professionals evaluate candidates for bariatric surgery? Survey results. Obes Surg. 2006;16:567–73.
5. Bauchowitz AU, Gonder-Frederick LA, Olbrisch ME, Azarbad L, Ryee MY, Woodson M, et al. Psychosocial evaluation of bariatric surgery candidates: a survey of present practices. Psychosom Med. 2005;67:825–32.
6. Sogg S, Mori DL. Revising the Boston interview: incorporating new knowledge and experience. Surg Obes Relat Dis. 2008;4:455–63.
7. Wadden TA, Sarwer DB. Behavioral assessment of candidates for bariatric surgery: a patient-oriented approach. Obesity. 2006;14(Suppl):S53–62.
8. Wadden TA, Foster GD. Weight and Lifestyle Inventory (WALI). Obesity. 2006;14(Suppl):S99–118.
9. Mitchell JE, Steffen KJ, de Zwaan M, Ertelt TW, Marino JM, Mueller A. Congruence between clinical and research-based psychiatric assessment in bariatric surgical candidates. Surg Obes Relat Dis. 2010;6:628–34.
10. Walfish S. Reducing Minnesota Multiphasic Personality Inventory defensiveness: effect of specialized instructions on retest validity in a sample of preoperative bariatric patients. Surg Obes Relat Dis. 2007;3:184–8.
11. Friedman KE, Applegate KL, Grant J. Who is adherent with preoperative psychological treatment recommendations among weight loss surgery candidates? Surg Obes Relat Dis. 2007;3:376–82.
12. Pawlow LA, O'Neil PM, White MA, Byrne TK. Findings and outcomes of psychological evaluations of gastric bypass applicants. Surg Obes Relat Dis. 2005;1:523–9.
13. Sarwer DB, Cohn NI, Gibbons LM, Magee L, Crerand CE, Raper SE, et al. Psychiatric diagnoses and psychiatric treatment among bariatric surgery candidates. Obes Surg. 2004;14:1148–56.
14. Heinberg LJ, Ashton K, Windover A. Moving beyond the dichotomous psychological evaluation: the Cleveland Clinic Behavioral Rating System for weight loss surgery. Surg Obes Relat Dis. 2010;6:185–90.
15. Merrell J, Ashton K, Windover A, Heinberg L. Psychological risk may influence drop-out prior to bariatric surgery. Surg Obes Relat Dis. 2012;8:463–9.
16. Allied Health Sciences Section Ad Hoc Behavioral Health Committee for the American Society for Metabolic and Bariatric Surgery. Suggestions for the pre-surgical psychological assessment of bariatric surgery candidates. Gainesville: American Society for Metabolic and Bariatric Surgery. 2004. Available from: http://www.asbs.org/html/pdf/PsychPreSurgicalAssessment.pdf. Accessed 8 May 2012.
17. White MA, Masheb RM, Rothschild BS, Burke-Martindale CH, Grilo CM. The prognostic significance of regular binge eating in extremely obese gastric bypass patients: 12-month postoperative outcomes. J Clin Psychiatry. 2006;67:1928–35.
18. Allison KC, Wadden TA, Sarwer DB, Fabricatore AN, Crerand CE, Gibbons LM, et al. Night eating syndrome and binge eating disorder among persons seeking bariatric surgery: prevalence and related features. Surg Obes Relat Dis. 2006;62:153–8.

19. Stunkard AJ, Allison KC. Two forms of disordered eating in obesity: binge eating and night eating. Int J Obes Relat Metab Disord. 2003;27:1–12.
20. Kalarchian MA, Marcus MD, Levine MD, Courcoulas AP, Pilkonis PA, Ringham RM, et al. Psychiatric disorders among bariatric surgery candidates: relationship to obesity and functional health status. Am J Psychiatry. 2007;164:328–34.
21. Sogg S. Assessment of bariatric surgery candidates: the clinical interview. In: Mitchell JE, de Zwaan M, editors. Psychosocial assessment and treatment of bariatric surgery patients. New York: Routledge; 2012. p. 15–35.
22. Heinberg LJ, Ashton K, Coughlin J. Alcohol and bariatric surgery: review and suggested recommendations for assessment and management. Surg Obes Relat Dis. 2012;8:357–63.
23. Peterson CB, Berg KC, Mitchell JE. Assessment of bariatric surgery candidates: structured interviews and self-report measures. In: Mitchell JE, de Zwaan M, editors. Psychosocial assessment and treatment of bariatric surgery patients. New York: Routledge; 2012. p. 37–60.
24. Beck AT, Steer RA, Brown GK. Beck depression inventory-second edition manual. San Antonio: Psychological Corporation; 1996.
25. Wadden TA, Butryn ML, Sarwer DB, Fabricatore AN, Crerand CE, Lipschutz PE, et al. Comparison of psychosocial status in treatment-seeking women with class III vs. class I-II obesity. Surg Obes Relat Dis. 2006;2:138–45.
26. Munoz DJ, Chen E, Fischer S, Roehrig M, Sanchez-Johnson L, Alverdy J, et al. Considerations for the use of the Beck Depression Inventory in the assessment of weight-loss surgery seeking patients. Obes Surg. 2007;17:1097–101.
27. Hamilton M. A rating scale for depression. J Neurol Neurosurg Psychiatry. 1960;23:56–62.
28. Kroenke K, Spitzer RL, Williams JB. Validity of a brief depression severity measure. J Gen Intern Med. 2001;16:606–13.
29. Spitzer RL, Yanovski S, Wadden T, Wing R, Marcus MD, Stunkard A, et al. Binge eating disorder: its further validation in a multisite study. Int J Eat Disord. 1993;13:137–53.
30. Derogatis LR. Symptom Checklist-90-R (SCL-90-R): administration, scoring, and procedures manual. 3rd ed. Minneapolis: National Computer Systems, Inc.; 1994.
31. Ransom D, Ashton K, Windover A, Heinberg L. Internal consistency and validity assessment of SCL-90-R for bariatric surgery candidates. Surg Obes Relat Dis. 2010;6:622–7.
32. Butcher JN, Dahlstrom WG, Graham JR, Tellegan A, Kaemmer B. The Minnesota Multiphasic Personality Inventory-2 (MMPI-2): manual for administration and scoring. Minneapolis: University of Minnesota Press; 1989.
33. Kinder BN, Walfish S, Scott Young M, Fairweather A. MMPI-2 profiles of bariatric surgery patients: a replication and extension. Obes Surg. 2008;18:1170–9.
34. Mechanick JI, Kushner RF, Sugerman HJ, Gonzalez-Campoy JM, Collazo-Clavell ML, Spitz AF, et al. American Association Of Clinical Endocrinologists, The Obesity Society, and American Society For Metabolic & Bariatric Surgery medical guidelines for clinical practice for the perioperative nutritional, metabolic, and nonsurgical support of the bariatric surgery patient. Obesity. 2009;17:S1–70.
35. Ashton K, Heinberg L, Windover A, Merrell J. Positive response to binge eating intervention enhances postoperative weight loss. Surg Obes Relat Dis. 2011;7:315–20.
36. West-Smith L, Sogg S. Creating a credential for bariatric behavioral health professionals: potential benefits, pitfalls, and provider opinion. Surg Obes Relat Dis. 2010;6:695–701.

Psychosocial Issues After Bariatric Surgery

Leslie J. Heinberg and Megan E. Lavery

Chapter Objectives

1. To appreciate the psychosocial issues of patients who have undergone bariatric surgery
2. To review studies that have examined specific psychosocial issues after bariatric surgery, including depression, suicide, eating pathology, and substance abuse
3. To understand the role of behavioral adherence and social support in optimizing postoperative outcomes

Introduction

Bariatric surgery is considered the most effective treatment for severe obesity (body mass index [BMI] ≥40 kg/m^2), resulting in an average weight loss of 25–35 % of initial body weight. As a result of this dramatic decrease in weight, as well as other significant reductions in medical comorbidity and increased longevity, bariatric surgery has become an increasingly common procedure. Unfortunately, despite successful outcomes for many bariatric surgery patients, there is considerable variability in outcome. A subset of patients struggles to lose the expected amount of weight, whereas others, although initially successful, regain a considerable amount of weight within the first few years following surgery. This regain can even reverse the improvement in comorbidities initially seen after surgery. Reasons for weight regain are generally not well understood. Although biological mechanisms such as metabolic changes, anatomical and physiological adaptations, and alterations in gut and adipocyte hormones have been posited, the majority of putative factors relate to behavior, compliance, and psychosocial factors.

As bariatric surgery procedures continue to grow, it is critical that clinicians and researchers better elucidate the psychosocial correlates related to weight loss and psychosocial outcomes following surgery. This chapter aims to synthesize the current literature regarding the association between bariatric surgery outcomes and psychosocial correlates in hopes of helping providers optimally facilitate postoperative behavior change. A number of psychosocial characteristics of bariatric surgery patients were reviewed in Chap. 1 by Sarwer and colleagues; this chapter will examine psychiatric comorbidities such as depression, suicide, eating pathology, and alcohol abuse that impact postoperative adjustment and management. Further, changes in psychosocial variables of interest such as quality of life and body image will be reviewed. Finally, behavioral and social factors, including adherence and social support, that impact postoperative outcome will be summarized.

Psychiatric Comorbidity

Depression

As noted in Chaps. 1 and 2, depression and obesity have been linked in a large number of studies. This suggests a vulnerability for depression in bariatric patients both preoperatively as well as postoperatively. Postoperatively, across a range of procedures, studies suggest that psychiatric comorbidity, particularly depression, is associated with less positive outcomes. For example, patients with two or more psychiatric disorders lost 10.8 BMI units after laparoscopic adjustable gastric banding (LAGB) compared to 16.1 BMI units in patients without a psychiatric diagnosis [1]. Similarly, poorer weight loss outcomes as measured by percent excess weight loss in laparoscopic sleeve gastrectomy (LSG) patients with a clinically diagnosed mood disorder

---

L.J. Heinberg, PhD (✉)
Behavioral Services, Bariatric and Metabolic Institute, Cleveland, OH, USA

Department of Medicine, Cleveland Clinic Lerner College of Medicine, Cleveland, OH, USA
e-mail: heinbel@ccf.org

M.E. Lavery, PsyD
Cleveland Clinic Foundation, 9500 Euclid Avenue/M61, Cleveland, OH 44195, USA

(e.g., major depression, bipolar affective disorder) were found at 1, 3, 6, and 9 months compared to those without a psychiatric diagnosis [2]. However, the groups were equivalent by 1 year post-LSG. Further, after removing patients with bipolar disorder from the analyses, no significant differences were found in the percentage of excess weight loss (%EWL) between patients with and without a lifetime history of depressive disorders [2]. Similar findings have been noted with Roux-en-Y gastric bypass (RYGB) patients. After adjusting for baseline BMI and other demographic covariates including gender, race, and age, a lifetime history of a mood disorder was associated with smaller decrease in BMI at 6-month follow-up [3]. Similarly, a lifetime history of an anxiety disorder was associated with poorer outcomes. Interestingly, current mood, anxiety, substance, and eating disorders were not associated with smaller weight losses [3]. Further, personality disorders (e.g., borderline personality disorder, narcissistic personality disorder, avoidant personality disorder) were not related to weight loss outcomes [3].

These studies have focused on the formal clinical diagnoses of major depression and other mood disorders. However, less robust predictive value has been demonstrated when examining depressive symptoms with paper and pencil questionnaires. Nevertheless, it is important to remember that while the presence of specific psychiatric diagnoses may be associated with smaller weight losses, these weight losses, and improvements in weight-related health problems, are still far more impressive than seen with more conservative weight loss treatments such as lifestyle modification and pharmacotherapy.

While the presence of preoperative depression may influence the magnitude of the postoperative weight loss, surgically induced weight loss has a clear, positive benefit on depressive symptoms as well as quality of life. Reductions of more than 50 % in Beck Depression Inventory scores have been demonstrated from baseline to 1 year post LAGB. Reductions on this measure as well as an interview-based assessment of depression also have been shown 1–2 years following RYGB. In a study of RYGB patients, the point prevalence of diagnosis of depression as measured by structured clinical interviews dropped from 33 % preoperatively to 16.5 % between 6 and 12 months postoperatively and to 14 % between years 2 and 3 [4]. However, no significant declines were demonstrated on point prevalence of anxiety disorders [4]. Of note, current or lifetime history of depressive disorders did not relate to weight loss outcomes. However, individuals with both depression and anxiety disorders—either currently or in their past—at baseline assessment had poorer weight loss outcomes [4]. A challenge to researchers and clinicians in understanding these findings is the high co-occurrence of mood disorders, such as depression and anxiety disorders. Indeed, many symptoms (e.g., sleep disturbance, negative cognitions) are present in both conditions. Future work that includes careful assessment of all types of psychiatric conditions may help illuminate the role of these disorders on postsurgical weight loss and the impact of weight loss on psychiatric symptoms.

A number of features of depression may make patients more vulnerable to poorer outcome and/or weight regain. Appetite disturbance is a key feature, as is avolition and a loss of energy. Further, there is a close association between binge eating disorder (BED) and depression, with the two disorders occurring together in approximately 50 % of patients. Finally, the majority of mood stabilizers, antidepressants, and atypical antipsychotics have obesogenic side effects. Preoperatively, almost three-quarters of patients report a lifetime history of psychotropic medication use whereas current psychotropic medication use is reported by approximately half of bariatric candidates. Long-term use of these medications holds the potential to negatively impact weight loss outcomes, a particularly relevant issue for younger surgery patients who may be on these medications for the rest of their lives and gain weight accordingly.

A related area of concern is the potential impact of a given procedure on the efficacy of psychotropic medications. Although many patients' medications related to metabolic illness are reduced or discontinued following surgery, many patients remain on their psychiatric medications. Unfortunately, the pharmacokinetics of psychotropic medications after surgery are not well understood. Dramatic changes in the absorption of medication may occur due to altered drug metabolism, reduced surface area of the gastrointestinal tract, and altered fat mass after surgery [5]. Studies modeling dissolution rates of antidepressants vary considerably. There is potential noted for dissolution to be increased, decreased, or to remain essentially unchanged [5]. Thus, there is a lack of evidence to inform clinicians with regard to differences in absorption, dissolution, and metabolism of medications after the different surgical procedures. Recently, a study compared post-RYGB patients to nonsurgical controls on sertraline (Zoloft) plasma levels. Both groups were matched on BMI, age, and gender [6]. Maximal plasma concentration and plasma concentration/time curve of the drug were significantly smaller than the nonsurgical controls [6].

For these reasons, it is recommended that patients be monitored closely by their prescribing providers—a concerning high percentage of whom are primary care physicians rather than psychiatrists—in the immediate postoperative period to assess potential problems with their psychotropic medications. Closer monitoring throughout the first year is warranted with examination of plasma levels for medications that have documented therapeutic ranges [5].

Suicide

Overall, the impact of weight loss on mood-related improvement is highly encouraging. However, for a subset of patients, there may be worsening of psychiatric symptoms. Over the past decade, there has been concern related to the observation of higher rates of suicide among bariatric patients postoperatively compared to the population as a whole or compared to obese individuals who do not undergo weight loss surgery [7]. Although longevity is largely increased by bariatric interventions, deaths by accident, drug overdose, and suicide have all been documented postoperatively [7, 8].

In the suicide literature, a number of risk factors for suicide have been repeatedly observed. These include psychopathology, depression, anxiety, personality disorders, eating disorders, alcohol and substance abuse, and chronic medical illness. All of these risk factors are more prevalent in persons with extreme obesity presenting for surgery. Indeed, although research data is somewhat equivocal regarding whether obesity is a risk, protective, or unrelated factor to suicide, a positive association between obesity and suicide has been observed most frequently in the literature [9]. Further, one study demonstrated that there is a 73 times greater prevalence of suicide history among bariatric patients when compared to the population. These past attempts are particularly concerning given that past suicide attempts are the strongest risk factor for future suicide deaths.

A number of possible explanations of the occurrence of suicide after bariatric surgery have been offered. For example, presurgical psychological distress could be exacerbated if the outcomes of surgery were disappointing, or failed to yield the improvements in quality of life that patients expected. Indeed a dramatic increase in rates of depressive and anxiety disorders and episodes, as late as 13–15 years post-bariatric surgery, have been observed. Additional putative factors include dissatisfaction with body image following dramatic weight loss, particularly with loose redundant skin, alterations in metabolic biomarkers such as a decrease in serum cholesterol, disinhibition and impulsivity secondary to altered absorption of alcohol, hypoglycemia, and changes in the pharmacokinetics of psychotropic drugs [9, 10].

In addition to identifying reasons why bariatric patients may be at risk of worsening depression and/or suicidal behavior, it is vitally important that clinicians involved in management of obesity, regardless of specialty, appreciate that depression and suicide are significant threats. Even after improvement or resolution of the obesity, the underlying psychopathology related to suicide likely remains for many individuals. Preoperative psychopathology remains one of the most parsimonious explanations for the recurrence of depression and suicidal behavior postoperatively in a psychiatrically vulnerable population. Thus, additional monitoring and treatment of at-risk patients may be the best strategy to prevent suicides in bariatric patients.

Disordered Eating

Because of variability in weight loss after bariatric surgery, a body of research has examined the prevalence and effects of disturbed eating on weight loss outcomes. This literature is reviewed in detail in Chap. 4. Patients with extreme obesity frequently report pathological eating habits, such as binge eating disorder (BED) and night eating syndrome (NES) [11]. BED is one of the most common psychiatric disorders endorsed by patients prior to surgery, present in approximately one in ten bariatric surgery candidates [12]. Preoperative BED patients do not differ significantly on BMI from non-BED patients. However, these patients often experience greater psychosocial distress and psychiatric comorbidities. Although binge eating episodes often decrease or cease immediately following surgery, long-term studies suggest symptoms can reemerge postoperatively. However, due to physical restrictions after surgery, it is often impossible for patients to eat the objectively large amounts of food typically characterizing binge eating.

For this reason, there has been discussion about the use of the formal diagnostic criteria for BED in persons who have undergone surgery. While some researchers have used the traditional Diagnostic and Statistical Manual of Mental Disorders (DSM) IV criteria to examine binge eating postoperatively, other investigators have utilized modified criteria that often exclude a specification of "an objectively large amount of food." Instead, several researchers have hypothesized that a subjective sense of loss of control (LOC) may be a critical component of disordered eating following surgery. Supporting this postulation, a growing body of literature reveals high rates of subjective LOC eating in bariatric surgery patients. For instance, Kofman and colleagues [13] examined disordered eating patterns in 437 gastric bypass patients between 3 and 10 years postsurgery. Surprisingly, half of participants (49.9 %) endorsed times when they felt they could not stop eating or control the amount they were eating. Using modified criteria for BED, which included the consumption of subjectively large quantities of food, 18 % of patients met the criteria for BED. In addition, 46 % of participants reported frequently consuming small quantities of food with LOC over an extended period (similar to "grazing" described in Chap. 4), with 72 % of patients reporting this pattern 2 or more days per week. These findings underscore the prevalence of eating with LOC following bariatric surgery. In order to more accurately capture patterns of disordered eating, it may be important to cultivate criteria that conceptualize LOC and number of eating episodes as vital components to disordered eating patterns after surgery.

Unfortunately, maladaptive eating patterns following surgery can have a negative impact on both surgical and psychological outcomes. LOC eating is often related to the consumption of more calories and a higher intake of carbohydrate and fat. As a result, postoperative disordered eating often has a negative impact on weight loss outcomes [14]. Several long-term outcome studies have highlighted a relationship between LOC eating and weight regain. Similar results have been found for patients who specifically engage in postoperative graze eating. Research also indicates that bariatric surgery patients with disordered eating report significantly lower quality of life [13]. Although the literature in this area is not conclusive, postsurgical LOC eating may represent both eating-specific and global distress.

Given the frequency of eating disorders among preoperative patients and the negative impact of disordered eating on psychosocial correlates, research has examined whether an eating disorder diagnosis prior to surgery is related to disordered eating postoperatively. (This literature also is reviewed in Chap. 4.) White and colleagues [14] have suggested that both preoperative objective and subjective LOC is highly predictive of LOC eating postsurgery. Saunders [15] also found that 80 % of patients who endorsed binge eating or grazing with LOC prior to surgery experienced LOC an average of 3–5 times per week 6 months postsurgery. Thus, these findings suggest that preoperative disordered eating is closely related to maladaptive eating patterns postsurgery.

However, whether preoperative eating disorders are related to poor prognosis remains highly debated. While some recommend that patients with eating disorders not undergo surgery until they receive targeted treatment, others contend that having binge eating, night eating, or graze eating should not disqualify patients from surgery. These diverging opinions accurately reflect the conflicting literature on the impact of preoperative eating disorders (namely, BED) on psychosocial outcomes. While some studies suggest that preoperative BED significantly predicts postoperative weight loss, other research suggests the opposite relationship or no relationship at all [14]. Findings around psychosocial correlates are also ambiguous. Some data indicate that patients with BED prior to surgery experience the most significant improvements in QOL and psychosocial functioning after surgery [14]. Other research suggests no significant difference in measures of QOL and overall distress in patients with and without preoperative BED/LOC eating. At the same time, a 2008 study suggests that patients with preoperative disordered eating may experience more body image distortion than patients without disordered eating despite similar weight reductions [16]. Therefore, at present, the association between preoperative disordered eating and psychosocial outcomes remains unclear. Encouragingly, brief cognitive-behavioral interventions for bariatric surgery candidates with BED have been shown to be highly efficacious, and responders to such treatment have been shown to lose more weight postoperatively than nonresponders. More specifically, when compared to nonresponders, patients categorized as positive responders have demonstrated significantly greater weight loss at both 6 and 12 months.

Although most studies have examined binge eating, graze eating, and night eating, clinical reports have documented the development of anorexia nervosa (AN) and bulimia nervosa (BN) postsurgery. Many case studies of AN or BN have involved self-induced vomiting, though laxative abuse, food restriction, and fasting have also been reported. At times, it is difficult to make a distinction between eating disorder behaviors associated with AN and BN and typical or less common postsurgical sequelae. The emergence of vomiting exemplifies this sentiment. Vomiting can occur in patients after surgery as a result of food intolerance or as a means to reduce discomfort. Data suggest that vomiting is common among postoperative patients (approximately 60 % of patients) with 12–15 % of patients admitting to vomiting to influence weight [15]. For a subgroup of patients, self-induced vomiting may become a method to hasten or maintain weight loss [17]. Given the likelihood of vomiting and other sequelae after surgery, some authors contend that the physical changes associated with surgery may contribute to the development of AN and BN. Arguably, the reinforcing effects of weight loss, a heightened focus on weight, and bodily changes inherent in the surgery process may all exacerbate eating disorder patterns.

Although bariatric surgery is a powerful tool, it is clear that eating disorders and pathological eating behaviors can emerge postoperatively. The literature suggests that LOC and graze eating are the most prominent disordered eating patterns among postsurgery patients. There remains a need to elucidate the diagnostic criteria for eating disorders after surgery, specifically in regard to BED. Furthermore, several studies suggest that a substantial portion of patients could benefit from targeted treatment. Future research is needed to clarify whether treatment of maladaptive eating patterns is most useful before or after surgery. Additional prospective, long-term studies examining changes in eating patterns over time could also help to identify factors that contribute to or maintain LOC eating postoperatively.

Alcohol and Substance Use

Alcohol and substance use are points of concerns both preoperatively and postoperatively in bariatric populations and, as a result, have received a significant amount of research and clinical attention. Current alcohol or substance abuse/dependence is seen as contraindications for bariatric surgery in a number of published guidelines, e.g., those set by the American Association of Clinical Endocrinologists/American Society for Metabolic and Weight Loss Surgery/The Obesity Society (AACE/ASMBS/TOS) and the National Institutes of Health (NIH). Further, the vast majority of bariatric surgery programs screen for and potentially delay and/or deny surgery based upon these issues. A lifetime history of any substance use disorder is significantly higher in weight loss surgery candidates (33.2 %) compared to the population at large (14.6 %) [12]. However, current alcohol and substance abuse is remarkably low (<1 %) compared to population norms (8.9 %) [12]. This lower rate has been consistently demonstrated, even in studies in which data collection is separate and confidential from the presurgical psychological evaluation. Regardless, the majority of bariatric programs require patients to reduce or eliminate problematic alcohol use prior to surgery.

In the last several years, the lay press has cited anecdotal information regarding "addiction transfer" in post-bariatric patients. In this reported phenomenon, patients who can no longer "abuse" food are theorized to develop other addiction problems. Although this has received a great deal of attention in the mass media, until recently little empirical data was available to understand the risk [18]. More recently, researchers have begun investigating the prevalence of problematic alcohol use after surgery. However, prevalence of substance abuse and other compulsive behaviors is almost nonexistent outside of case reports. A Web-based questionnaire indicated that 83 % of self-selected respondents continued to consume alcohol after RYGB. Among those who continue to drink alcohol, 84 % drank one or more alcoholic beverages a week and 28.4 % indicated a problem controlling alcohol. This was in contrast to only 4.5 % of the sample of patients identifying problems managing alcohol prior to surgery. However, while 14 % of the sample drank considerably more alcohol after surgery, 15 % of respondents noted that they drank considerably less.

More recently, longitudinal data across ten bariatric programs and more than 2,000 patients demonstrated a significant increase in alcohol use disorders in the second postoperative year [19]. Specifically following RYGB, rates of alcohol use disorders were higher in the second year compared to the year prior to and immediately following surgery. In more than half of the cases, alcohol use disorders were not reported in the year prior to surgery. A number of related risk factors were found including male gender, younger age, smoking, regular preoperative alcohol use, recreational drug use, and lower scores on social support [19]. In a smaller study of longer-term outcomes (13–15 years), Mitchell and colleagues [20] found an increase in alcohol abuse over time (2.6 % presurgery to 5.1 % postsurgery) but a decline in alcohol dependence (10.3 % presurgery vs. 2.6 % postsurgery). In another long-term study (6–10 years post-RYGB), 7.1 % of the population had alcohol abuse or dependence before surgery, which was unchanged postoperatively, whereas 2.9 % endorsed alcohol dependence after surgery while not endorsing alcohol problems preoperatively [21]. Others have found an alcohol use disorders prevalence of almost 12 % in patients who were at least 2 years post-weight loss surgery and that current problems were significantly more likely in patients with a lifetime history of alcohol use disorders and those who underwent an RYGB. In a study examining substance abuse treatment center admissions, 2–6 % of admissions were positive for a bariatric surgery history [22].

However, in this and many of the other reviewed studies, it is unclear whether reported events are the result of increased use in those who were already misusing or abusing alcohol prior to surgery, relapse in persons with a history of addiction problems who were in remission prior to surgery, or new onset cases. Follow-up studies with longer duration were associated with higher rates of alcohol use disorders. This is concerning as it may point to patients worsening over time. Although the majority of studies demonstrate an increased risk, particularly with RYGB, it is also important to note that most studies do not show prevalence rates significantly higher than population norms.

Interestingly, two studies have demonstrated better weight loss outcomes—at least in the first 2 years—among patients with a past substance abuse history as compared to those patients without past problems with alcohol or other substances [23, 24]. It was hypothesized in both studies that individuals who have successfully resolved alcohol or substances problems may utilize similar skills in making lifestyle changes following surgery. Research has yet to elucidate how long an individual should ideally be abstinent before undergoing bariatric surgery. Many programs require 12 months of documented sobriety, a defensible recommendation given that substance abuse relapse rates fall dramatically after 12 months.

Physiological changes following surgery may change vulnerability to problematic alcohol use. The pharmacokinetics of alcohol differ post-RYGB relative to presurgery and nonsurgical control comparison groups [25, 26]. Pharmacokinetic findings in these studies, like those of psychiatric medications previously described, have varied, likely as a result of significant differences in methodology and assessment. Most obviously, the significant weight loss patients experience results in a higher concentration of ethanol for each drink consumed. However, other pharmacokinetic changes reported to occur post-RYGB are accelerated alcohol absorption as demonstrated by a shorter time to reach maximum concentration, higher maximum alcohol concentration, longer time to eliminate alcohol, rapid emptying of the gastric pouch facilitating faster absorption of alcohol, and the reduced volume of the stomach resulting in less alcohol dehydrogenase, which partially metabolizes alcohol.

For example, in a case-crossover study of RYGB patients [26], blood alcohol content (BAC) was measured using breathalyzer recordings (BrAC) preoperatively and 3 and 6 months after RYGB. The peak BrAC in patients after consuming 5 oz of red wine at 6 months (0.088 %) was more than 3.5 times greater than preoperatively (0.024 %), and differential symptoms of intoxication were noted [26]. This level is also above the legal limit of intoxication for driving in most states. Similar findings of higher maximum alcohol concentration have been demonstrated in a prospective study of patients who have undergone laparoscopic sleeve gastrectomy.

Preoperative assessment and treatment recommendations have been offered that focuses on standardized assessment methods, preoperative education, and the use of behavioral contracts to better inform patients that there is a potential for increased risk of alcohol use disorders [27]. In general, patients should be educated as part of their preoperative assessment/preparation about the changes that will occur in how they will absorb and metabolize alcohol and that some patients (e.g., those with a past history of alcohol use disorders) may be at higher risk for problematic use after surgery. This increased risk points to the importance of education, informed consent, and continued monitoring. Patients should be informed that the best way to mitigate the risk of problematic alcohol use disorders is to drink in considerable moderation. For those who are concerned about this risk or who have multiple risk factors, abstinence from alcohol is the best course of action. Unfortunately, far less is known about how to manage patients if problems with alcohol or substances develop. Future research should examine the sensitivity and specificity of assessment techniques and the efficacy of risk management strategies and develop interventions for patients who exhibit problematic alcohol use following surgery. Further, the rates of substance abuse and dependence (both illicit and prescription) and other compulsive behaviors (e.g., gambling, sexual behaviors, etc.) following weight loss surgery should be explored.

Psychosocial Issues

Quality of Life

Chapter 3 provides a detailed discussion of quality of life in bariatric surgery. Here we provide a brief overview of changes in quality of life after surgery. Within the first year after surgery, many bariatric surgery patients experience rapid improvements in health-related quality of life (HRQOL) [28]. For example, 1 year after LAGB, patients demonstrate important improvements within physical, psychosocial, and sexual functioning domains [29]. Surprisingly, the most significant gains have been documented in the first few months postsurgery [28]. However, one recent study [30] suggests that these rapid improvements may not be consistent across the multiple domains of quality of life. More specifically, at 3 months post-laparoscopic gastric bypass or LAGB, Vincent and colleagues [30] found that patients endorsed significant improvements within physical domains on the Medical Outcomes Study short-form 36-item instrument (SF-36). Similar increases were not observed on the mental component score of the SF-36. These results suggest that within a short period after surgery, the physical domain of HRQOL may be affected to a greater degree than psychological correlates. It is likely that this pattern reflects the quick improvement in medical comorbidities often seen soon after surgery. Social, occupation, and emotional functioning may improve more gradually as patients begin to progressively engage in life experiences after surgery. Although Sarwer and colleagues [31] found significant improvements in several domains of quality of life within a few months following surgery, their data also suggests differences in quality of life scores across groups. In particular, while males experienced continued improvements in SF-36 mental health subscale and SF-36 mental health summary scores, females began to experience a decline in SF-36 mental health summary scores after 20 weeks and at 92 weeks endorsed SF-36 mental health subscale scores that were not significantly different than preoperative values. Ultimately, regardless of its initial trajectory, studies suggest that improvements in HRQOL tend to plateau 1–2 years postsurgery and may reach levels akin to values seen in nonobese populations.

The mechanisms underlying these significant improvements in HRQOL values have been the subject of increasing interest. Several investigations have explored the role of degree of weight loss on HRQOL. Although a few studies have established a relationship between excess weight loss (EWL) and HRQOL [28], overall % EWL has not been shown to be predictive of HRQOL values [29]. In fact, despite differences in mean EWL, RYGB, and LAGB, patients have demonstrated comparable improvements in HRQOL. Similar findings have been documented between LSG and LAGB patients. Therefore, it appears that the difference in typical EWL between bariatric surgery procedures has little impact on HRQOL postsurgery.

Given the restricted influence of weight loss, researchers have begun to examine other potential determinants of HRQOL. Investigators have postulated that presurgical comorbidities may impact the magnitude of HRQOL improvements after surgery. However, the data thus far do not support a relationship between these variables [29]. Furthermore, although bariatric surgeries can result in significant food intolerance, nausea, and vomiting, studies indicate that gastrointestinal side effects are minimally related to HRQOL [28]. In an attempt to further clarify factors associated with HRQOL, Pilone and colleagues recently explored the impact of level of HRQOL prior to surgery, self-perceived effects of surgery, and hunger/satiety cues on HRQOL in 334 postoperative LAGB patients 1 year after surgery. Patients with the most impaired levels of HRQOL at baseline experienced the greatest improvements in HRQOL. In addition, higher satiety after meals and a higher perceived efficacy of the band were related to larger increases in physical and mental components of HRQOL [28]. These findings suggest that patients with markedly impaired HRQOL prior to surgery may experience the largest improvements. In addition, it appears that patients' perceptions of the power of the intervention may impact an overall sense of quality of life. It is possible that patients who view their procedure as highly effective may experience increased self-efficacy regarding their ability to control their eating and EWL.

In addition to examining correlates of HRQOL, the stability of HRQOL improvements has been the focus of some research. Unfortunately, studies examining the long-term course of HRQOL after surgery have yielded conflicting results. Some findings suggest that the early improvements in HRQOL are maintained long-term regardless of weight regain. However, evidence from a 10-year prospective study suggests that variations in HRQOL are consistent with changes in weight [32]. More specifically, researchers observed peak improvements in HRQOL during the first year following surgery. A gradual decline in HRQOL was documented from 1 to 6 years post-op. This pattern appeared to correspond with typical weight regain. From 6 to 10 years after surgery, both HRQOL and weight stabilized. These findings underscore the need to clarify the role of weight regain in HRQOL after surgery.

Body Image

As noted in Chap. 3, body image is a multidimensional psychological construct that includes perception of body size, satisfaction with weight/shape/appearance, and behavioral aspects (e.g., avoidance of wearing revealing clothing, avoidance of activities such as swimming). Relatively little is known about the body image experiences of severely obese persons across the age spectrum, in part as the majority of psychometrically validated measures of body image do not necessarily and appropriately capture the body image experiences of those with extreme obesity or those who experience the massive weight loss seen with bariatric surgery.

Regardless of these methodological issues, bariatric patients have been shown to experience significant improvements in body image in the first 2 years following surgery [31]. These changes are correlated with percent weight loss and the postoperative values are comparable to published norms. However, there is considerable variability in body image, and greater preoperative body image dissatisfaction has been shown to predict psychological distress 1 year following surgery [33].

A fairly sizable literature has examined body image in postoperative patients as it relates to the common problem of excess skin and the resulting interest in body contouring surgery. Rapid and substantial weight loss is often associated with hanging, redundant skin, which is aesthetically displeasing to patients; it often leads to skin irritation and skin breakdown, infection, and ulcerations. Further, patients often note its effects on physical functioning, sexual functioning, posture, and difficulties with urination. Although overall body image improves postoperatively, some men and women remain dissatisfied with specific body areas associated with redundant skin.

Adherence to Postoperative Guidelines

Inadequate adherence to the dietary and behavioral recommendations required of bariatric surgery can have significant consequences. Perhaps most notably, nonadherence to postsurgical instructions has been associated with lower EWL. Limited adherence to the postoperative diet has specifically been linked to malnutrition and weight regain, including folic acid, vitamin B12, and iron deficiencies. Poor nutritional adherence can also lead to unpleasant gastrointestinal symptoms (e.g., nausea, vomiting, "plugging," and gastric dumping). In addition, nonadherence to follow-up care recommendations has been identified as a significant factor in the development of postsurgical complications. Missing appointments can also result in a reduced support network and less behavioral reinforcement. Thus, it is clear that poor adherence to postsurgical recommendations can have significant consequences for patients within several domains.

Given the potential "costs" of not following recommendations, one might expect rates of nonadherence to be low within the context of bariatric surgery. In an attempt to elucidate the extent of nonadherence, Toussi and colleagues [34] examined several facets of adherence in 112 gastric bypass patients, including appointment attendance, exercise, food choices, medication compliance, and weight loss plan adherence. Both pre- and postsurgery patients experienced the most difficulty attending appointments. In fact, 65 % patients missed at least one appointment before surgery, while another 72 % missed at least one postoperative visit. Similarly, nonadherence to exercise and weight loss instructions (e.g., eating large portions, grazing, etc.) rose after surgery, with rates increasing from 39 to 51 % and 42 to 57 %, respectively. Although poor food choices were not a considerable issue prior to surgery (11 %), nonadherence to dietary guidelines multiplied within 2 years following surgery (37 %). Despite the potential consequences of these choices, the findings imply that rates of nonadherence generally increase postsurgery [34]. It is possible that this pattern reflects greater motivation to adhere to recommendations preoperatively due to surgery serving as a primary incentive for behavior change.

As a result of the prevalence and potential impact of nonadherence, a recent emphasis has been placed on identifying factors affecting compliance. In a retrospective study of 375 bariatric surgery patients, Wheeler and colleagues [35] found that several characteristics were significantly correlated with postoperative adherence. More specifically, results indicate that a greater BMI prior to surgery is a significant predictor of postoperative nonadherence. Younger patients also were significantly less likely to adhere with postoperative appointments [35]. The investigators postulate that younger patients may be more likely to be the primary caregivers of young children, which may interfere with appointment attendance. This hypothesis appears supported by the additional finding that being single significantly improves adherence [35].

In addition to demographic characteristics, studies have also investigated the association between psychological correlates and adherence. Unfortunately, there is no universal agreement regarding the role of psychiatric conditions on postoperative compliance. Some research suggests that psychological comorbidities serve as barriers to adherence. For example, within a retrospective study, researchers examined the medical records of 149 RYGB patients during the first 4 years after surgery [36]. Results indicate that a diagnosis of depression is correlated with insufficient weight loss and poor dietary adherence. Similarly, self-esteem, depressive symptoms, and affect were all associated with adherence to nutritional guidelines [11]. At the same time, other studies suggest a limited relationship between psychiatric disorders and postoperative adherence. For example, depressive symptoms were unrelated to attending follow-up visits [35]. Further, using structured diagnostic interviews, one investigation found that most Axis I and Axis II disorders were not associated with compliance with diet, exercise, and appointment recommendations. However, there was evidence of a negative relationship between narcissistic personality disorder and adherence.

Considering the conflicting state of the research, it is possible that differences in the measurement of psychiatric disorders between studies account for some of the inconsistency. In addition, this body of literature may be restricted by the fact that many studies considered severe uncontrolled depression or other psychiatric disorders to be a contraindication to surgery. Therefore, patients with more severe psychiatric symptoms may not undergo surgery and subsequently would not be included in postoperative adherence studies.

Furthermore, it has been hypothesized that preoperative eating disorders may interfere with dietary adherence. While several studies indicate that eating disorders are related to nonadherence with the postoperative diet, other investigations suggests little to no relationship. For example, a study by Sarwer and colleagues examined the relationship between preoperative cognitive restraint (one's ability to intentionally control food intake) and self-reported adherence to dietary guidelines in 200 RYGB patients [11]. Participants who endorsed higher levels of cognitive restraint at baseline reported greater adherence to the postoperative diet and experienced more weight loss 2 years postoperatively. These results imply that preoperative eating patterns and cognitive strategies may continue to influence dietary adherence after surgery. However, the relationship between maladaptive eating prior to surgery and compliance with dietary guidelines postsurgery remains unclear.

Memory and executive functioning deficits in severely obese populations have been consistently demonstrated in the literature. As a result, a body of research has begun to examine the influence of cognitive deficits on adherence. Within a sample of 84 patients, Spitznagel and colleagues [36] found that 16 % of preoperative patients evidenced clinically impaired performance on components of attention/executive and verbal memory functioning. Such deficits could lead to reduced adherence to postoperative lifestyle changes, including poor meal planning, difficulties resisting foods, and trouble accurately recalling dietary and exercise guidelines. Although the association between cognitive deficits and adherence has yet to be examined empirically within a bariatric surgery population, the relationship between cognitive impairments and poor adherence to other medical regimens has been well established. However, in light of the fact that cognitive performance may improve as a result of the weight loss surgery, it is difficult to ascertain how baseline cognitive performance may affect patients' abilities to adhere to lifestyle changes. Thus, much remains unknown about the specific factors related to postsurgical adherence. Unfortunately, many of the current studies examining adherence are limited by their retrospective nature. In addition, the definition of adherence varies widely across studies, thus making it difficult to truly compare results. It is critical that future research continue to identify factors associated with adherence while addressing current limitations. Additional research is needed in order to improve providers' understanding of barriers to adherence following bariatric surgery. Ultimately, this understanding could result in the development of interventions to improve adherence and enhance outcomes for bariatric surgery patients.

Social Support

Social support is hypothesized to enhance patients' ability to cope with the drastic lifestyle changes associated with bariatric surgery. Social support can come in many forms, including family cohesiveness, online forums, and program supports. In particular, support groups are thought to be an integral component of the weight management process for many patients. Several empirical studies demonstrate improved weight loss outcomes in patients who attend support groups following weight loss surgery [37]. This growing body of evidence suggests that patients should be encouraged to attend support groups, though differences in weight loss may not be seen until several months postsurgery due to the initial strength of surgical interventions.

Given the relationship between support group attendance and EWL, it is important to evaluate whether there is a critical number of support group meetings that patients must attend in order to obtain significant benefit. Livhits et al. [37] suggest that attendance at even one support group postsurgery is one of the strongest predictors of weight loss. This assertion implies that support group attendance in and of itself may be related to more significant EWL. However, some research supports the notion that more than a few meetings are needed to achieve greater weight loss. For example, after accounting for time since surgery, a 1998 study found that the number of support group meetings attended accounted for a significant amount of variance in weight loss values. Similarly, other research has demonstrated a linear relationship between number of group meetings attended and weight loss after controlling for baseline BMI. In addition, an investigation found that at 12 months postsurgery, patients who attended five support group meetings had an average of 55.5 % EWL versus 47.1 % EWL in patients who attended fewer than five support group meetings. This group of studies highlights how number of support group meetings may influence the relationship between attendance and EWL. However, additional research is needed to clarify the ideal amount of meetings attended and other related factors, including group cohesiveness.

Unfortunately, this body of literature suffers from several limitations. For one, the operational definition of support group attendance varies widely across studies. While one study required attendance at one postoperative support group, another investigation only accepted attendance at 50 % or more meetings over a specific span of time. In addition, studies examining the relationship between participation in support groups and weight loss are limited by their observational and prospective natures. A causal association between support groups and weight loss cannot be demonstrated without the rigor of randomized trials. However, several investigators have expressed concerns around withholding support group attendance. Given that most patients lose a significant portion of their weight within the first year after surgery, some researchers argue that assigning patients to a control group could markedly impact their weight loss. Therefore, several concerns and factors would need to be taken into account when constructing future control trials studying support group attendance.

Research examining other aspects of social support is less consistent than the literature on support groups. Surprisingly, only one known study has found a significant relationship between other forms of social support and EWL. More specifically, married bariatric surgery patients had more than 2.6 times greater risk of achieving suboptimal weight loss when compared to unmarried counterparts. Nevertheless, other studies have failed to find significant results. Although one investigation found a relationship between perceived social support and weight loss within a behavioral weight loss program, similar results were not demonstrated for the surgery group. In addition, using semi-structured interviews, a 1995 study examined the potential influence of several components of social support (emotional support and number of close friends and relatives) over the first 2 years after surgery in gastric bypass patients. No aspect of social support was associated with postoperative EWL. However, facets of social support were found to be related to several other outcome variables. For example, lower emotional support and affection scores were related to significantly stronger feelings that life had not changed as much as expected following surgery. In addition, participants with higher positive interaction scores were less likely to endorse a preoccupation with food. Thus, although general correlates of social support may not directly relate to EWL, these findings imply that social support may impact important aspects of life after surgery.

Conclusion

There is significant evidence that bariatric surgery is the most effective and durable treatment for severe obesity. In addition to significant weight loss and resolution of many medical comorbidities, after surgery psychological and psychosocial difficulties often improve significantly. This is especially striking given that severely obese persons often have greater psychological vulnerabilities than population base rates. However, there is considerable variability in bariatric surgery outcomes. A number of psychosocial factors such as body image, adherence, and social support may play a role in this variability. Further, although psychiatric symptoms often decrease, a subset of patients may have continued difficulties with eating behaviors, alcohol use, and/or mood symptoms. Continued monitoring and treatment of psychological factors by multidisciplinary teams may help optimize outcomes and decrease negative psychosocial sequelae.

Question and Answer Section

Questions

1. Typically modified criteria for binge eating disorder (BED) for post-op patient:
   A. Emphasize frequency of eating
   B. Are no different than the traditional criteria for BED
   C. Exclude a criterion for loss of control
   D. Exclude a criterion for the consumption of an objectively large amount of food

2. Studies examining support group attendance suggest that:
   A. Support group attendance is unrelated to outcomes.
   B. Patients who attend support groups often lose less weight.
   C. Patients who attend support groups typically have better weight loss outcomes.
   D. The effects of support group attendance on outcomes are unknown.
3. Toussi et al.'s (2009) study on adherence suggests that both before and after surgery patients experience the most difficulty…
   A. Following dietary guidelines
   B. Following general weight loss instructions
   C. Following exercise guidelines
   D. Attending appointments

Answers

1. **D**. Post-op BED criteria typically excludes a criterion for the consumption of an objectively large amount of food.
2. **C**. Patients who attend support groups typically have better weight loss outcomes.
3. **D**. Pre- and postsurgery, patients have the most difficulty attending appointments.

References

1. Kinzl JF, Schrattenecker M, Traweger C, Mattesich M, Fiala M, Biebl W. Psychosocial predictors of weight loss after bariatric surgery. Obes Surg. 2006;16:1609–14.
2. Semanscin-Doerr D, Windover A, Ashton K, Heinberg LJ. Mood disorders in laparoscopic sleeve gastrectomy patients: does it affect early weight loss? Surg Obes Relat Dis. 2010;6:191–206.
3. Kalarchian MA, Marcus MD, Levine MD, Soulakova JN, Courcoulas AP, Wisinski MSC. Relationship of psychiatric disorders to 6-month outcomes after gastric bypass. Surg Obes Relat Dis. 2008;4:544–9.
4. de Zwaan M, Enderle J, Wagner S, Mühlhans B, Ditzen B, Gefeller O, et al. Anxiety and depression in bariatric surgery patients: a prospective, follow-up study using structured clinical interviews. J Affect Disord. 2011;133:61–8.
5. Sarwer DB, Faulconbridge LF, Steffen KJ, Roerig JL, Mitchell JE. Managing patients after surgery: changes in drug prescription, body weight can affect psychotropic prescribing. Curr Psychiatry. 2011;10:3–9.
6. Roerig JL, Steffen K, Zimmerman C, Mitchell JE, Crosby RD, Cao L. Preliminary comparison of sertraline levels in postbariatric surgery patients versus matched nonsurgical cohort. Surg Obes Relat Dis. 2012;8:62–6.
7. Tindle HA, Omalu B, Courcoulas A, Marcus M, Hammers J, Kuller LH. Risk of suicide after long-term follow-up from bariatric surgery. Am J Med. 2010;123:1036–42.
8. Adams TD, Gress RE, Smith SC, Halverson RC, Simper SC, Rosamond WD, et al. Long-term mortality after gastric bypass surgery. N Engl J Med. 2007;357(8):753–61.
9. Heneghan H, Heinberg LJ, Windover A, Rogula T, Schauer PR. Weighing the evidence for an association between obesity and suicide risk. Surg Obes Relat Dis. 2012;8:98–107.
10. Mitchell JE, Crosby R, deZwaan M, Engel S, Roerig J, Steffen K et al. Possible risk factors for increased suicide following bariatric surgery. Obesity. 2013;21(4):665–72.
11. Sarwer DB, Wadden TA, Moore RH, Baker AW, Gibbons LM, Raper SE, et al. Preoperative eating behavior, postoperative dietary adherence and weight loss following gastric bypass surgery. Surg Obes Relat Dis. 2008;4(5):640–6.
12. Mitchell JE, Selzer F, Kalarchian MA, Devlin MJ, Strain G, Elder KA et al. Psychopathology before surgery in the Longitudinal Assessment of Bariatric Surgery-3 (LABS-3) psychosocial study. Surg Obes Relat Dis. 2012;8(5):533–41.
13. Kofman MD, Lent MR, Swencionis C. Maladaptive eating patterns, quality of life, and weight outcomes following gastric bypass: results of an internet survey. Obesity. 2010;18:1938–43.
14. White MA, Kalarchian MA, Masheb RM, Marcus MD, Grilo CM. Loss of control over eating predicts outcomes in bariatric surgery: a prospective 24-month follow-up study. J Clin Psychiatry. 2010;71(2):174–84.
15. Saunders R. "Grazing": a high-risk behavior. Obes Surg. 2004;14:98–102.
16. Morrow J, Gluck M, Lorence M, Flancbaum L, Geliebter A. Night eating status and influence on body weight, body image, hunger, and cortisol pre- and post- Roux-en-Y Gastric Bypass surgery. Eat Weight Disord. 2008;13(4):e96–9.
17. Mitchell JE. Bulimia with self-induced vomiting after gastric stapling. Am J Psychiatry. 1985;142:656.
18. Sogg S. Alcohol misuse after bariatric surgery: epiphenomenon or "Oprah" phenomenon? Surg Obes Rel Dis. 2006;3:366.
19. King WC, Chen J, Mitchell JE, Kalarchian MA, Steffen KJ, Engel SG, et al. Prevalence of alcohol use disorders before and after bariatric surgery. JAMA. 2012;307(23):1–10.
20. Mitchell JE, Lancaster KL, Burgard MA, Howell LM, Krahn DD, Crosby RD, et al. Long-term follow-up of patients' status after gastric bypass. Obes Surg. 2001;11:464–8.
21. Ertelt TW, Mitchell JE, Lancaster K, et al. Alcohol abuse and dependence before and after bariatric surgery: a review of the literature and report of a new data set. Surg Obes Rel Dis. 2008;4:647–50.
22. Saules KK, Wiedemann A, Ivezaj V, Hopper JA, Foster-Hartsfield J, Schwarz D. Bariatric surgery history among substance abuse treatment patients: prevalence and associated features. Surg Obes Relat Dis. 2010;6:615–21.
23. Clark MM, Balsiger BM, Sletten CD, Dahlman KL, Ames G, Williams DE, Abu-Lebdeh HS, Sarr MG. Psychosocial factors and 2-Year outcome following bariatric surgery for weight loss. Obes Surg. 2003;13:739–45.
24. Heinberg LJ, Ashton K. History of substance abuse relates to improved postbariatric body mass index outcomes. Surg Obes Relat Dis. 2010;6:417–21.
25. Hagedorn JC, Encarnacion B, Brat GA, Morton JM. Does gastric bypass alter alcohol metabolism? Surg Obes Rel Dis. 2007;3:543–8.
26. Woodard GA, Downey J, Hernandez-Boussard T, Morton JM. Impaired alcohol metabolism after gastric bypass surgery: a case-crossover trial. J Am Coll Surg. 2011;212:209–14.
27. Heinberg LJ, Ashton K, Coughlin JW. Alcohol and bariatric surgery: a review and suggested recommendations for assessment and management. Surg Obes Relat Dis. 2012;8(3):357–63.
28. Pilone V, Mozzi E, Schettino AM, Furbetta F, Di Maro A, Giardiello C, et al. Improvement in health-related quality of life in first year after laparoscopic adjustable gastric banding. Surg Obes Relat Dis. 2012;8(3):260–8.
29. Dixon JB, Dixon ME, O'Brien PE. Quality of life after lap-band placement: influence of time, weight loss, and comorbidities. Obes Res. 2001;9(11):713–21.
30. Vincent HK, Ben-David K, Conrad BP, Lamb KM, Seay AN, Vincent KR. Rapid changes in gait, musculoskeletal pain, and quality of life after bariatric surgery. Surg Obes Relat Dis. 2012;8(3):346–54.

31. Sarwer DB, Wadden TA, Moore RH, Eisenberg MH, Raper SE, Williams NN. Changes in quality of life and body image after gastric bypass surgery. Surg Obes Relat Dis. 2010;6:608–14.
32. Karlsson J, Sjöström L, Sullivan M. Swedish obese subjects (SOS)–an intervention study of obesity. Two-year follow-up of health-related quality of life (HRQL) and eating behavior after gastric surgery for severe obesity. Int J Obes Relat Metab Disord. 1998;22(2):113–26.
33. Ortega J, Fernandez-Canet R, Àlvarez-Valdeita S, Cassinello N, Buguena-Puigcerver MJ. Predictors of psychological symptoms in morbidly obese patients after gastic bypass surgery. Surg Obes Relat Dis. 2012;8(6):770–6.
34. Toussi R, Fujioka K, Coleman KJ. Pre- and postsurgery behavioral compliance, patient health, and postbariatric surgical weight loss. Obesity. 2009;17:996–1002.
35. Wheeler E, Prettyman A, Lenhard MJ, Tran K. Adherence to outpatient program postoperative appointments after bariatric surgery. Surg Obes Relat Dis. 2008;4:515–20.
36. Spitznagel MB, Garcia, S, Miller, LA, Strain G, Devlin, M, Wing R, et al. Cognitive function predicts weight loss after bariatric surgery. Surg Obes Relat Dis. 2013;9(3):453–9.
37. Livhits M, Mercado C, Yermilov I, Parikh JA, Dutson E, Mehran A, Ko CY, et al. Is social support associated with greater weight loss after bariatric surgery? A systematic review. Obes Rev. 2011;12:142–8.

Technology to Assess and Intervene on Weight-Related Behaviors with Bariatric Surgery Patients

J. Graham Thomas and Dale S. Bond

Chapter Objectives

1. To describe the shortcomings of retrospective self-report measures for studying weight-related behaviors
2. To describe the use of ecological momentary assessment (EMA) and objective monitors for studying weight-related behaviors
3. To describe the use of Internet, text-messaging, smartphone, and virtual reality technology for intervening on weight-related behaviors

Introduction

Advances in technology have undoubtedly contributed to the obesity epidemic that is now affecting most developed countries [1]. Developments in agriculture, manufacturing, and food science technology have made it possible to produce highly palatable, high-calorie food at very low cost. Labor-saving devices have led to dramatic reductions in the need to perform physical activity at home and in the workplace. Sedentary leisure time activities such as television, video games, and Internet browsing have gradually replaced more traditional exercise-intensive activities. However, technology can also be applied in ways that facilitate healthy weight control by studying and intervening upon eating and physical activity behaviors.

This chapter describes a variety of ways in which technology has been used to facilitate healthy weight control in both research and clinical settings. The first section is focused on the measurement of weight-related behaviors using ecological momentary assessment (EMA) and mobile sensors. Particular emphasis is placed on studies of the eating and physical activity behaviors of bariatric surgery patients. The second section describes ways in which technology such as Internet-connected computers and mobile smartphones has been used to deliver behavioral weight loss treatment. Technology-based interventions for bariatric surgery patients are being developed and tested, but much of the work is in the preliminary stages. Therefore, most of the treatments described in the second section have not been tested with bariatric patients, but the lessons learned from them are still applicable to individuals undergoing weight loss surgery. Current and future applications of this technology for bariatric patients are discussed in the third and final section.

Technology to Measure Weight-Related Behaviors

Why Use Technology to Measure Behavior?

Effective healthcare intervention typically depends on an accurate understanding of the underlying condition(s) that is the focus of treatment. Eating and physical activity behaviors are an integral part of the etiology of obesity and its treatment in all forms, including bariatric surgery. Thus, it is important to understand the eating and physical activity behaviors of patients prior to surgery and changes that do (or more often, do not) occur after surgery, in order to optimize the effectiveness of treatment.

Historically, the assessment of eating and physical activity behaviors has involved some form of retrospective

J.G. Thomas, PhD (✉)
Weight Control and Diabetes Research Center, The Miriam Hospital, The Warren Alpert Medical School of Brown University, 196 Richmond Street, Providence, RI 02903, USA
e-mail: john_g_thomas@brown.edu

D.S. Bond, PhD
Department of Psychiatry and Human Behavior,
The Weight Control and Diabetes Research Center,
Brown Alpert Medical School, The Miriam Hospital,
196 Richmond Street, Providence, RI 02903, USA
e-mail: dbond@lifespan.org

self-report measure, such as questionnaires and/or clinical interviews. When these methods are used, patients are typically asked to recall their experiences, behaviors, and/or symptoms over the previous days, weeks, or months. These approaches come with an unspoken, but critically important, assumption: that patients are able to accurately recall their experiences and behavior over the specified time period. There is now an abundance of evidence that this assumption is unfounded in many, if not most, instances [2].

Research suggests that humans are relatively skilled at remembering unique events, especially those that are highly emotionally charged, such as the birth of a child or the occurrence of a serious injury. However, humans have particular difficulty recalling events that are routine and of little long-term significance, which describes most eating, physical activity, and sedentary behavior. Awareness of the fallibility of memory is limited because the human brain has a capacity to fill gaps in memory by using heuristics (i.e., mental shortcuts) to make educated guesses about what *must have happened* based on whatever information is available [3].

Decades of research have identified many types of heuristics and memory bias that could influence the ability of a bariatric surgery patient to accurately recall their weight-related behaviors and other obesity-related experiences. For example, when a patient is asked to describe behaviors that are too far in the past to be accurately remembered, consistency bias may lead to the inaccurate assumption that past behavior must resemble current behavior. If the patient was asked to report on his eating habits or physical activity behaviors, she may provide a response that is based on her *recent* behavioral patterns, which may no longer resemble his behavior during the time period that she can no longer accurately recall. Likewise, mood-congruent memory bias may lead a patient to recall emotionally positive memories (e.g., instance of good compliance with prescribed postoperative eating and physical activity behaviors) when the patient is in a "good" mood and emotionally negative memories (e.g., poor behavioral compliance) when the patient is in a "bad" mood.

Diaries and journals are an alternative form of assessment that does not rely on retrospective recall. Typically, patients are given paper forms to complete at predetermined times and/or when certain events occur (i.e., record food intake after eating). Unfortunately, compliance to paper diaries is often very low. Furthermore, patients may complete the diary retrospectively, unbeknownst to the clinician or researcher, thereby masking poor compliance. For example, one study investigated self-reported versus actual diary compliance by concealing a light sensor in a paper diary. Self-reported compliance was 90 %, while actual compliance was only 11 % [4]. This suggests that patients completed the diary retrospectively, which again makes the data susceptible to the simple forgetting and bias that affects retrospective self-report.

Collecting Better Self-Report Data: Ecological Momentary Assessment Using Mobile Technology

Ecological momentary assessment (EMA) is an alternative data collection approach that is thought to be less affected by memory bias because it involves measurement of *currently occurring* experiences, behaviors, and environmental conditions in real time and in patients' natural environment [5]. Modern EMA is typically implemented via mobile smartphone or some other electronic handheld device that allows patients to respond to predetermined sets of questions. Unlike paper diaries, the device logs *when* a patient has responded, so that adherence to the EMA protocol can be objectively verified. An additional benefit of EMA is that data are collected in patients' natural environment (rather than an artificial setting such as a physician's office or research laboratory), which eliminates another type of bias associated with the setting for the data collection.

Compared to questionnaires and clinical interviews, the typical EMA protocol contains relatively fewer questions, but they are asked repeatedly (e.g., several times per day over several days or weeks). Patients may be asked to answer questions at random times throughout the day or in response to specific events (e.g., before/after eating and/or exercise; at the start and/or end of the day). While patients may answer only a few questions each time they use the device, the questions that are presented may be tailored to the time of day, the events that are currently occurring, and the patients' recent responses. Thus, EMA can be a highly efficient assessment method; fewer questions are asked, but the information that is collected is more targeted. Furthermore, because patients answer the same questions repeatedly, it is possible to observe patterns of change over time and to make causal inferences (e.g., if environmental condition X repeatedly precedes behavior Y, it may be inferred that X contributes to Y).

EMA has been used extensively to study eating disorders, addictive behaviors, chronic pain, and other medical conditions. One notable study found that individuals who denied binge eating during a gold-standard clinical interview were found to be engaging in substantial binge eating behavior when measured via EMA [6]. Few studies have used EMA to study obese populations, and only one has used EMA to study bariatric surgery patients. Nonetheless, the findings from this study are directly relevant to the care of the bariatric patient.

We recently studied the eating and physical activity behavior of 21 patients who underwent gastric bypass or laparoscopic gastric banding approximately 6 months prior to the study [7]. Patients used an electronic handheld device to answer questions upon waking, after eating, and at the end of the day for six consecutive days. While measurement of adherence to published postoperative eating and physical activity behaviors was a particular focus of the research, patients were not aware of this aspect of the study and were told only that the investigators were measuring the eating and physical activity patterns of patients.

Compliance with several of the recommended behaviors was good. All of the patients reported that they almost always stopped eating upon the onset of satiation, and nearly all patients indicated that they avoided drinking while eating and abstained from consuming alcohol. However, the patients' frequency of eating, size of meals, and speed of eating raised cause for concern. On average, patients reported eating only 3.4 times per day—much less than the recommendation to eat at least five times per day, which was consistently met by only one of the 21 patients. Given the low frequency of eating, it is not surprising that patients' meals were approximately 3× as large as recommended (≤8 oz recommended) and that none of the patients consistently met the recommendation for meal size. Furthermore, only 25 % of patients routinely spent at least 20 min eating their meals, which may not be enough time to trigger feelings of satiation. About half of the sample consistently consumed at least five servings (1.5 oz each) of fruits and vegetables per day and avoided concentrated sweets/snacks. Only about one-third of the sample routinely avoided consuming caloric beverages.

Physical activity behaviors were also studied [8]. At the start of each day, patients were asked whether they intended to perform physical activity (PA) that day and for how long. At the end of the day, patients were asked to answer questions about any structured physical activity performed for at least ten continuous minutes. On average, patients reported an intention to perform physical activity on 65.9 % of days, for an average of 53.7 min per day. These intentions were at least partially met (i.e., at least 10 min of physical activity was performed) on 60.5 % of days that physical activity was planned, but patients reached their full goal on only 18.5 % of days. Averaging across all days that they intended to be active (including those when PA was not performed), patients performed 34.0 min of PA. The average discrepancy between intended and actual PA was a deficit of 19.6 min. More physical activity tended to be performed on days that more physical activity was planned.

This research highlights the benefits of using EMA to study bariatric surgery patients, and it suggests several avenues for behavioral intervention that may improve surgical outcomes. First, it suggests that bariatric patients could benefit from additional intervention on their eating behavior to facilitate more frequent eating of smaller meals, which are consumed more slowly. Second, it suggests that bariatric surgery patients perform more physical activity when they plan to be active and when they set higher goals for the duration of their physical activity. In contrast, physical activity is almost never performed when the patient does not articulate a plan to be active at the start of the day.

Beyond Self-Report: Objective Measures of Eating and Physical Activity

There are clear advantages of using EMA as compared to traditional behavioral assessment tools such as questionnaires, clinical interviews, and diaries. However, EMA shares a notable shortcoming with these other tools, which is reliance on patient self-report. Mobile sensors such as accelerometers and cameras are now being used to address this limitation. These tools reduce the need for patients to describe their experiences, behaviors, and environment because they are measured automatically. Sensors are often used in conjunction with advanced computing tools that allow complex data to be analyzed and summarized to facilitate intervention.

Accelerometers are a well-established tool for objectively monitoring physical activity [9]. These devices measure the direction and intensity of movement in up to three dimensions several times per second. The device is typically worn on the upper arm or at the waist. Several studies have demonstrated that accelerometers provide very accurate counts of various physical activity parameters such as steps taken and calories burned through voluntary physical activity. Many accelerometer devices now also incorporate other physiologic sensors such as skin temperature, heat flux, and galvanic skin response. When paired with sophisticated computer algorithms, these multi-sensor devices can recognize specific types of physical activity and have the potential to provide more accurate estimates of caloric expenditure.

Several studies have now used accelerometers to measure the physical activity of bariatric surgery patients before and after surgery. On average, patients tend to engage in very little physical activity preoperatively, with as much as 81 % of their time spent in sedentary behavior (i.e., sitting or reclining during waking hours) [10]. Fewer than 20 % of patients have been observed to accrue the recommended ≥10,000 steps per day [11]. When compared to normal-weight controls, bariatric surgery patients spend about half as much time performing moderate-to-vigorous physical activity [12].

Preoperative to postoperative changes in physical activity are of particular interest because of evidence suggesting that patients who become more active after surgery achieve superior weight losses and improvements in health and quality of life (see Chap. 22). When these changes were measured using retrospective self-report questionnaires such as the Paffenbarger Physical Activity Questionnaire, patients reported a fivefold increase in the minutes of structured moderate-to-vigorous physical activity they performed 6 months after surgery [13]. When these same changes were measured using an RT3 accelerometer, no preoperative to postoperative changes in this level of physical activity were detected. These findings highlight the limitations of the aforementioned retrospective self-report measures and the potential importance of intervening on patients' postoperative physical activity behaviors to maximize weight loss outcomes after surgery.

Compared to physical activity, the objective measurement of dietary intake is substantially more complex and requires more sophisticated devices and computer processing software. Despite the enormous challenge, several highly creative solutions have been developed. Much of the early work involved wearable devices that measured chewing and swallowing to estimate the amount of food consumed. A second generation of wearable device uses a forward-facing camera to record the user's daily activities, including any food the user consumes [14]. This system also includes sophisticated software to help a dietician identify food and calculate caloric content. The most recent solutions for objectively estimating food intake involve smartphones, which allow users to take photos of the food that they eat and automatically analyze the composition of the food including caloric content [15]. When compared to traditional paper diaries, use of the smartphone-based tools has been shown to dramatically increase the accuracy of estimates of caloric intake, when measured using doubly labeled water.

Future Directions in Technology-Based Measurement Approaches

Considerable effort is currently devoted to the development and miniaturization of many types of sensors. In the near future, it will likely be possible to measure multiple behavioral and physiological parameters accurately and in real time, with the option to make this information immediately available to healthcare providers. As the volume and complexity of the information we are able to collect grows, we will also need more sophisticated techniques for summarizing and analyzing data. One promising approach involves machine learning, which is a type of artificial intelligence in which computers are able to detect patterns in complex data and make predictions about future events. As more data is collected, the computer "learns" and is able to make more accurate predictions. Similar technology is currently being used in substance abuse research to detect when a patient in recovery is at high risk of relapse (e.g., when his GPS-equipped smartphone detects that he is entering a region where he has previously purchased illicit substances).

Technology to Intervene on Weight-Related Behaviors

As previously mentioned, the ultimate aim of measuring weight-related behaviors is often to collect information that will be used to craft more effective interventions. Many of the unique characteristics of technology-based measurement approaches also lend themselves to treatment.

Why Use Technology to Deliver Behavioral Intervention?

Compared to in-person treatment, technology-based interventions may have advantages related to convenience, reach, cost, and efficacy. Convenience is a factor that is often of great importance to patients. When patients receive treatment via their personal computer or smartphone, for example, they avoid barriers to conventional in-person treatments such as the need to take time off of work, find childcare, travel to the clinic, and possibly feel embarrassed about their weight and/or behaviors. Furthermore, unlike most healthcare providers, technology-based interventions are typically available whenever, and as often as, a patient wishes to use them.

The scalability of technology-based treatments is often superior to in-person treatments. Nutrition and physical activity counseling is often provided individually or in groups, and the number of patients who can receive treatment is limited by the number of providers available. While the initial cost of developing technology-based interventions may be high, they can often be deployed to a very large number of patients for very little additional incremental cost. This is particularly advantageous in regions where access to healthcare providers is limited.

As discussed later, the efficacy of technology-based weight control interventions has historically been lower than similar in-person treatments. However, because the cost per patient of delivering technology-based interventions can be very low, the cost effectiveness (i.e., the amount of benefit obtained per unit of treatment cost) may be higher. Furthermore, as the science of technology-based intervention advances, there are signs that these interventions may become at least as or even more effective than exclusively in-person treatments.

Behavioral Weight Loss Treatment: The Foundation of Technology-Based Interventions

More than 35 years of effort has been invested in developing behavioral treatment programs that produces weight loss by helping patients develop healthy eating and physical activity habits [16]. In the absence of bariatric surgery, these programs routinely produce weight losses of 5–10 % of patients' initial body weight, which is associated with improvements in health, risk of disease, and quality of life (see Chap. 15). While bariatric surgery patients expect much larger weight losses, the skills taught in behavioral weight loss programs substantially overlap with the skills that are needed to comply with postoperative recommendations for diet and physical activity. When these programs are administered to bariatric surgery patients (preoperatively *or* postoperatively), they can improve weight loss outcomes.

All behavioral weight loss programs provide basic diet and physical activity education, but most patients already understand that they need to eat less and exercise more in order to lose weight. Thus, behavioral weight loss programs focus on teaching skills to help patients make, and sustain, healthy changes to their eating and activity habits. Many of these skills are based on social cognitive theory and other basic principles of learning. Most programs start with setting explicit goals for weight loss (including the rate in addition to the ultimate amount), diet (calories and macronutrient content), and physical activity (usually includes time, type, frequency, and intensity).

Once goals have been set, participants typically record their daily weight, caloric intake, and time spent performing physical activity using paper diaries. Self-monitoring is a crucial part of behavioral weight loss programs and is perhaps the strategy that is most strongly and consistently associated with weight loss. Feedback on these diaries is often provided as part of treatment and has been shown to improve weight loss outcomes. Unfortunately, and as previously noted, compliance with self-monitoring is often very low and diaries are often not completed in a timely manner, which largely negates the benefit.

Behavioral weight loss programs also include training in a variety of other strategies such as stimulus control, which involves limiting cues for unhealthy behavior (e.g., removing high-calorie foods from the home, taking the television out of the bedroom) and adding cues for healthy behavior (e.g., putting a bowl of fresh fruit in the kitchen, putting a treadmill in front of the television). Other strategies include the development of social support, assertiveness training, emotional coping skills, building rewards for "good" behavior, and breaking associations between routine behaviors and unhealthy eating and sedentary behaviors (e.g., consuming high-calorie snacks while watching television). Most programs also include a component focused on weight loss maintenance and relapse prevention, although the development of effective maintenance programs has proven to be a substantial challenge.

Web-Based Behavioral Weight Control Interventions

The Web was one of the first, and continues to be one of the most popular, technologies used to deliver behavioral weight loss interventions [17]. Web-based interventions usually include some type of education and skills training, which was historically delivered via static Web pages but may now be delivered via more engaging modalities such as videos and podcasts. As with weight loss programs delivered in person, self-monitoring continues to be a crucial part of Web-based, behavioral weight loss programs. While many participants in Web-based programs still use paper diaries for their self-monitoring, they are typically encouraged to enter summary information, such as daily weight, calories, and physical activity minutes, into the intervention Web site. In early programs, brief written human feedback on this summary information was provided via e-mail or the Web to support patients, give them some additional guidance, and foster a sense of accountability. In recent Web-based programs, sophisticated computer algorithms that provide highly tailored feedback have been substituted for human feedback as they are less costly and more scalable. Web-based interventions may include other features such as message boards where patients may support each other and share weight loss tips.

Early Web-based programs produced very modest weight losses of approximately 4 kg in non-bariatric patients after 6 months of treatment. However, these early studies are very important because they are some of the first to demonstrate that the Internet can be used to improve patients' eating and physical activity behaviors with very little contact with human treatment providers. More recent Web-based programs have achieved larger weight losses of approximately 6 kg in 3 months, which is still less than the 10 kg produced by some traditional in-person treatment programs.

Research on Web-based interventions in non-bariatric populations suggests that the overall Web site usage is strongly associated with weight loss success [18]. This is not surprising, as individuals who used the Web site more often received a greater dose of intervention and may represent a group that is particularly high in motivation and readiness for behavior change. Feedback is a specific feature of Web-based programs that is associated with weight loss success, especially during the early phase of a treatment program. During maintenance, Web site features that facilitate social support (e.g., message boards and the availability of contact information for other patients in the program) may facilitate long-term weight control.

Mobile Phone and Smartphone Technology

At the time of this writing, nearly 100 % of the US population owns a mobile phone and over 50 % of the population owns a smartphone such as an iPhone or Android. Furthermore, smartphones are more commonly owned by racial minorities than Whites. Thus, an intervention delivered via smartphone has potential to reach populations that have been disproportionately affected by the obesity epidemic.

Several text message-based interventions have been developed and tested for improving the eating and physical activity behaviors of non-bariatric patients. In some instances, text messaging was used in conjunction with some other type of treatment modality such as in-person or Web-based intervention. Almost anyone can receive a text on almost any mobile phone, so these interventions have the potential for tremendous reach. Unfortunately, text messages are a very limited type of technology, and the results of these studies tend to be very modest. One of the best text message-based weight loss treatments produced weight loss of about 4 kg after 4 months [19].

Smartphones are handheld computers with advanced functionality that makes it possible to deliver behavioral weight control intervention in powerful new ways [20]. These devices are typically carried with their owners at all times, which means that intervention can be delivered almost anywhere at any time. Likewise, it is possible for patients to access intervention resources when they need them most—in their natural environment when facing challenges to their healthy eating and physical activity habits. Because most smartphones have a persistent Internet connection, engaging multimedia intervention content may be developed that includes audio, video, and interactive elements.

Smartphones also have the potential to facilitate adherence to self-monitoring by automating this very important, but repetitive and sometimes tedious, task. Instead of needing to carry paper diaries and a calorie reference book, patients may use their smartphone to record the foods that they consume. Calories and other nutritional information can be calculated automatically, along with a running total of calories consumed relative to the participants' daily goal. Some apps also use engaging graphics and automatic feedback messages to summarize patients' progress and prompt them to engage in healthy behavior.

A potentially powerful, and controversial, feature of smartphones is the ability for healthcare providers to monitor their patients' behavior in near real time. For example, a patient may choose to allow their healthcare provider to monitor their daily weight, diet, and physical activity patterns. If the patient knows that her healthcare providers can choose to see her behavior at any given time, it may motivate her to make healthy choices more consistently. However, this can put healthcare providers in the untenable position of being responsible for monitoring their patient's behaviors in near real time and taking immediate action to preserve their health if the patient reports unhealthy behaviors (e.g., a bout of binge drinking). The situation is further complicated by the rapid pace of technology development. A large number of health-related smartphone applications and mobile devices are always under development, with new functions and abilities that may have unanticipated consequences. Thus, it is a substantial challenge for regulating bodies to monitor and provide guidelines for appropriate use, for developing technologies.

Very little research has been conducted thus far to test smartphones as a medium for delivering behavioral weight loss intervention. In one pilot study, 20 participants received a smartphone-based behavioral weight loss program that included brief instructional videos and self-monitoring of daily weight, food intake, and structured physical activity minutes [21]. Participants were also allowed to self-monitor their progress on up to three additional tailored behavioral goals and receive tailored prompts to facilitate compliance. For example, an individual who consistently ate a high-calorie lunch from a fast-food restaurant might set the goal to prepare a healthy lunch at home instead. In the morning, they would receive a reminder to prepare their lunch and an adherence check (i.e., they indicated if they met their behavioral goal that day). Approximately once per week, a human interventionist reviewed patients' most recent self-monitoring records (retrieved in real time from their smartphones) and provided brief written feedback and encouragement. A weekly weigh-in with an interventionist and brief printed weight loss lessons were used to supplement the smartphone-based tools. After an initial 12 weeks of intervention, participants were given the option of continuing for another 12 weeks.

The results of the pilot study were very promising. All 20 participants completed the initial 12-week treatment, and 15 choose to continue for an additional 12 weeks. Of the five who did not continue, four reached their weight loss goal in the first 12 weeks and/or did not want additional treatment and one was diagnosed with a serious medical condition. The weight losses were 9.0 kg (9.1 % of initial body weight) at 12 weeks and 11.9 kg (12.2 % of initial body weight) at 24 weeks, which compares very favorably to the weight losses of 5–10 % of initial body weight that are routinely produced by in-person treatments. These good outcomes are at least partially attributable to the high rates of compliance with the self-monitoring protocol, which averaged 90.8 % during the first 12 weeks and 84.9 % during the second 12 weeks (compared to 40 % or less in some in-person treatment programs) [21]. In addition, the treatment received the highest possible ratings for satisfaction. This study suggests that a smartphone-based weight loss program may be very effective and well liked.

Virtual Reality (VR) Technology

Virtual reality is one of the newest forms of technology that is being used to deliver behavioral weight control treatment [22]. VR technology can take many forms, including the traditional fully immersive "rigs" with three-dimensional (3D) goggles and other sophisticated sensory inputs. These setups are particularly good at giving the user a very realistic experience, which can be beneficial when the goal is to elicit a strong emotional and/or behavioral response. While fully immersive VR has been used very successfully to treat conditions such as drug addiction and post-traumatic stress disorder, it is only beginning to be applied to obesity treatment. It may be very useful for exposing obese patients to powerful cues for eating, such as highly palatable food. Repeated presentations of highly palatable food in VR could help desensitize patients to these cues so that they have a less powerful effect on consumptive behavior.

"Desktop VR" is an alternative implementation of this technology that does not require any special equipment other than a standard desktop computer. Rather than wearing goggles, the user views a virtual scene through the "window" of their monitor. This technology has several applications for weight control that are currently being tested. One such application capitalizes on the "Proteus effect," which is the theory that a patient is more likely to engage in a behavior after viewing an avatar (i.e., virtual model) that resembles herself performing that behavior in a virtual setting. For example, a patient that views a virtual model of herself going to the gym and exercising may be more likely to exercise herself.

Another application of Desktop VR involves placing the user in a virtual scenario, such as a party at a friend's house, and presenting them with situations that challenge their healthy eating and physical activity habits. For example, the user may face peer pressure to eat high-calorie food and may have to make difficult choices about what food to eat at the party. A virtual "coach" may accompany the user to suggest and even model weight control strategies and help the user understand the consequences of their decisions. This allows the user to learn and practice weight control strategies in safe, realistic, settings, which may ultimately lead to greater confidence and commitment for practicing these strategies in the real world. This approach may be especially beneficial when used in conjunction with a Web-based weight loss intervention, as described previously. Such a system is currently under development and will be tested in the near future.

Still another application of VR is to deliver traditional behavioral weight control interventions in virtual settings. Instead of attending group treatment sessions at a clinic in the real world, a virtual group treatment session may be held in a VR environment such as Second Life (a Web-based virtual world). Much as in a traditional group treatment session, an instructor leads the group by speaking to the attendees (text or actual audio) with accompanying visual aids (e.g., handouts, slides). Each patient controls an avatar that attends the treatment session and can view and interact with the instructor and other attendees. This is a novel approach to delivering an already empirically validated behavioral weight loss treatment that may reduce barriers to treatment such as needing to travel to the clinic. It may also provide opportunities to practice weight loss skills in virtual settings, much as described in the previous paragraph.

Behavioral Technology for Use with Bariatric Populations

At present, few of the technologies described in this chapter have existing applications that are specially designed for bariatric surgery patients. It can be quite challenging to develop these tools for a number of reasons. First, bariatric surgery tends to be highly effective for many patients even in the absence of intensive behavioral intervention. Thus, there is not always a sufficient appreciation for the role of behavioral intervention with bariatric surgery patients, despite evidence that the eating and physical activity behaviors of many patients are suboptimal. Second, while behavioral weight loss interventions for nonsurgical patients have been extensively researched, there is still a relatively limited understanding of the best behavioral strategies for weight control among bariatric surgery patients. It is not known to what degree the strategies that are known to be effective for nonsurgical patients should be modified (or may be used as is) for bariatric surgery patients. Third, bariatric surgery patients are a subpopulation of individuals affected by obesity. Thus, specialized knowledge is required to develop technology-based interventions for this group, and the ultimate market for consumer products is smaller than products developed for the general obese population.

Despite the challenges, technology-based interventions for bariatric surgery patients *are* under development. One obvious application that is particularly relevant for bariatric surgery patients involves using remote devices to monitor postoperative recovery (e.g., wound healing, early detection of infection) and compliance with postoperative self-care routines (e.g., medication compliance, diet progression, performance of physical activity). Depending on the type of device that is used, this information may be automatically transmitted to the patients' healthcare providers where summary reports can be generated, and action can be taken to initiate further intervention, if needed. This technology has an obvious potential to increase the efficiency of healthcare services by identifying problem situations early and directing resources toward the patients who will receive the most benefit.

Until bariatric-focused tools become available, there are a variety of tools intended for general use that can be applied to bariatric surgery patients. While not specifically intended for use with bariatric populations, many of these technologies are still relevant and useful to bariatric populations.

Many technology-based tools for behavior measurement, such as EMA and accelerometers, can be used with bariatric patients with very little modification. While EMA tends to be a research tool and is less used for clinical purposes, all that is needed to conduct EMA with bariatric patients is a device that is programmed with a relevant set of questions. Physical activity measurement devices such as armband accelerometers are used for research and clinical intervention. Potential users should be aware that these devices must be attached to the body, and some devices may be more comfortable than others for severely obese users due to their design and where they are worn (e.g., an armband or shoe accelerometer may be more comfortable than one worn at the waist). Additionally, the algorithms that many devices and their associated software programs use to classify types of physical activity and energy expenditure may not have been developed and/or tested using severely obese samples, and the accuracy of the results may be negatively affected. Even so, devices such as the bodybugg®, which measures physical activity and sleep, can be very useful for helping motivation patients to become more physically active and to monitor their progress toward their physical activity goals. Commercial accelerometers vary in price and sophistication, with the more expensive devices (such as the bodybugg) providing better accuracy and a more detailed analysis of activity.

There are very few, if any, commercial Web sites that deliver empirically validated behavioral weight loss treatment, as most of the existing sites have been developed in the context of research studies and are not available for a general audience. However, there are an abundance of excellent Web sites that facilitate self-monitoring of body weight, food intake, and physical activity. These Web sites can be very useful in clinical practice, as they make self-monitoring easier for patients and they also often include a timestamp of when entries were made so that healthcare providers can feel confident that the diaries were completed at the appropriate times. Some Web sites also include message boards and other opportunities for social support, which is known to be helpful for maintaining a weight loss. Example sites include www.MyFitnessPal.com, www.SparkPeople.com, and www.LIVESTRONG.com. It should be noted that some of these Web sites include features to help users set goals for dietary intake, weight loss, and other parameters. The recommendations provided by these Web sites may be appropriate for the general population but not bariatric surgery patients. Any healthcare provider who recommends these tools to their patients should help their patients set appropriate goals.

Ethicon Endo-Surgery, which manufactures devices for bariatric surgery, formerly offered a Web site, www.realizemysuccess.com, that provided self-monitoring tools and weight loss tips specifically for bariatric surgery patients. One small study was conducted that suggested that use of the Web site was associated with weight loss success. However, the site was closed, reportedly because a variety of high-quality self-monitoring Web sites are available.

At the time of this writing, there are a handful of smartphone applications intended specifically for use by bariatric surgery patients. Most of these applications provide very basic educational information about bariatric surgery and/or are poorly designed and therefore of little use. However, much like the Web sites described previously, there are some excellent smartphone applications for self-monitoring of weight, dietary intake, and physical activity. Some applications have functions that further simplify self-monitoring, such as the ability to scan barcodes of packaged foods to add them to the food diary. Some of the Web sites previously listed also have a smartphone application. Other popular smartphone applications include Lose It! and DailyBurn. As when recommending Web sites for self-monitoring, it is important for the healthcare provider to ensure their patients set appropriate goals for dietary intake, physical activity, and weight loss.

At present, commercial applications of VR technology for intervening on weight loss behaviors are under development, but there are few, if any, that are currently available. In the near future, it may become popular to conduct dietary counseling in a virtual office and/or provide bariatric surgery patients with VR scenarios that teach patients weight loss behaviors and challenge them to implement them effectively. While VR holds great promise for improving weight loss outcomes, research will be needed to best understand how to use this largely untapped resource.

Conclusion

In conclusion, there are a variety of approaches for using technology to intervene on weight-related behaviors. Excellent self-monitoring technologies are commercially available via the Web, smartphones, and accelerometer-based devices. Many new tools are in development that may ultimately help patients make the behavioral changes that facilitate weight loss after bariatric surgery. However, no matter how sophisticated the technology becomes, it will never be a substitute for care from medical professionals. Behavioral technology is best thought of as a tool to help extend the care offered by healthcare providers. In the near future, we may look forward to seeing a diversity of powerful tools that will allow us to improve the care we deliver to our patients and empower them to make healthy choices in their behavior.

Question and Answer Section

Questions

1. Advantages of using technology to intervene on weight-related behaviors include all except:
   A. Reduces barriers to treatment
   B. Simplifies tasks such as self-monitoring
   C. Facilitates communication between patient and healthcare provider
   D. Requires no special equipment or devices

2. A variety of inexpensive, high-quality Web sites and smartphone applications are currently available to assist patients with:
   A. Learning weight loss strategies
   B. Self-monitoring their weight and weight-related behaviors
   C. Communicating with healthcare providers
   D. Viewing their medical records

Answers

1. **D**. While using technology to deliver behavioral intervention may be advantageous, it often requires special equipment and/or devices such as computers and smartphones.
2. **B**. Many weight control technologies are being developed and researched, but only self-monitoring technologies are currently available and ready for widespread use.

References

1. Hill JO, Peters JC. Environmental contributions to the obesity epidemic. Science. 1998;280:1371–4.
2. Stone AA, Shiffman S, Atienza AA, Nebeling L. Historical roots and rationale of Ecological Momentary Assessment (EMA). In: Stone AA, Shiffman S, Atienza AA, Nebeling L, editors. The science of real-time data capture: self-reports in health research. New York: Oxford University Press; 2007. p. 3–10.
3. Gorin AA, Stone AA. Recall biases and cognitive errors in retrospective self-reports: a call for momentary assessments. In: Baum A, Revenson T, Singer J, editors. Handbook of health psychology. Mahwah: Lawrence Erlbaum Associates; 2001. p. 405–13.
4. Stone AA, Shiffman S, Schwartz JE, Broderick JE, Hufford MR. Patient non-compliance with paper diaries. BMJ. 2002;324(7347):1193–4.
5. Shiffman S, Stone AA, Hufford MR. Ecological momentary assessment. Annu Rev Clin Psychol. 2008;4:1–32.
6. le Grange DL, Gorin A, Catley D, Stone AA. Does momentary assessment detect binge eating in overweight women that is denied at interview? Eur Eat Disord Rev. 2001;9(5):309–24.
7. Thomas JG, Bond DS, Ryder BA, Leahey TM, Vithiananthan S, Roye GD, et al. Ecological momentary assessment of recommended postoperative eating and activity behaviors. Surg Obes Relat Dis. 2011;7(2):206–12.
8. Bond DS, Thomas JG, Ryder BA, Vithiananthan S, Pohl D, Wing RR. Ecological momentary assessment of the relationship between intention and physical activity behavior in bariatric surgery patients. Int J Behav Med. 2013;20(1):82–7.
9. Butte NF, Ekelund U, Westerterp KR. Assessing physical activity using wearable monitors: measures of physical activity. Med Sci Sports Exerc. 2012;44(1 Suppl 1):S5–12.
10. Bond DS, Unick JL, Jakicic JM, Vithiananthan S, Pohl D, Roye GD, et al. Objective assessment of time spent being sedentary in bariatric surgery candidates. Obes Surg. 2011;21(6):811–4.
11. King WC, Belle SH, Eid GM, Dakin GF, Inabnet WB, Mitchell JE, Longitudinal Assessment of Bariatric Surgery Study, et al. Physical activity levels of patients undergoing bariatric surgery in the Longitudinal Assessment of Bariatric Surgery study. Surg Obes Relat Dis. 2008;4(6):721–8.
12. Bond DS, Jakicic JM, Vithiananthan S, Thomas JG, Leahey TM, Sax HC, et al. Objective quantification of physical activity in bariatric surgery candidates and normal-weight controls. Surg Obes Relat Dis. 2010;6(1):72–8.
13. Bond DS, Jakicic JM, Unick JL, Vithiananthan S, Pohl D, Roye GD, et al. Pre- to postoperative physical activity changes in bariatric surgery patients: self-report vs. objective measures. Obesity. 2010;18(12):2395–7.
14. Sun M, Fernstrom JD, Jia W, Hackworth SA, Yao N, Li Y, et al. A wearable electronic system for objective dietary assessment. J Am Diet Assoc. 2010;110(1):45–7.
15. Martin CK, Han H, Coulon SM, Allen HR, Champagne CM, Anton SD. A novel method to remotely measure food intake of free-living individuals in real time: the remote food photography method. Br J Nutr. 2009;101(3):446–56.
16. Butryn ML, Webb V, Wadden TA. Behavioral treatment of obesity. Psychiatr Clin North Am. 2011;34(4):841–59.
17. Tate DF, Wing RR, Winett RA. Using Internet technology to deliver a behavioral weight loss program. JAMA. 2001;285(9):1172–7.
18. Krukowski RA, Harvey-Berino J, Ashikaga T, Thomas CS, Micco N. Internet-based weight control: the relationship between web features and weight loss. Telemed J E Health. 2008;14(8):775–82.
19. Patrick K, Raab F, Adams MA, Dillon L, Zabinski M, Rock CL, et al. A text message-based intervention for weight loss: randomized controlled trial. J Med Internet Res. 2009;11(1):e1.
20. Tufano JT, Karras BT. Mobile eHealth interventions for obesity: a timely opportunity to leverage convergence trends. J Med Internet Res. 2005;7(5):e58. 20.
21. Thomas JG, Wing RR. Health-E-Call, a smartphone-assisted behavioral obesity treatment: pilot study. JMIR Mhealth Uhealth. 2013;1(1):e3.
22. Coons MJ, Roehrig M, Spring B. The potential of virtual reality technologies to improve adherence to weight loss behaviors. J Diabetes Sci Technol. 2011;5(2):340–4.

Psychosocial Issues in Adolescent Bariatric Surgery

Meg H. Zeller and Jennifer Reiter-Purtill

Chapter Objectives

1. To illustrate how the adolescent bariatric patient presents with unique psychosocial challenges that may differ from the adult patient
2. To outline what is known versus unknown about the psychosocial health and outcomes of bariatric surgery for an adolescent patient

Introduction

An alarming 6 % of today's teenagers face the day-to-day challenge of being extremely obese—body mass index (BMI) ≥99th percentile [1, 2]—and thus, carry a heightened risk of obesity-related medical comorbidities once only seen as "adult" diseases. Given that extreme obesity is blatantly visible, physically challenging, and highly stigmatized, it has the potential to impact an adolescent's day-to-day quality of life independent of, or prior to, any palpable health effects. Thus, the greater, more immediate impact of extreme obesity in adolescence is likely psychosocial, not medical. Existing evidence would suggest youth with extreme obesity have great difficulty achieving and maintaining sufficient weight loss via lifestyle modification, or with adjunctive pharmacologic agents, as both treatments typically produce a 5–10 % weight loss. The concern for these youth is further compounded given that the period from adolescence to adulthood (ages 18–25) is largely overlooked in the weight management literature. Accordingly, the vast majority of teens who are extremely obese today will carry forward their excess weight and disease burden into adulthood.

The beginning of this century marked the emergence of a new and growing literature characterizing the psychosocial health of the subpopulation of adolescents with extreme obesity, those seeking surgical weight loss, and the initial psychosocial outcomes. As detailed elsewhere in this volume, early studies support the safety and short-term efficacy of bariatric surgery for adolescents with associated improvements in physical as well as psychosocial health (e.g., quality of life, depressive symptoms, self-concept).

Unfortunately, preliminary studies that include a psychosocial focus suffer from methodological challenges related to the reliance on small sample sizes and patients from single institutions. Thus, current knowledge is limited not only in terms of generalizability of published data, but also the statistical power available to test more complex and informative questions. Further, with few exceptions [3], our understanding of psychosocial outcomes of adolescent bariatric surgery is limited to the first postoperative year. Nonetheless, these early studies provide a vital foundation from which clinical guidelines and adolescent care models can begin to have a more age-salient empirical basis versus our initial reliance on the adult bariatric experience. The aim of this chapter is to summarize the current knowledge base about the psychosocial health of the adolescent bariatric patient with consequent and critical directions for future clinical research.

It is important to note that, unlike the adult patient, adolescent bariatric surgery occurs at a critically important time in psychosocial development—a period of rapid change in emotional, interpersonal, social, and educational and vocational domains, when good adaptation bodes well for continued positive transition into young adulthood [4]. Further, the postoperative course co-occurs with a challenging developmental transition. The distinct period between adolescence and young adulthood, "emerging adulthood" (ages 18–25),

M.H. Zeller, PhD (✉)
Department of Behavioral Medicine and Clinical Psychology,
Cincinnati Children's Hospital Medical Center,
University of Cincinnati College of Medicine,
3333 Burnet Avenue MLC3015, Cincinnati, OH 45215, USA
e-mail: meg.zeller@cchmc.org

J. Reiter-Purtill, PhD
Department of Behavioral Medicine and Clinical Psychology,
Cincinnati Children's Hospital Medical Center, 3333 Burnet Avenue MLC3015, Cincinnati, OH 45215, USA
e-mail: jennifer.reiter_purtill@cchmc.org

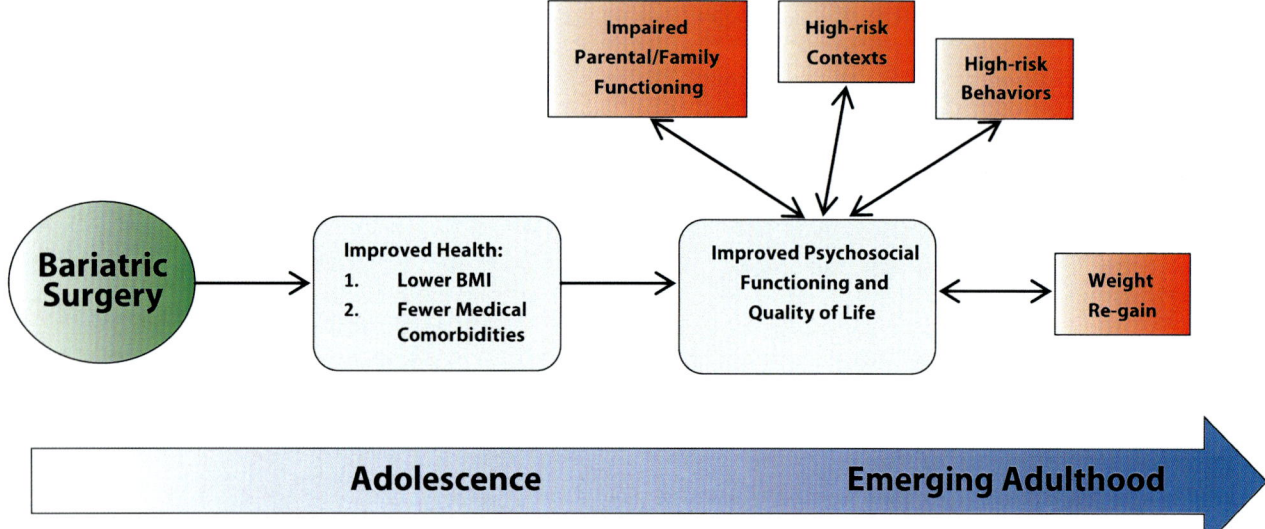

Fig. 8.1 Organizational framework used in this chapter

is seen as one of the most "volitional" periods of life [5], characterized by increasing independence (financial, residential) and exploration in relationships (e.g., peers, family, romantic relationships). Thus, understanding of the adolescent patient must occur within an age-salient psychosocial context. For example, there is growing evidence that in addition to the "usual psychosocial suspects" most often the focus of the adult bariatric literature (e.g., depression, binge eating disorder, and quality of life), there are key age-salient psychosocial factors (versus psychopathology) affected by extreme obesity in adolescence that may be positively impacted by surgical weight loss (e.g., perceived competence, body image, the social network). There are also contextual factors known to negatively affect psychosocial functioning for *any* adolescent, regardless of weight status (e.g., impaired parent/family functioning, engagement in high-risk behaviors, high-risk contexts), that also must be considered. This basic framework presented in Fig. 8.1 will be used to organize this review.

Key Domains of Adolescent Psychosocial Health

Health-Related Quality of Life (HRQOL)

Health-related quality of life (HRQOL) describes the impact of a particular condition/disease or intervention on the daily functioning of individuals across physical, emotional, and social domains. Generic measures of HRQOL (e.g., PedsQL™[6]) allow for cross-disease comparisons, while disease or condition-specific instruments measure aspects of daily functioning that are specific to a disease (e.g., asthma, cancer, diabetes). The field of obesity has progressed to include condition-specific measures allowing the characterization of how weight and weight change specifically affect day-to-day functioning in adolescents (e.g., weight-related quality of life or WRQOL:IWQOL-Kids [7], Sizing Them Up [8]). Given that HRQOL has emerged as a critical patient-reported outcome (PRO) recommended for use in clinical trials and prospective observational research, it follows that this domain of adolescent psychosocial health is perhaps the best described in the adolescent bariatric literature to date.

Obese youth report significant impairments in both HRQOL and WRQOL and across all domains of functioning (i.e., physical, social, emotional, school, body-esteem) and increasing impairment with increasing BMI [9]. Further, adolescents at extreme levels of obesity (BMI ≥40) presenting for bariatric surgery have exhibited the greatest global impairments in HRQOL and WRQOL reported to date [10]. An emerging adolescent literature suggests significant improvements in HRQOL and WRQOL across the first and/or second postoperative years following laparoscopic gastric banding [11] and Roux-en-Y gastric bypass [3].

Our investigative team provided some of these first prospective and preliminary data noting critical areas for further exploration [3]. First, while the net BMI change at 2 years postoperatively was approximately 35 %, the overwhelming majority remained clinically obese. Interestingly HRQOL and WRQOL improvements were dramatic, being more typical of nonclinical or non-overweight adolescent samples, suggesting more "normative" quality of life of healthy non-overweight youth despite not achieving nonobese body weight. It may be that experiencing a change in weight has more impact on quality of life than an actual weight achieved. In addition, analyses revealed a deceleration in the rate of change and a slight decline in quality-of-life domains in parallel with weight regain. Interestingly, these initial adolescent findings are consistent with the adult literature reviewed in Chap. 3.

Psychopathology

Remarkably less represented in the adolescent bariatric literature specifically, and the adolescent extreme obesity literature more broadly, are studies that describe the presence of psychopathology. As detailed in Chap. 2, adult bariatric patients often present with one or more psychiatric disorders preoperatively, most commonly with mood disorders and binge eating disorder (BED). While a link between adolescent obesity and depression is often spoken of, the empirical data remains equivocal, whether assessing community or treatment-seeking samples. In fact, the majority of obese adolescents exhibit subclinical range or minimal depressive symptomatology, with only a subset having clinically significant symptoms or meeting diagnostic criteria for a depressive disorder [12–16]. For example, Goodman and colleagues [17] recently demonstrated that adolescents with extreme obesity were no more likely to report greater depressive symptoms than youth of healthy weight.

For the adolescent bariatric patient, the evidence is consistent with the broader adolescent obesity literature: only a minority (16–30 %) of adolescents present with clinical range depressive symptomatology, whether at the initial preoperative psychological evaluation (e.g., prior to approval for surgery) [10, 11, 18] or when assessed post-approval within the month prior to their surgery in the context of research [19]. Further evidence suggests little change in symptom presentation between these pre- and post-approval [20] negating the possible interpretation that adolescents underreport depressive symptoms at first contact in an effort to present well ("impression management") in their pursuit of surgery. Encouragingly, initial outcome data suggest a statistically significant reduction in depressive symptoms across the first postoperative year [19, 21] with some preliminary evidence of a significant increase in symptoms during the second year in the context of weight regain [3]. Arguably, whether these changes are clinically meaningful to the patient remains unknown. Recognizing there is some variability in depressive symptom presentation prior to surgery, future studies powered to examine symptom severity differences (i.e., comparing trajectories of those with/without clinical range depressive symptoms) over time are imperative. However, these data are consistent with the adult literature, in which initial improvements in depressive symptoms may erode 18–24 months post-surgery or that new onset of depressive symptoms may occur over time.

Unfortunately, no prevalence studies of BED in adolescents with extreme obesity exist. However, the broader adolescent obesity literature suggests less than 3 % of obese adolescents meet diagnostic criteria for the disorder [22], with the prevalence of subthreshold binge eating considerably higher, and particularly for those in clinical samples and seeking weight loss (20–30 %) [23, 24]. Two studies [11, 18] have reported on disordered eating behaviors in extremely obese adolescents, although both notably describe clinical samples of teens presenting for bariatric surgery. Disordered eating behaviors were not infrequent, albeit not characteristic of the majority of patients, and included binge eating episodes (25 % [11], 48 % [18]), night eating (36.3 % [11]) as well as rapid eating (44 %), having guilt associated with eating (36 %), eating until uncomfortably full (36 %), loss of control (24 %), and eating without hunger (24 %) [18]. To date, there are no outcome data characterizing the impact of bariatric surgery and its associated weight loss on disordered eating behaviors in adolescents. This is an important area for future research given the adult experience suggests binge eating behaviors can reemerge following surgery and are associated with weight regain.

A recent investigation by Sysko and colleagues [11] took a broader approach to examine psychiatric symptoms in a group of extremely obese adolescents approved for laparoscopic gastric banding. Using statistical methods (i.e., latent class analysis), the investigators reduced their comprehensive preoperative psychological assessment protocol (e.g., self-report measures of depression, disordered eating, and anxiety, as well as the clinical interview) into three distinct subgroups of adolescents: those with "low" psychopathology (50 %), those with "nonspecific" or "intermediate" psychopathology (36.3 %), and those with "eating pathology" in combination with other psychiatric symptoms (13.7 %). This small "eating pathology" group was characterized as being more likely to report binge eating episodes or night eating, as well as more depressive symptoms, anxiety symptoms, and present Diagnostic and Statistical Manual of Mental Disorders (DSM)-IV diagnoses. Thus, a consistent preliminary pattern has begun to emerge across the early literature: The adolescent bariatric patient population at the time of surgery is variable, although generally low, in terms of prevalence of presenting psychopathology. This being said, there may be a small subgroup with a more problematic psychiatric profile that may include eating pathology.

Self-Concept

An adolescent's self-concept is based on their perceived competence across multiple age-salient dimensions (i.e., physical appearance, social acceptance, global self-esteem, as well as athletic, academic, romantic, and job competence). These competencies have consistently been shown to be associated with better psychosocial health [25, 26].

A relatively large literature [27] has demonstrated that obese youth report lower self-concept than youth of healthy weight. Furthermore, adolescents whose obesity has persisted from middle childhood report lower self-concept compared to those with obesity onset in adolescence.

Our understanding of self-concept in extremely obese youth who undergo bariatric surgery is limited to one study [3]. Based on the broader adolescent obesity literature, it was not unexpected to find that adolescents prior to bariatric surgery self-reported lower perceived competence across all domains (i.e., global self-esteem, physical appearance, social acceptance, as well as athletic, academic, romantic, and job competence) as compared to the normative sample for the measure [28]. Arguably, in the context of the aforementioned findings with the sample (e.g., improvements in HRQOL, WRQOL, depressive symptoms paralleled weight loss and regain), significant improvements in all perceived competencies over time is consistent and would also be expected. However, while some domains showed a subsequent slight decline in functioning (e.g., appearance, close friendship, and social acceptance) in the second postoperative year, others showed continued improvement over time (e.g., global self-esteem, athletic, job competence, and romantic appeal). While these findings are indeed preliminary and in need of replication, they do suggest a broader psychosocial impact (i.e., beyond psychopathology and quality of life) of surgical weight loss for the adolescent patient as they mature and manage new age-salient roles (e.g., work, romantic relationships).

Body Image Dissatisfaction

Body image dissatisfaction (BID) is a known correlate of psychosocial distress for adults presenting for bariatric surgery and which lessens with both surgical and nonsurgical weight loss [29]. A noted finding to post-surgical weight loss is that some bariatric patients continue to report BID due to sagging excess skin [30]. Only one study to date has assessed BID in extremely obese adolescents and is limited to the first postoperative year. Ratcliff and colleagues [20] examined BID by calculating the discrepancy between adolescents' figure ratings of their current and ideal body size at baseline/presurgery and again at 6 and 12 months after bariatric surgery. BID was significantly reduced over time, particularly within the first 6 months post-surgery. Additional work needs to examine how body image may change as a result of surgical weight loss beyond the first postoperative year. Knowing excess skin is not unique to adult bariatric patients, and that anecdotally, some adolescent patients progress to seeking body-contouring surgery, BID a critical area for further investigation.

Interpersonal Relations

Positive peer relations are central to healthy social and emotional development in youth. Unfortunately, there is solid evidence that obese adolescents are less liked by peers and socially marginalized in their school peer network [31, 32]. In addition, obese adolescents report more peer victimization than adolescents of average weight, including name-calling and teasing about their weight and appearance [33–35]. These experiences are concerning given that negative peer relations for any adolescent (i.e., independent of weight status) are predictive of greater psychopathology and poorer school/job performance and interpersonal relations in adulthood [4]. Further, appearance-related teasing has been linked to a number of concurrent issues including greater BID, low self-concept, binge eating behaviors, and greater depressive symptoms, including suicidal ideation and suicide attempts [36].

To date, there is no literature that characterizes the social networks of adolescents with extreme obesity, and more specifically, the social relationships of adolescents who undergo bariatric surgery and if/how these relations change postoperatively. Clinical experience suggests that a majority of patients report some distress regarding their peer status prior to surgery. Encouragingly, many patients experience notable changes in their peer contact and relationships postoperatively and in a generally positive direction. Certainly the aforementioned evidence [3] provided by self-report measures (e.g., subscales of HRQOL/WRQOL or self-concept measures) that capture their perceptions of impaired social life and subsequent improvements sheds some light on perceived changes in social status and romantic appeal postoperatively.

Factors That May Negatively Impact Adolescent Psychosocial Functioning

Parent/Family Functioning

Unlike adult care models, the practice of pediatric medicine proves unique due to the presence and influence of caregivers [37]. The broader pediatric literature demonstrates an association between impaired caregiver and family functioning and poorer treatment outcomes in pediatric conditions reliant on regimen adherence, lifestyle change, and/or treatment intensity (i.e., surgery). Childhood obesity develops within a family environment. Accordingly, an adolescent undergoing bariatric surgery functions within a family environment that has contributed to their presurgery health and psychosocial impairment. Unfortunately, the literature is only beginning to identify the parent and family characteristics of the obesogenic family environment and specifically that of the adolescent with extreme obesity considering or undergoing bariatric surgery.

A glimpse into what may be key family factors to consider comes from several cross-sectional studies that have described families of obese youth presenting to nonsurgical multidisciplinary weight management programs. The majority (66–90 %) of female caregivers of treatment-seeking obese youth were also obese (BMI ≥ 30 kg/m^2) [38–40], with many self-reporting clinical levels of psychological distress (28–50 %) [16, 39, 40], elevated levels of parenting stress (18 %) [41], and problematic family functioning [3, 11]. Further, mothers who reported their own psychological distress were more likely to have obese adolescents who reported greater depressive symptoms [16]. Thus, the family environment may be characterized not only by a shared disease (obesity) but potentially dysfunction.

Two studies to date have examined family factors in the context of adolescent bariatric surgery [3, 11]. While direct comparisons of these findings prove difficult due to use of different assessment tools, both suggest that the degree of general family dysfunction is variable and certainly not universal for the adolescent patient. For example, Sysko and colleagues [11] utilized presurgery psychiatric evaluation data and found that for a small group of adolescents presenting with high levels of psychopathology (e.g., BED, depressive and anxiety symptoms), there was also high levels of self-reported family conflict and lower cohesion among family members. In contrast, a second study [3] found limited family or caregiver dysfunction at the time of surgery and no detectable change in these family factors across the initial 12 months following surgery. Thus, as the adolescent undergoes significant change in weight and psychosocial health, the family appears to remain stable. Remarkably absent in the adolescent bariatric literature are assessment tools that would allow the characterization of more "condition-specific" family factors that may impact bariatric surgery outcomes, be they physical or psychosocial. For example, understanding aspects of emotional and instrumental social support that promote the adolescent patient's adherence to the postoperative medical and lifestyle regimen is critically needed.

Not surprisingly, the overwhelming majority (86 %) of female caregivers at the time of their adolescents' surgeries were obese themselves, if not extremely obese (47 % BMI >40 kg/m^2) [3]. Further, of those "bariatric caregivers" who were *not* extremely obese at the time of their adolescent's surgery, 25 % had undergone bariatric surgery within the previous 3 years, with another caregiver undergoing bariatric surgery between the adolescent's 6- and 12-month postoperative visits. The adult literature has demonstrated a strong family history for extreme obesity among adult family members [42, 43]. At the same time, a recent study suggested that bariatric surgery may render an additional benefit (e.g., "halo effect") of weight loss for family members who did not undergo surgery, including children in the home [44]. Future research needs to explore whether bariatric surgery will emerge as a family weight loss tool and whether having a caregiver who has also undergone bariatric surgery presents unique benefits and/or challenges for the adolescent patient.

High-Risk Contexts

Childhood Trauma

Increasing evidence suggests an association between childhood trauma, including child abuse and neglect, and the development of obesity [45–47]. Noll and colleagues presented the first evidence for the prospective longitudinal association of childhood sexual abuse with the subsequent development of obesity by young adulthood [45]. Retrospective reports of childhood sexual abuse history from adult bariatric candidates have ranged from 16 % [48] to 69 % [49]. To date, there have been no studies that have addressed the impact of childhood trauma on the psychosocial functioning of obese youth or the prevalence of childhood trauma in adolescents who undergo bariatric surgery. The broader developmental literature suggests there are several psychosocial impairments that are both sequelae of childhood trauma and correlates of childhood and adolescent obesity (e.g., depression, BED, difficulties with peers, poor self-esteem, BID) [50, 51]. Further, high-risk behaviors such as substance abuse and dependence, delinquency, and high-risk sexual behaviors have also been cited as short- and long-term sequelae of childhood trauma [52, 53]. Thus, the consequences of abuse may amplify or exacerbate the psychosocial risks associated with extreme obesity and be negatively related to the level of psychosocial improvement that follows bariatric surgery.

Socioeconomic Status

Socioeconomic status, at the family or even neighborhood level, has great potential to negatively affect adolescent health. Childhood obesity has been linked to a number of related family socioeconomic factors, including lower family household income, single-parent status, lower parental education, poor living conditions, and lack of neighborhood safety [54]. However, these types of associations have not been assessed or are less consistent for obese adolescents [55, 56]. The range of socioeconomic status of youth presenting for laparoscopic gastric banding at one institution suggests variability, with a reported median family income of approximately $49,000, with 14.5 % of patients below poverty level [11]. What role socioeconomic status plays in an obese teen's psychosocial improvements post-surgery remains unknown and is an important context for further study.

High-Risk Behaviors

Adolescence is a developmental period characterized by an increased willingness to engage in behaviors considered to be risky, harmful, or even antisocial. Alcohol, tobacco, and illicit drug use are often initiated during this time period, as is sexual activity. Adolescence is also a developmental period known for increased risk for the first onset of nonfatal suicidal behaviors (e.g., ideation, attempts) [57]. While arguably the initiations of such behaviors are seen as "normative," these behaviors are not always benign. For example, adolescence/emerging adulthood is also a period of risk for progression to abusing or becoming dependent on substances [58, 59] or acquiring a sexually transmitted infection [60, 61]. Suicide is also the third leading cause of death in this age group [61].

Until quite recently, prevalence rates of these high-risk behaviors in extremely obese adolescents were unknown. Ratcliff and colleagues [62] utilized a nationally representative school-based sample (Youth Risk Behavior Surveillance Survey [YRBSS]) demonstrating that, with few exceptions, adolescents with extreme obesity engage in high-risk behaviors (alcohol/tobacco/drug use, sexual behaviors) at rates comparable to their healthy weight peers (i.e., no greater or less risk than a "typical" adolescent). However, there were some unique and concerning exceptions. Specifically, these national data suggested that while adolescent girls with extreme obesity were *less* likely than healthy weight girls to have had sexual intercourse, if they had, it was more likely to have happened under the influence of alcohol or drugs, a known context of increasing risk (e.g., unprotected sex). Also, extreme adolescent obesity was associated with greater likelihood of smoking, and for boys, initiation of smoking before the age of 13, a known predictor of increased risk of tobacco dependence.

We recently used the YRBSS to gain a better understanding of suicidal behaviors (e.g., suicidal ideation and nonfatal attempts) of adolescents who fall into different excess weight categories (overweight, obese, extreme obesity), taking into consideration whether they also perceived themselves to be "overweight" [63]. These national data suggest that relative to healthy weight youth who accurately perceived their weight, adolescents at any level of excess weight who also accurately perceived themselves as "overweight" had greater odds of engaging in suicidal ideation, whereas if inaccurate, had no greater odds. Findings regarding actual nonfatal suicide attempts were less straightforward and varied based on actual weight/weight perception accuracy and race/ethnicity.

To fully understand the impact of bariatric surgery on the psychosocial health outcomes of adolescents, the frequency of their engagement in such high-risk behaviors must be considered. Furthermore, in light of an emerging adult bariatric literature examining links between bariatric surgery and alcohol use/abuse or other addictive behaviors, as well as associations with increased risk of death by suicide, understanding the high-risk behaviors of the adolescent patient becomes increasingly paramount.

Conclusion

There are many known age-salient factors (e.g., family functioning, high-risk contexts and behaviors) that contribute to the psychosocial health (e.g., psychopathology, quality of life, interpersonal relations, self-concept, body image dissatisfaction) of the adolescent in general, those with obesity, and those whose obesity has progressed to extreme levels. From a developmental perspective, evidence of psychosocial health impairments without effective intervention places an adolescent who carries their obesity burden forward at risk for continued poor psychosocial health and development as they transition to adulthood. Certainly the available adult obesity literature leads us to predict an otherwise bleak picture of health and well-being. Initial adolescent bariatric psychosocial outcome data indicating improvements in multiple domains are impressive, although as previously mentioned are limited to single-site studies of small sample size, with follow-up extending to only the 24-month time-point. It is likely that the significant improvement in health and psychosocial functioning following bariatric surgery creates conditions for changing the developmental course of these at-risk adolescents in a positive direction. However, whether new risk factors emerge or whether improvements erode over time remains unknown.

A broad developmentally based approach is needed to help explain the positive as well as any negative adolescent bariatric outcomes, thereby preventing simple explanations (i.e., "bariatric surgery is the cause") from permeating the literature. These age-salient psychosocial and contextual factors, however, have never been included in the same analytic model, nor examined as they relate to the significant weight loss following adolescent bariatric surgery. Furthermore, no studies to date have examined preoperative psychosocial predictors of adolescent outcomes. These types of modeling would require the power of a large sample of adolescents, followed prospectively and in a standardized manner, with minimal cohort attrition, compared to a similar group of adolescents with extreme obesity not undergoing bariatric surgery over the same course of time. Ongoing studies within the Teen-Longitudinal Assessment of Bariatric Surgery (Teen-LABS) Consortium [64] and its associated ancillary studies will provide the necessary conditions for this kind of modeling to be achieved.

The adolescent bariatric surgery literature is in its infancy but also occurring in the context of medical progress. While gaps in the psychosocial literature are previously described, there are several additional areas worth noting at the present time. For example, future studies are needed to examine if there are psychosocial indicators or outcomes for different bariatric procedures newly offered to adolescents such as the laparoscopic gastric band or sleeve gastrectomy versus the more invasive Roux-en-Y gastric bypass (RYGB). Given the seminal, longer-term, prospective, and controlled study of adults (Swedish Obesity Study) suggests that a "significant minority" demonstrates weight regain as early as the second year [65]. Understanding weight regain trends and their impact on the psychosocial health of the adolescent patient is imperative. Finally, we lack any empirical examination of the role of medical comorbidities and their resolution as they relate to the psychosocial health of the adolescent patient over time.

However, an important caveat must be included herein. This chapter is in no way to be seen as "prescriptive" in terms of what should be included in an adolescent pre-surgical psychological evaluation. Such an evaluation would prove quite burdensome (e.g., time, cost) to both the patient and the provider. Further, and unfortunately, until the adolescent bariatric surgery literature adequately "ages," we will lack an empirically derived understanding of the predictive value of any psychosocial domain in terms of determining adolescent candidacy and better or worse health and psychosocial outcomes. This chapter is written with a more developmental perspective highlighting age-salient considerations of the adolescent patient population, with critical areas for research. This is not to suggest preoperative psychological evaluations are not necessary for an adolescent patient; based on the present literature review, it is quite to the contrary. It is consistently recommended that a clinical bariatric team providing care to an adolescent patient include a licensed mental health professional as a participating team member (versus a community provider) with expertise in adolescent mental health, *as well as* experience working with adolescent patients and their families in the context of lifestyle change and adherence to medical regimens. The initial reliance on the adult model of preoperative psychological evaluations (see Chap. 5) is both prudent and appropriate, with the addition of the evaluation of age-salient factors that may either support or pose barriers to the adolescent's engagement in the preoperative and/or postoperative regimen (e.g., school schedule and performance, peer relations and support, family functioning and commitment to lifestyle change, history of adherence to medical regimens, limited resources, use of tobacco/alcohol/drugs). Such factors can be adequately obtained via a solid pediatric clinical interview. With the exception of an active substance abuse disorder, none of these factors would be considered exclusion criterion for an adolescent's candidacy but rather as contextual factors to consider in the execution of clinical care to each individual adolescent patient and their family.

Question and Answer Section

Questions

1. Fill in the blank. The psychosocial health profile of the adolescent with extreme obesity undergoing bariatric surgery is likely_____that of the typical adult bariatric patient.
   A. Different than
   B. Similar to
2. The adolescent bariatric surgery literature has advanced to a level that provides clear guidelines of which psychosocial factors are seen as supportive and which are barriers (i.e., contraindications) to surgical candidacy.
   A. True
   B. False

Answers

1. Answer **A**. The psychosocial health profile of an adolescent patient undergoing bariatric surgery is different than an adult. Adolescents undergo surgery during a transitional developmental period, known for change and including the emergence of high-risk behaviors, and changing family contexts due to increasing emotional and physical independence over time. This is normative, but it is unclear how an adolescent patient navigates such changes in the context of surgical weight loss.
2. Answer **B**. The adolescent bariatric surgery literature is in its infancy and limited by single-site and small sample studies, limiting the ability to test true predictors of positive versus negative surgical outcomes.

References

1. Freedman DS, Khan LK, Serdula MK, Ogden CL, Dietz WH. Racial and ethnic differences in secular trends for childhood BMI, weight, and height. Obesity. 2006;14(2):301–8.
2. Koebnick C, Smith N, Coleman KJ, Getahun D, Reynolds K, Quinn VP, et al. Prevalence of extreme obesity in a multiethnic cohort of children and adolescents. J Pediatr. 2010;157(1):26–31.e2.
3. Zeller MH, Reiter-Purtill J, Ratcliff MB, Inge TH, Noll JG. Two-year trends in psychosocial functioning after adolescent Roux-en-Y gastric bypass. Surg Obes Relat Dis. 2011;7(6):727–32. Pubmed Central PMCID: 21497142.
4. Roisman GI, Masten AS, Coatsworth JD, Tellegen A. Salient and emerging developmental tasks in the transition to adulthood. Child Dev. 2004;75(1):123–33. PubMed PMID: 15015679.
5. Arnett JJ. Emerging adulthood: a theory of development from the late teens through the twenties. Am Psychol. 2000;55(5):469–80. PubMed PMID: 2000-15413-004.
6. Varni JW, Seid M, Kurtin PS. PedsQL 4.0: reliability and validity of the pediatric quality of life inventory version 4.0 generic core scales

in healthy and patient populations. Med Care. 2001;39:800–12. PubMed PMID: 11468499.
7. Kolotkin RL, Zeller MH, Modi AC, Samsa GP, Polanichka Quinlan N, Yanovski JA, et al. Assessing weight-related quality of life in adolescents. Obesity. 2006;14(3):448–57.
8. Modi AC, Zeller MH. Validation of parent-proxy, obesity-specific quality of life measure: sizing them up. Obesity. 2008;16(12):2624–33.
9. Tsiros MD, Olds T, Buckley JD, Grimshaw P, Brennan L, Walkley J, et al. Health-related quality of life in obese children and adolescents. Int J Obes. 2009;33(4):387–400.
10. Zeller MH, Roehrig HR, Modi AC, Daniels SR, Inge TH. Health-related quality of life and depressive symptoms in adolescents with extreme obesity presenting for bariatric surgery. Pediatrics. 2006;117(4):1155–61.
11. Sysko R, Zakarin EB, Devlin MJ, Bush J, Walsh BT. A latent class analysis of psychiatric symptoms among 125 adolescents in a bariatric surgery program. Int J Pediatr Obes. 2011;6:289–97.
12. Britz B, Siegfried W, Ziegler A, Lamertz C, Herpertz-Dahlmann BM, Remschmidt H, et al. Rates of psychiatric disorders in a clinical study group of adolescents with extreme obesity and in obese adolescents ascertained via a population based study. Int J Obes. 2000;24:1707–14.
13. Erermis S, Cetin N, Tamar M, Bukusoglu N, Akdeniz F, Goksen D. Is obesity a risk factor for psychopathology among adolescents? Pediatr Int. 2004;46(3):296–301. PubMed PMID: 15151546.
14. Goodman E, Whitaker RC. A prospective study of the role of depression in the development and persistence of adolescent obesity. Pediatrics. 2002;110:497–504. PubMed PMID: 12205250.
15. Lamertz CM, Jacobi C, Yassouridis A, Arnold K, Henkel AW. Are obese adolescents and young adults at higher risk for mental disorders? A community survey. Obes Res. 2002;10(11):1152–60. PubMed PMID: 12429879.
16. Zeller MH, Saelens BE, Roehrig HR, Kirk S, Daniels S. Psychological adjustment of obese youth presenting for weight management treatment. Obes Res. 2004;12(10):1576–86.
17. Goodman E, Must A. Depressive symptoms in severely obese compared with normal weight adolescents: results from a community-based longitudinal study. J Adolesc Health. 2011;49(1):64–9.
18. Kim RJ, Langer JM, Baker AW, Fitter DE, Williams NN, Sarwer DB. Psychosocial status in adolescents undergoing bariatric surgery. Obes Surg. 2008;18:27–33.
19. Zeller MH, Modi AC, Noll JG, Long JD, Inge TH. Psychosocial functioning improves following adolescent bariatric surgery. Obesity. 2009;17(5):885–90. Pubmed Central PMCID: PMC2713017.
20. Ratcliff MB, Eshleman KE, Reiter-Purtill J, Zeller MH. Prospective changes in body image dissatisfaction among adolescent bariatric patients: the importance of body size estimation. Surg Obes Relat Dis. 2012;8(4):470–5. PMID: 22154271.
21. Messiah SE, Lopez-Mitnik G, Winegar D, Sherif B, Arheart KL, Reichard KW, et al. Changes in weight and co-morbidities among adolescents undergoing bariatric surgery: 1-year results from the bariatric outcomes longitudinal database. Surg Obes Relat Dis. 2012 (0). Epub 28 Mar 2012.
22. Johnson JG, Cohen P, Kasen S, Brook JS. Childhood adversities associated with risk for eating disorders or weight problems during adolescence or early adulthood. Am J Psychiatry. 2002;159(3):394–400. PubMed PMID: 11870002.
23. Decaluwe V, Braet C, Fairburn CG. Binge eating in obese children and adolescents. Int J Eat Disord. 2003;33(1):78–84. PubMed PMID: 12474202.
24. Glasofer DR, Tanofsky-Kraff M, Eddy KT, Yanovski SZ, Theim KR, Mirch MC, et al. Binge eating in overweight treatment-seeking adolescents. J Pediatr Psychol. 2007;32(1):95–105. PubMed PMID: 16801323.
25. Jacquez F, Cole DA, Searle B. Self-perceived competence as a mediator between maternal feedback and depressive symptoms in adolescents. J Abnorm Child Psychol. 2004;32(4):355–67.
26. Tram JM, Cole DA. Self-perceived competence and the relation between life events and depressive symptoms in adolescence: mediator or moderator? J Abnorm Psychol. 2000;109(4):753–60.
27. Griffiths LJ, Parsons TJ, Hill AJ. Self-esteem and quality of life in obese children and adolescents: a systematic review. Int J Pediatr Obes. 2010;5:282–304.
28. Harter S. The self-perception profile for adolescents. Unpublished manuscript. University of Denver, Department of Psychology. Denver; 1988.
29. Sarwer DB, Wadden TA, Moore RH, Eisenberg MH, Raper SE, Williams NN. Changes in quality of life and body image after gastric bypass surgery. Surg Obes Relat Dis. 2010;6(6):608–14. Pubmed Central PMCID: PMC3031862.
30. Sarwer DB, Allison KC, Berkowitz RI. Assessment and treatment of obesity in the primary care setting. In: Hass LJ, editor. Handbook of primary-care psychology. Oxford/New York: Oxford University Press; 2004. p. 435–54.
31. Zeller MH, Reiter-Purtill J, Ramey C. Negative peer perceptions of obese children in the classroom environment. Obesity. 2008;16(4):755–62.
32. Strauss RS, Pollack HA. Social marginalization of overweight children. Arch Pediatr Adolesc Med. 2003;157(8):746–52. PubMed PMID: 12912779.
33. Storch EA, Milsom VA, DeBraganza N, Lewin AB, Geffken GR, Silverstein JH. Peer victimization, psychosocial adjustment, and physical activity in overweight and at-risk-for-overweight youth. J Pediatr Psychol. 2007;32(1):80–9.
34. Janssen I, Craig WM, Boyce WF, Pickett W. Associations between overweight and obesity with bullying behaviors in school-aged children. Pediatrics. 2004;113(5):1187–94.
35. Pearce MJ, Boergers J, Prinstein MJ. Adolescent obesity, overt and relational peer victimization, and romantic relationships. Obes Res. 2002;10(5):386–93. PubMed PMID: 12006638.
36. Eisenberg ME, Neumark-Sztainer D, Story M. Associations of weight-based teasing and emotional well-being among adolescents. Arch Pediatr Adolesc Med. 2003;157(8):733–8. PubMed PMID: 12912777.
37. American Academy of Pediatrics. Family pediatrics: report of the task force on the family. Pediatrics. 2003;111(6):1541–71.
38. Modi AC, Guilfoyle SM, Zeller MH. Impaired health-related quality of life in caregivers of youth seeking obesity treatment. J Pediatr Psychol. 2009;34(2):147–55.
39. Zeller MH, Reiter-Purtill J, Modi AC, Gutzwiller J, Vannatta K, Davies WH. Controlled study of critical parent and family factors in the obesogenic environment. Obesity. 2007;15(1):126–36.
40. Janicke DM, Marciel KK, Ingerski LM, Novoa W, Lowry KW, Sallinen BJ, et al. Impact of psychosocial factors on quality of life in overweight youth. Obesity. 2007;15(7):1799–807.
41. Guilfoyle SM, Zeller MH, Modi AC. Parenting stress impacts obesity-specific health-related quality of life in a pediatric obesity treatment-seeking sample. J Dev Behav Pediatr. 2010;31(1):17–25. Pubmed Central PMCID: PMC2821720.
42. Crerand CE, Wadden TA, Sarwer DB, Fabricatore AN, Kuehnel RH, Gibbons LM, et al. A comparison of weight histories in women with class III vs class I-II obesity. Surg Obes Relat Dis. 2006;2:165–70.
43. Slotman GJ. Gastric bypass: a family affair—41 families in which multiple members underwent bariatric surgery. Surg Obes Relat Dis. 2011;7(5):592–8.
44. Woodard GA, Encarnacion B, Peraza J, Hernanadez-Boussard T, Morton J. Halo effect for bariatric surgery. Arch Surg. 2011;146(10):1185–90.

45. Noll JG, Zeller MH, Trickett PK, Putnam FW. Obesity risk for female victims of childhood sexual abuse: a prospective study. Pediatrics. 2007;120:61–7.
46. Felitti VJ. Long-term medical consequences of incest, rape, and molestation. South Med J. 1991;84(3):328–31. PubMed PMID: 2000519.
47. Williamson DF, Thompson TJ, Anda RF, Dietz WH, Felitti V. Body weight and obesity in adults and self-reported abuse in childhood. Int J Obes Relat Metab Disord. 2002;26(8):1075–82. PubMed PMID: 12119573.
48. Gustafson TE, Gibbons LM, Sarwer DB, Crerand C, Fabricatore AN, Wadden TA, et al. History of sexual abuse among bariatric surgery candidates. Surg Obes Relat Dis. 2006;3:369–74.
49. Grilo CM, Masheb RM, Brody M, Toth C, Burke-Martindale CH, Rothschild BS. Childhood maltreatment in extremely obese male and female bariatric surgery candidates. Obes Res. 2005;13(1): 123–30. PubMed PMID: 15761171.
50. Grilo CM, Masheb RM. Childhood psychological, physical, and sexual maltreatment in outpatients with binge eating disorder: frequency and associations with gender, obesity, and eating-related psychopathology. Obes Res. 2001;9:320–5. PubMed PMID: 11346674.
51. Trickett PK, Noll JG, Reiffman A, Putnam FW. Variants of intrafamilial sexual abuse experience: implications for short- and long-term development. Dev Psychopathol. 2001;13(4):1001–19. PubMed PMID: 11771904.
52. Kilpatrick DG, Acierno R, Saunders BE, Resnick HS, Best CL, Schnurr PP. Risk factors for adolescent substance abuse dependence: data from a national sample. J Consult Clin Psychol. 2000;68:19–30.
53. Noll JG, Trickett PK, Putnam FW. A prospective investigation of the impact of childhood sexual abuse on the development of sexuality. J Consul Clin Psychol. 2003;71(3):575–86. Pubmed Central PMCID: PMC3012425.
54. Ogden CL, Lamb MM, Carroll MD, Flegal KM. Obesity and socioeconomic status in children and adolescents: United States, 2005–2008. NCHS Data Brief. 2010;(51):1–8. PubMed PMID: 21211166.
55. Haas JS, Lee LB, Kaplan CP, Sonneborn D, Phillips KA, Liang S. The association of race, socioeconomic status, and health insurance status with the prevalence of overweight among children and adolescents. Am J Public Health. 2003;93(12):2105–10.
56. Goodman E, Slap GB, Huang B. The public health impact of socioeconomic status on adolescent depression and obesity. Am J Public Health. 2003;93(11):1844–50.
57. Nock MK, Borges G, Bromet EJ, Cha CB, Kessler RC, Lee S. Suicide and suicidal behavior. Epidemiol Rev. 2008;30(1): 133–54.
58. Winters KC, Lee C-YS. Likelihood of developing an alcohol and cannabis use disorder during youth: association with recent use and age. Drug Alcohol Depend. 2008;92(1–3):239–47. Pubmed Central PMCID: PMC2219953.
59. Brown SA, McGue M, Maggs J, Schulenberg J, Hingson R, Swartzwelder S, et al. A developmental perspective on alcohol and youths 16 to 20 years of age. Pediatrics. 2008;121 Suppl 4:290–310. Pubmed Central PMCID: PMC2765460.
60. Centers for Disease Control and Prevention. Trends in reportable sexually transmitted disease in the United States, 2006. National surveillance data for chlamydia, gonorrhea, and syphilis [cited 2011 May 23]. Available from: www.cdc.gov/std/stats06/trends2006.htm.
61. Centers for Disease Control and Prevention. HIV Surveillance Report, 2009, vol. 21. [cited 2011 May 23]. Published Feb 2011. Available from: http://www.cdc.gov/hiv/topics/surveillance/resource/reports/.
62. Benoit Ratcliff M, Jenkins TM, Reiter-Purtill J, Noll JG, Zeller MH, Benoit Ratcliff M, Jenkins TM, Reiter-Purtill J, Noll JG, Zeller MH. Risk-taking behaviors of adolescents with extreme obesity: normative or not? Pediatrics. 2011;127:827–34. Pubmed Central PMCID: 21518723.
63. Zeller MH, Reiter-Purtill J, Jenkins TM, Ratcliff MB. Adolescent suicidal behavior across the excess weight status spectrum. Obesity (in press).
64. Inge TH, Zeller MH, Harmon CM, Helmrath MA, Bean J, Modi AC, et al. Teen-longitudinal assessment of bariatric surgery: methodological features of the first prospective multicenter study of adolescent bariatric surgery. J Pediatr Surg. 2007;42(11): 1969–71.
65. Sjostrom L, Lindroos AK, Peltonen M, Torgerson J, Bouchard C, Carlsson B, et al. Lifestyle, diabetes, and cardiovascular risk factors 10 years after bariatric surgery. N Engl J Med. 2004;351(26): 2683–93. PubMed PMID: 15616203.

Part II

Nutrition

Perioperative Nutrition Assessment of the Bariatric Surgery Patient

Laura Lewis Frank

Chapter Objectives

1. To describe the key components of the nutrition care process including nutrition assessment, diagnosis, intervention and monitoring, and evaluation
2. To describe the role of nutrition assessment as an ongoing, nonlinear dynamic process of objective and subjective data gathering in order to determine potential nutrition problems of the bariatric patient
3. To describe the perioperative role of the nutrition professional, namely, the registered dietitian (RD), in improving patient outcomes

Introduction

Bariatric surgery appears to be a safe and feasible treatment to achieve long-term weight loss and improvements in cardiovascular risk factors, symptoms, and quality of life in obese individuals [1]. Moreover, surgical weight loss strategies are more successful than diet alone in achieving and maintaining weight loss [1, 2]. However, the long-term success of bariatric surgery relies on the patients' ability to make sustained lifestyle changes in the areas of nutrition and physical activity [3]. To obtain the best patient outcomes, a comprehensive, multidisciplinary team approach provides the best care to any bariatric patient and the food and nutrition professional, or registered dietitian (RD), plays an integral role in the nutrition assessment and follow-up process across the care continuum [4]. Indeed, due to the continuing trend of obesity and utilization of bariatric surgery for the treatment of obesity, there will undoubtedly be a growing role for the registered dietitian [5]. The RD possesses the knowledge and skills in the overall management of the bariatric surgical patient as well as proficiency in bariatric nutrition education and counseling [4].

Modifying eating behaviors is mandatory for the long-term success of the bariatric patient [6]. The dietitian can help facilitate improvements in food- and nutrition-related knowledge and assist patients with decision-making regarding desirable food choices for each surgery type [3, 4]. Researchers have reported that despite the significant weight loss and dramatic improvements in comorbidities associated with bariatric surgery, a significant minority of patients appear to experience suboptimal weight loss [7]. Although the reasons for this are not well understood, suboptimal weight loss is often attributed to preoperative psychosocial characteristics and/or eating behaviors [6], as well as poor adherence to the recommended postoperative diet [7]. These results emphasize the need for perioperative dietary counseling to improve surgical weight loss outcomes [6, 7], underscoring the dietitian's vital role in the nutrition care process [8] unique to the bariatric patient.

Nutrition Care Process

The *nutrition care process* (NCP) is designed to improve the consistency and quality of individualized care for patients as well as the predictability of patient outcomes [8]. The term "patient" will be used in this chapter; however, note that the "patient" can also be referred to as a client, a group, and/or a surrogate to patient care including family members or caregivers. There are four steps to the NCP: (1) nutrition assessment, (2) nutrition diagnosis, (3) nutrition intervention, and (4) nutrition monitoring and evaluation and are outlined in Fig. 9.1.

L.L. Frank, PhD, MPH, RD, CD (✉)
Coordinated Program in Dietetics, Program in Nutrition & Exercise Physiology (NEP), MultiCare Health System, College of Pharmacy, Washington State University, Tacoma, WA, USA

Frank Nutrition & Exercise Consulting, LLC, Gig Harbor, WA, USA
e-mail: FrankL@wsu.edu

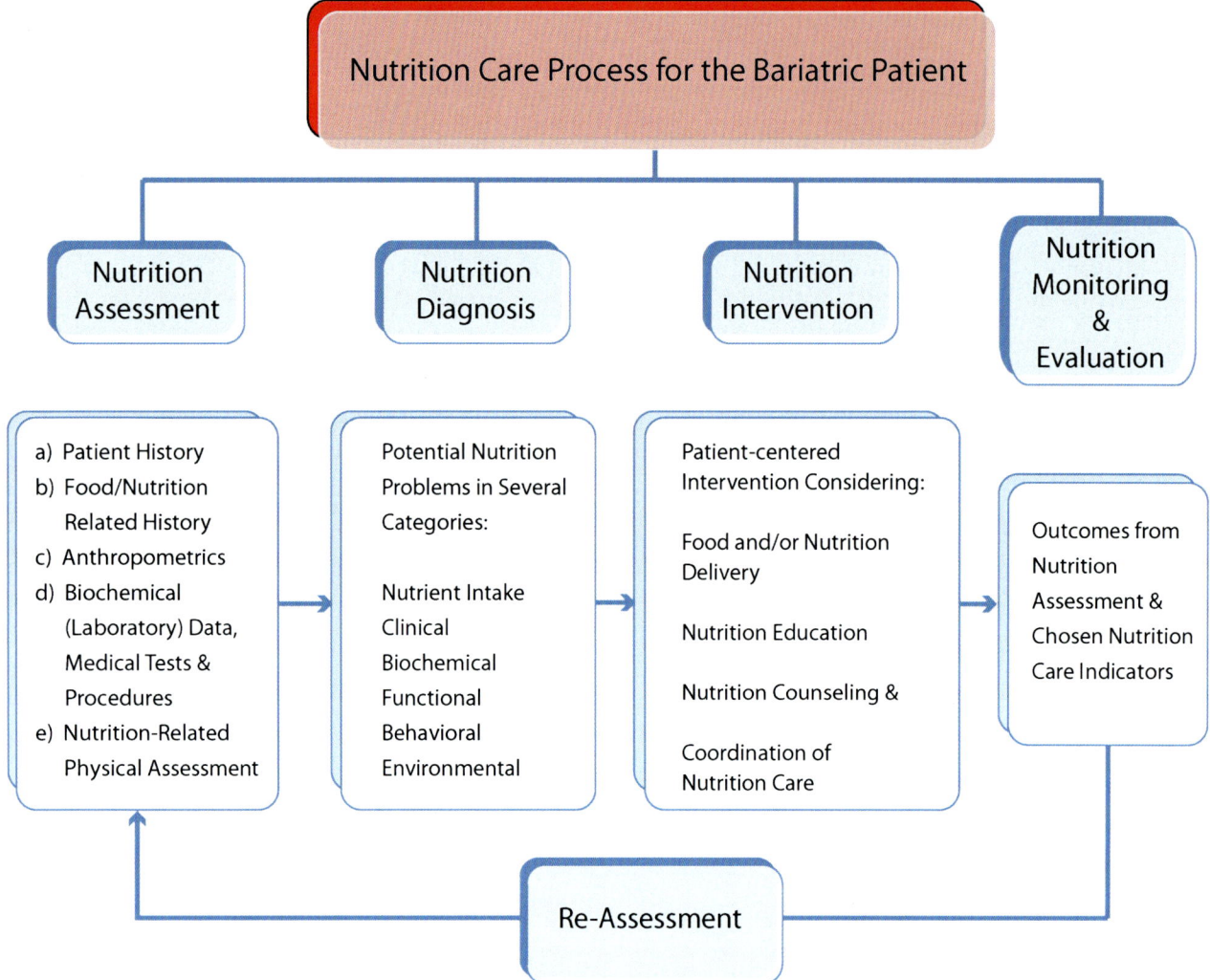

Fig. 9.1 Nutrition care process integrating key components: nutrition assessment, nutrition diagnosis, nutrition intervention, monitoring and evaluation, and reassessment. As this is an ongoing, cyclic process meant to improve bariatric patient outcomes, continual monitoring and reassessment of outcome measures are required perioperatively (Permission from publisher: American Dietetic Association)

Nutrition Assessment

Nutrition assessment is step one of the NCP [8]. The nutrition assessment is a systematic method for obtaining, verifying, and interpreting data needed to identify nutrition-related problems, the associated etiology(ies) related to the problem, and the significance and signs and symptoms manifested by the nutrition-related problem. The nutrition assessment process is an ongoing, dynamic process involving objective and subjective data gathering from the patient and the patient's medical record. Nutrition assessment indicators are then compared to criteria, relevant norms, and standards for interpretation. From this data, the food and nutrition professional can determine whether a nutrition diagnosis or nutrition problem exists.

Nutrition assessment terms are identified and grouped into five domains: (1) *food/nutrition-related history*; (2) *anthropometrics*; (3) *biochemical data, medical tests, and procedures*; (4) *nutrition-focused physical findings*; and (5) *patient/client history* (Fig. 9.2) [8]. For individual patients, nutrition-related data can be derived from patient interviews, observation and measurement, medical records, or from the referring health provider. For groups, data may come from surveys, administrative data sets, or epidemiological data or research studies.

The nutrition assessment is initiated after a patient is referred to the dietitian and leads to the appropriate determination of whether a nutrition diagnosis or problem exists. Referral to the nutrition professional will be different, depending upon whether there is an outpatient or inpatient

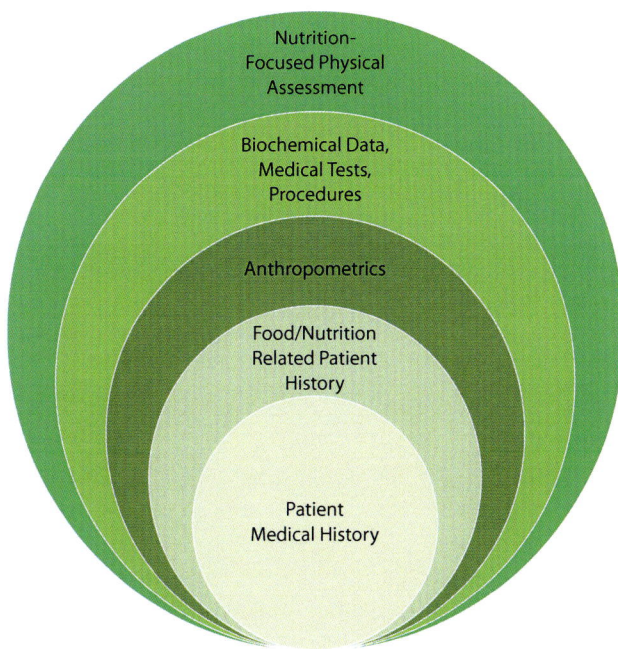

Fig. 9.2 Key categories of nutrition assessment used to obtain, verify, and interpret needs for the bariatric patient. The nutrition assessment process is an ongoing, dynamic process involving objective and subjective data gathering from the patient and the patient's medical record. Bariatric patients should undergo nutrition assessments across the care continuum (Permission from publisher: American Dietetic Association)

emphasis. For example, the bariatric outpatient is generally referred to the food and nutrition professional or registered dietitian as part of bariatric "pathway" where the patient is preparing for surgery. Presurgically, the patient may be seeking nutrition-intervention strategies to meet weight loss goals that are either self-imposed or mandated by third-party payers or weight loss surgery programmatic criteria. In contrast, a postsurgical inpatient referred to the RD as part of the nutrition screening process would imply that the patient was deemed at high nutrition risk, and therefore, the nutrition assessment process would require a different set of nutrition-related problem statements requiring different intervention strategies to meet outcome goals. An example of these differences can be seen in Table 9.1.

The specific domains associated with the data-gathering task of the nutrition assessment are important for the clinician to identify potential areas of nutrition-related problems. *Food/nutrition-related history* includes information regarding the patient's food and nutrient intake [8]. For the bariatric patient, this will be a key data point when assessing the pre- and postsurgical patient. This information can help identify inadequate or excessive energy or nutrient intakes. Also included in this category are food and nutrient administration, medication/herbal supplement use, knowledge/beliefs/ attitude of food and supplements, eating and food behaviors, factors affecting access to food and/or food/nutrition-related supplies, and physical activity and function. For the bariatric patient, the food/nutrition-related history section is a key arena for the nutrition professional to exercise many models of cognitive-change theories shown effective at improving metabolic syndrome risk variables and weight loss with lifestyle modification [9].

Anthropometric measurements includes information about the patient's height, weight, weight history, body mass index (BMI), growth pattern indices, and percentile ranks (important for pediatric nutrition assessment). Comparative standards for anthropometrics are encouraged to be used [8]. In the bariatric patient, BMI is typically used to determine whether a patient meets eligibility requirements. The 1991 National Institutes of Health (NIH) Consensus Development Conference Panel [10] established general eligibility criteria for bariatric surgery. Individuals could be considered surgical candidates if they possessed either a BMI ≥ 40 kg/m^2 or a BMI ≥ 35 kg/m^2 if they had one or more high-risk comorbid conditions. These conditions include, but are not limited to, coronary artery disease (CAD) or obesity-related cardiomyopathy, severe obstructive sleep apnea (OSA), obesity hypoventilation syndrome (OHS), Pickwickian syndrome (combination of OSA and OHS), nonalcoholic fatty liver disease (NAFLD), nonalcoholic steatohepatitis, hypertension, dyslipidemia, pseudotumor cerebri, gastroesophageal reflux disease (GERD), asthma, venous stasis disease, severe urinary incontinence, debilitating arthritis, and uncontrolled type 2 diabetes mellitus (T2DM). Surgery may also be indicated among patients with a BMI between 35 and 40 if they have impaired quality of life (QOL) including but not limited to body size problems precluding or severely interfering with employment, family function, and ambulation. The consensus panel also determined that surgery must be performed in a setting of multidisciplinary practitioners and that presurgically the patient should undergo both psychiatric and nutritional evaluation and education. Due to the metabolic changes associated with bariatric surgery, the Food and Drug Administration (FDA) has approved the use of the laparoscopic adjustable gastric band (LAGB) for patients with a BMI of 30 to 35 kg/m^2 with Type 2 Diabetes (T2DM) or other obesity-related comorbidities [11].

Other anthropometric measures important to the bariatric patient is *percent excess weight loss (%EWL)*. *Percent excess weight loss*—defined as a percentage of preoperative weight minus postoperative weight divided by preoperative weight minus ideal body weight (IBW)—is typically used to measure outcomes from the various types of bariatric surgeries. Reported weight loss as percentage of EWL comparing dif-

Table 9.1 Differences in nutrition assessment of outpatient versus inpatient bariatric patients

Outpatient	Inpatient
Example: preoperative nutrition assessment for weight loss	*Example*: postoperative nutrition assessment screened at high nutrition risk
Goal: to initiate healthy meal plan for weight loss	*Goal*: to assess nutrition deficiency and treat
Referral source: surgical program process, third-party payer mandates, self-referred for weight loss, referred by primary care provider (PCP)	*Referral source*: hospital admission criteria, MD consult, nursing assessment, diet technician referral from nutrition screen
Assessment: 47-year-old female, BMI: 43 kg/m²	*Assessment*: 47-year-old female, BMI: 47 kg/m²
PMH: type 2 diabetes, hypertension, hyperlipidemia, nonalcoholic fatty liver disease	*Signs/symptoms*: ~4 weeks of persistent nausea and retching q 2–3 h, productive of saliva only, persistent abdominal pain, anorexia, altered mental status (AMS), severe loss of memory, confabulation, ataxia
Labs: blood pressure 130/90, glucose 180, cholesterol 300, triglycerides 320	*PMH*: type 2 diabetes, hypertension, hyperlipidemia, major depression
Physical assessment: obese female, no gross abnormalities, low physical mobility, skin/eyes/nail beds intact with no lesions or abnormalities	*PSxH*: Roux-en Y gastric bypass 4 weeks ago, uncomplicated Sx. Presurgical BMI: 53 kg/m²
Food/nutrition-related history: patient reports eating "constantly" throughout the day and evening, craves crunchy/salty foods such as potato chips, dislikes vegetables except corn and potatoes, and eats fast food at least 5 days per week due to work schedule. Patient does not exercise and is not physically active	*Labs*: potassium 2.7(L), lactate 3.2(H), glucose 124(H), C-reactive protein >150(H), albumin 2.7(L)
Knowledge/beliefs: patient is very motivated to "do what it takes" to get bariatric surgery and is willing to change her lifestyle (diet and exercise) for improved outcomes	*Physical assessment*: obese female, no gross abnormalities, bedridden (patient states she is not stable to walk), numbness and tingling in feet that radiates to above-the-knee (peripheral neuropathy), eyes present with nystagmus
	Food/nutrition-related history: patient reports no appetite since surgery, abdominal pain, nausea, and vomiting (productive of saliva only), not able to take nutrition supplements
Nutrition diagnosis: obesity (problem) related to disordered eating pattern, excessive energy intake, physical inactivity (etiologies or causes) as evidenced by obesity grade III (BMI 40+), overconsumption of high-fat and/or calorie-dense food or beverages, estimated excessive energy intake, infrequent physical activity (signs/symptoms)	*Nutrition diagnosis*: inadequate vitamin intake (thiamin) (problem) related to decreased ability to consume sufficient amounts of vitamin due to nausea, vomiting, and malabsorption due to gastric bypass surgery (etiology) as evidenced by symptoms associated with thiamin deficiency: peripheral neuropathy, ataxia, nystagmus, and altered mental status (confabulation) consistent with Wernicke's encephalopathy
Nutrition education and counseling intervention: patient-centered goals generated for utilization of "plate method" for one-quarter plate starch, one-quarter plate lean meat, and one-half plate of vegetable (patient agreed to have salad daily). Patient agreed to try baked potato chips and pretzels vs. potato chips or other deep-fried, salty snacks. Patient agreed to limit these snacks to one per day. Patient agreed to aim for five servings of fruits and vegetables per day	*Intervention*: assess status of thiamin, preferably by using erythrocyte transketolase lab (confirmed deficiency if >1.20 µg/mL/h) and provide IV thiamin therapy: up to 500 mg thiamin one to three times daily for 3 days [12]
	Refer patient to neurologist for further follow-up with peripheral neuropathy. Refer patient for follow-up with bariatric surgeon due to abdominal pain, nausea, and vomiting since surgery 4 weeks ago
Food diary given to patient to discuss next follow-up	Refer patient to outpatient RD for further nutrition education regarding vitamin and mineral supplementation and meal planning
Monitoring and evaluation: patient will follow up with dietitian in 4 weeks to discuss eating behaviors, food choices (food diary)	*Monitoring and evaluation*: RD will follow up with patient prior to discharge to assess tolerance and outcomes of thiamin repletion
Goal: patient will choose five servings of fruits and vegetables daily. Patient's weight: lose at least 8 lb in 4 weeks	Goal: for patient's signs and symptoms of thiamin deficiency to improve

ferent types of surgeries over a 1–2 year, 3–6 year, and a 7–10 year follow-up has been previously described [2]. Comparing follow-up data at 7–10 years, the gastric band, the Roux-en Y gastric bypass (RYGB), and the biliopancreatic diversion (BPD) ± duodenal switch (DS) and the banded RYGB resulted in a 14–60, 25–68, and 60–70 % excess weight loss, respectively. Comparing individualized patient outcomes to published norms can help determine whether patients are within weight loss standards after surgery.

Biochemical data, medical tests, and procedures include laboratory data and medical tests [8]. Laboratory data is an important tool in the nutrition professional's toolbox and helps define a nutrition diagnosis or problem including nutrient deficiencies and/or toxicities. Medical tests and procedures are important for the presurgical patient in objectively determining whether a patient meets surgical criteria and is fit for surgery. For the postsurgical patient, medical tests and procedures are important in determining whether the patient is qualified to begin oral feeds or in ruling out possible surgical complications.

Nutrition-focused physical findings include information about the patient's physical appearance, apparent muscle and fat wasting (a clinical manifestation of protein–calorie malnutrition), swallow function, functional status (handgrip strength, ability to perform activities of daily living [ADLs], and physical performance), appetite, affect, and signs and symptoms of micronutrient deficiencies [8]. These signs and symptoms will be further reviewed in this textbook. For a more detailed overview of micronutrient deficiencies associated with bariatric surgery, the reader is encouraged to refer to Aills et al. [12].

Patient/client history includes the personal history, medical/health/family/social history, treatments, and complementary/alternative medicine use [8]. Past and present medical history is an important tool in the nutrition professional's toolbox to help complete the nutrition care process. The nutrition professional will be required to exercise critical thinking skills in determining appropriate data to collect from both objective and subjective sources. Clinical judgment will need to be utilized to determine whether there is a need for additional data gathering in order to diagnose nutrition problems and generate nutrition-intervention strategies accordingly. Indeed, distinguishing between relevant/important versus irrelevant/unimportant data is a skill well orchestrated by the food and nutrition expert such as the registered dietitian.

Nutrition Diagnosis

Nutrition diagnosis is step two of the NCP [8]. The nutrition diagnosis is a critical step between the nutrition assessment and nutrition intervention. Standardization of the nutrition diagnosis language has been proposed by the Academy of Nutrition and Dietetics and has been published elsewhere [8]. The nutrition diagnosis includes a nutrition problem utilizing standardized nutrition diagnosis terminology, associated etiology(ies) [9], or "root" cause(s), the significance, and signs and symptoms associated with the problem. The nutrition professional can then create a PES (Problem, Etiology, Signs/Symptoms) statement, which can then target specific nutrition-intervention strategies. The PES statement is derived from the clustering and synthesis of data gathering obtained from objective and subjective information during the nutrition assessment process. Nutrition professionals should critically evaluate whether they can resolve or improve the selected nutrition diagnosis, determine the "root cause" of the nutrition problem, and then determine measurable signs and symptoms that will best indicate that the nutrition problem has resolved or improved. Furthermore, it is imperative that the practitioner use all domains and nutrition diagnostic categories to recognize potential areas of nutrition intervention. Table 9.1 provides two examples of possible PES statements that may be used for the bariatric patient in two different clinical scenarios.

There are essentially three domains where the nutrition problems may fall: *intake*, *clinical*, and *behavioral/environmental*. To date, more than 70 nutrition diagnosis/problems have been identified [8]. The *intake* domain is defined as the "actual problems related to intake of energy, nutrition, fluids, bioactive substances, either through oral diet or nutrition support. As mentioned, this area of nutrition diagnosis is key for the RD to identify potential pitfalls in the bariatric patient's energy, fluid, and nutrient balance. Knowledge of a patient's nutrition intake from food records, calorie counts (utilized in the inpatient bariatric patient only), and dietary supplement intake records can help identify the following potential nutrition-related problems: increased/decreased nutrient needs, malnutrition, imbalance of nutrients, and inadequate/excessive/inappropriate intake of fats, protein, carbohydrate/fiber, vitamins, and minerals as well as bioactive substances such as dietary supplements.

The *clinical* domain is defined as "nutrition findings/problems identified that relate to medical or physical conditions" including *functional, biochemical, and weight* categories [8]. The post-bariatric patient would qualify for use of the nutrition diagnosis of altered gastrointestinal (GI) function, found under the functional category of the clinical domain. An example of a PES statement for the post-bariatric patient would then be: altered GI function (P: Problem) related to alteration in GI structure and/or function (E: Etiology) as evidenced by gastric bypass (S: Sign/Symptom or defining characteristic).

The *biochemical* category found within the *clinical* domain is defined as the "change in capacity to metabolize nutrients as a result of medications, surgery or as indicated by altered laboratory values" [8]. The bariatric patient's potential for impaired nutrient utilization, food avoidance, and food and nutrition supplement intolerance after surgery [14] can translate into abnormal laboratory findings, however, other patients may present with subclinical laboratory outcomes where clinical signs and symptoms of deficiency exists while laboratory data may be within normal limits [13].

The *weight* category found within the *clinical* domain is defined as chronic weight or changed weight status when compared to comparative norms, usual body weight, ideal body weight (IBW), or desirable body weight (DBW) [8]. Note that at this time in the bariatric community, there is no consensus or best-practice standard for determining ideal or desirable body weight. This potential category of nutrition-related problems can help the food and nutrition professional identify bariatric patients who are overweight/obese and/or presenting with unintentional weight gain (or weight regain after surgery). Furthermore, post-bariatric patients may also be diagnosed with underweight and/or unintentional weight loss. For example, unintentional and/or rapid weight loss may be associated with protein–calorie malnutrition or vitamin/mineral deficiencies such as thiamin deficiency [13].

The *behavioral/environmental* domain of the nutrition diagnosis terminology is defined as nutritional problems identified that relate to knowledge, attitudes/beliefs, physical environment, access to food and food supplies, or food safety [8]. Categories found under the behavioral/environmental domain include knowledge and beliefs, physical activity and function, and food safety and access. Focusing on the bariatric patient's food- and nutrition-related knowledge deficits, potential harmful beliefs or attitudes about food or nutrition-related topics, readiness for diet/lifestyle change, potential disordered eating beliefs and patterns, level of adherence to bariatric nutrition guidelines, and assessment of undesirable food choices are areas of emphasis that the RD can problem-shoot and counsel the patient for improved outcomes [4]. It is also important to evaluate other issues that could affect nutrient status including readiness for change; realistic goal setting; general nutrition knowledge; as well as behavioral, cultural, psychosocial, and economic issues [13].

The RD can also work as part of the multidisciplinary team to address a bariatric patient's level of physical activity, inability or lack of desire to manage self-care, and potential self-feeding difficulties or impaired ability to function. By working closely with exercise specialists and physical therapists, the nutrition professional can help identify potential areas of nutrition-related problems that may negatively impact the success of the bariatric patient in managing an exercise regimen. Moreover, researchers have shown that weight loss is improved by patients who attend structured events and motivational forums provided by exercise specialists [15, 16].

Nutrition Intervention

Nutrition intervention is step 3 in the NCP [8]. Nutrition interventions are specific actions used to remedy a nutrition diagnosis or problem. Therefore, the intervention can target individual patients, groups, or communities. The nutrition intervention most likely targets the "E" or etiology of the nutrition problem; however, in specific circumstances, the nutrition intervention is directed at reducing/eliminating the "S" or the signs/symptoms. The four domains of nutrition intervention that have been identified include *food and/or nutrient delivery*, *nutrition education*, *nutrition counseling*, and *coordination of nutrition care*. Nutrition interventions should be based on evidenced-based practice guidelines and referenced accordingly. For each nutrition intervention or plan prescribed by the nutrition professional, appropriate patient-centered goals should be set for improved patient outcomes.

Nutrition Monitoring and Evaluation

Nutrition monitoring and evaluation is the fourth step in the NCP [8]. The purpose of this step is to quantify progress made by the patient in meeting the nutrition care goals and outcomes from the nutrition assessment and chosen nutrition care indicators. Furthermore, nutrition monitoring and evaluation should entail the review of progress from specific, measurable, attainable, realistic, and time-bound (S.M.A.R.T.) patient-centered goals generated through the nutrition-intervention step of the NCP. The monitoring and evaluation of the bariatric patient is meant to be an opportunity to reassess objective and subjective data, which may allow the practitioner to detect new potential nutrition problems while evaluating the progress on previously diagnosed nutrition problems.

Preoperative Nutrition Assessment and Follow-Up

A comprehensive nutrition assessment should be conducted preoperatively to identify the patient's nutritional and educational needs [13]. Dietitians begin to educate patients preoperatively and continue their instruction across the care continuum [3]. Presurgery, the RD can help screen the patient's presurgical preparedness for surgery, provide presurgical diet evaluation and instruction, and help in the development of patient-centered goals and objectives to result in desirable patient outcomes following weight loss surgery. Aills et al. [13] have further described the suggested preoperative nutrition assessment and education for the bariatric surgical patient.

The dietitian can assist the patient to obtain preoperative weight loss, often mandated by third-party payer criteria and by the surgeon. Physician-mandated weight loss may be undertaken in individual patients to evaluate a patient's ability to adhere to dietary changes and to comply with treatment, to decrease surgical risk, and/or to reduce the size of the liver and visceral fat load to improve the technical aspects of surgery [2]. The nutrition professional plays a critical role in the medical nutrition therapy associated with obesity-related diseases such as hyperlipidemia, hypercholesterolemia, hypertension, hypothyroidism, and cardiovascular disease. If patients have comorbid conditions such as T2DM, the dietitian (especially those with specialty expertise as a certified diabetes educator) can help the patient obtain glycemic control prior to surgery. However, a protocol for perioperative glycemic control should be reviewed *before* the patient undergoes bariatric surgery [2]. Therefore, if a patient has been medically diagnosed with these comorbid conditions, the nutrition professional can educate the patient on diet and lifestyle behaviors that may improve the patient's presurgical health.

A psychosocial–behavioral evaluation, which assesses environmental, familial, and behavioral factors, should be considered for all patients before bariatric surgery [2]. Any patient considered for bariatric surgery with a known or suspected psychiatric illness should undergo a formal mental health evaluation before performance of the surgical procedure and may not be appropriate candidate for surgery. Overall, patients should undergo evaluation of their ability to incorporate nutritional and behavioral changes before and after bariatric surgery.

Preoperative Nutrition Deficiencies

Preoperative nutrition deficiencies have been reported [2, 13, 17]. The RD can identify and describe a specific nutrition problem such as a preexisting nutrient deficiency as well as develop appropriate nutrition interventions for correction of these preexisting nutritional deficiencies [13]. In such, it is imperative that the nutrition professional recognize signs and symptoms, physical findings, and aberrant laboratory results associated with micronutrient deficiencies. One study retrospectively analyzed the preoperative values of several labs, including serum albumin, calcium, 25-OH vitamin D, iron, ferritin, hemoglobin, vitamin B12, and thiamin in 379 consecutive patients (320 women and 59 men; mean BMI: 51.8 ± 10.6 kg/m2; 25.8 % white, 28.4 % African-American, 45.8 % Hispanic) undergoing bariatric surgery between 2002 and 2004 [17]. Preoperative deficiencies were noted for iron (43.9 %), ferritin (8.4 %), hemoglobin (22 %; women 19.1 %, men 40.7 %), thiamin (29 %), and 25-OH vitamin D (68.1 %). Low ferritin levels were more prevalent in females (9.9 % versus 0 %; $P=0.01$); however, anemia was more prevalent in males (19.1 % versus 40.7 %; $P<0.005$). Patients younger than 25 years were more likely to be anemic than patients over 60 years (46 % versus 15 %; $P<0.005$). This correlated with iron deficiency, which was more prevalent in younger patients (79.2 % versus 41.7 %; $P<0.005$). Whites (78.8 %) and African-Americans (70.4 %) had a higher prevalence of vitamin D deficiency than Hispanics (56.4 %, $P=0.01$). Whites were the least likely group to be thiamin deficient (6.8 % versus 31.0 % African-Americans and 47.2 % Hispanics; $P<0.005$). These authors concluded that presurgical nutritional deficiencies are common in patients undergoing Roux-en-Y gastric bypass, and these deficiencies should be detected and corrected early to avoid postoperative complications.

It is prudent that all patients undergo an appropriate nutritional evaluation, including selective micronutrient measurements and assays, before any bariatric surgical procedure. Unfortunately, there are no standards of care or screening for all surgical candidates. However, nutritional guidelines for laboratory tests before and after surgery have been published [13]. According to these authors, established baseline values are important when trying to distinguish between postoperative complications, deficiencies related to surgery, noncompliance with recommended nutrient supplementation, or nutritional complications arising from preexisting deficiencies. Recommended routine preoperative nutrition screens include protein (albumin, prealbumin), the minerals iron and zinc, as well as the vitamins B12, folate, pyridoxine (vitamin B6), thiamin (vitamin B1), and the fat-soluble vitamins A, D, E, and K.

According to other guidelines [2], all patients should undergo an appropriate nutritional evaluation, including micronutrient assessments before any bariatric procedure. These authors recommend preoperative assessment of iron (using an iron panel), vitamin B12 (optional methylmalonic acid [MMA] and homocysteine), erythrocyte or red blood cell folate, vitamin D (25-OH vitamin D), and optional thiamin. Furthermore, in comparison with purely restrictive procedures, a more extensive perioperative nutrition evaluation is required for malabsorptive procedures. Preoperative assessment of vitamins A and D (vitamin E and K optional) as well as intact parathyroid hormone (iPTH) is recommended for individuals planning to undergo BPD with or without DS. Routine chemistry studies (fasting blood glucose, liver profile, and lipid profile), urinalysis, prothrombin time (INR), blood type, and complete blood cell count are usually recommended. If patients present with elevated mean corpuscular volume (MCV) values, it is also prudent to assess MMA in order to distinguish between vitamin B12 and folate deficiency [2].

Postoperative Nutrition Assessment and Follow-Up

The management of postoperative nutrition begins preoperatively with a thorough assessment of nutrient status, a strong educational program, and follow-up to reinforce important principles associated with long-term maintenance of weight loss [13]. Postoperative nutritional management of the post-bariatric patient has been previously described [2–4, 6, 13]. After bariatric surgery, dietary counseling aimed at modifying eating behavior is crucial for obtaining successful results [6]. Sarwer et al. [7] reported that baseline cognitive restraint and adherence to the recommended postoperative diet were associated with the percentage of weight loss after gastric bypass surgery. Therefore, the goals of dietary management in the postoperative period are to facilitate weight loss and reduce the risk of nutritional deficiencies [3] as well as to prevent and/or control potential postoperative complications [4]. Nutrition management of common medical issues after bariatric surgery has been described previously [3, 4]. These complications include, but are not limited to, vomiting,

Table 9.2 Suggested laboratory assessment values for the pre- and post-bariatric patient

Fasting blood glucose
Complete blood count
Liver function tests
Lipid profile
Protein: albumin, prealbumin, total protein
Minerals: iron (iron panel), zinc, selenium, copper
Vitamins: thiamin (vitamin B1), cyanocobalamin (vitamin B12), folate, pyridoxine (vitamin B6), vitamin A, vitamin D (25-OH vitamin D)
Optional vitamin E and K
Intact parathyroid hormone (iPTH)
Prothrombin time

bilious vomiting, diarrhea, steatorrhea, dumping syndrome, hypoglycemia, gallstones, intestinal obstruction, stomal complications, GI bleeding, and incisional hernias [3]. More discussion of potential complications will be further described in this textbook.

Frequent monitoring and adjustments in diet or nutritional supplements may be needed during both the postsurgical weight loss and weight maintenance periods [5], in which the dietitian plays a key role. A systematic review of the literature suggests that bariatric surgery patients are at risk for deficiency of the following nutrients after surgery: vitamins B12, B1, C, folate, A, D, and K, along with the trace minerals iron, selenium, zinc, and copper [12]. Therefore, prudent nutrition assessment of these and other nutrient deficiencies is a mandatory part of the integrated health care in the postsurgical bariatric patient [2, 11]. Further discussion of micronutrient deficiencies following weight loss surgery will be provided within this textbook. An overview of suggested laboratory assessment measures to assess and monitor through the nutrition care and bariatric surgery process both pre- and postoperatively is found in Table 9.2.

Although there are no published standards on the best-practice nutrition follow-up schedule for bariatric patients, studies show that patients who are lost in medical and nutritional follow-up have less success in weight reduction and maintenance and are at greater risk of developing nutritional deficiencies [14, 15]. Furthermore, it has been shown that a positive relationship between the frequency of patient–provider contact during the postoperative period and the promotion of long-term success of weight loss in the postsurgical weight loss patient exists [2, 7]. In contrast, failure to attend follow-up appointments is associated with poor weight loss and postoperative complications [18]. Therefore, regular, timed follow-up appointments integrating medical nutrition therapy are needed to improve bariatric patient outcomes [13]. A consensus for the follow-up nutrition and metabolic consultations after bariatric surgery, stratified by type of procedure performed and presence of comorbidities, has been published [2], recommending more frequent monitoring during the first year after surgery (every 2–3 months) and then biyearly or annually thereafter. Other practitioners recommend evaluations 4–6 weeks after surgery, then quarterly for 1 year and annually thereafter or according to the patient's need [3].

General Nutrition Guidelines Following Bariatric and Metabolic Surgery

General nutrition guidelines following surgery include several diet modifications including food texture and consistency, volume of liquids and solids consumed, frequency and duration of meals, and adjustments for food intolerance and malabsorption. Common food intolerances include bread, rice, pasta, tough meat, milk, dairy, and carbonated beverages [3]. Food textures tolerated poorly may include dry, sticky, or stringy foods, while concentrated sweets may induce dumping syndrome [13]. Therefore, dietary recommendations should be based on the overall nutrition assessment of the patient and should promote improved patient outcomes and quality of life.

For each diet stage, patients should be encouraged to follow beneficial eating behaviors. When introducing beverages or liquids into the diet after surgery, the patient should be encouraged to sip slowly; to avoid use of a straw (which might increase air into the GI tract); and to avoid carbonation, sugar, caffeine, and/or alcohol. Concentrated sweets should be avoided in post-bariatric patients for several reasons: to reduce caloric intake, to avoid "empty calories," to avoid elevated blood glucose concentrations, and to avoid dumping syndrome among bypass patients whose pyloric sphincter had been removed during the surgical procedure. If the patient chooses to drink fruit juice, it should be diluted 50:50 with water to decrease the sugar content.

Patients should be encouraged to take small bites and thoroughly chew to "applesauce" consistency when solid food is introduced into the diet. Foods in general should be nutrient dense and low in saturated fat and sugar in order to optimize the nutritional adequacy and improve tolerance to solid food. Patients should be encouraged to eat slowly (planning on approximately 30 min per meal) and to avoid consuming liquids with solids. Some investigators recommend 8 oz of liquid over a 30–60 min period [3]. When patients reach advanced diet-progression stages, they should be advised to adhere to a balanced meal plan that consists of more than five servings of fruits and vegetables daily for optimal fiber consumption, colonic function, and phytochemical consumption [2].

Table 9.3 Suggested diet-progression stages following bariatric surgeries

Stage	Amount, frequency	Diet-stage duration	Examples
I: Clear liquid	1–2 oz every hour as tolerated	24–48 h (1–2 days)	Ice chips; water; broth; sugar-free gelatin; non-caffeinated, sugar-free herbal tea; diluted fruit juice; clear-liquid nutrition supplements
II: Full liquid	2 oz every hour as tolerated	10–14 days	Non-/low-fat milk and milk alternatives, non-/low-fat and sugar-free pudding, non-/low-fat creamed soups, full-liquid nutrition supplements
III: Blenderized/pureed	6 small meals per day consisting of 2–3 oz of pureed food	10–14 days	Strained, pureed, or blenderized foods low in fat and sugar; scramble eggs and egg substitute; pureed meats and meat alternatives (tofu, tempeh); flaked fish; lentils and beans; pureed fruits and vegetables; soft cheeses and hot cereal
IV: Soft	3–6 meals per day consisting of ½ to ¾ cup	4 weeks	Eggs, ground or chopped meats, meat alternatives, flaked fish, lentils and beans, canned fruit and vegetables in own juice, soft-cooked non-stringy vegetables, and well-tolerated cooked grains
V: Regular	3 meals per day consisting of 1–1/2 cups of food	For life	Foods of any texture and consistency. Patient should prioritize high-quality protein at each meal and choose foods low in saturated fat and concentrated sweets

Diet-Progression Recommendations

A protocol-derived staged-meal-progression, based on the type of surgical procedure, should be provided to the patient. *To date, there are no evidenced-based standards of practice for the type and duration of staged-meal-progression that should be implemented after surgery, and most bariatric centers have adopted their own recommendations.* Although there are no standards published regarding the diet progression after each type of surgery, examples of prudent, acceptable stage-progressions have been published [2, 3, 6, 13]. Furthermore, there are no standards adopted in the bariatric community for the length of time that an individual stays in a respective diet stage; however, the patient should advance diet as tolerated and when medically feasible. Aills et al. [13] reported results from an online survey conducted by the ASMBS of 68 dietitians (50 % of the RD membership) regarding texture and diet advancement of the postsurgical patient. Most respondents stated that multiple phases or stages were used as part of their program protocol. Most programs reported the following stages: clear-liquid (95 %), full-liquid (94 %), puree (77 %), and ground or soft diet (67 %). In addition, each progressive or advanced stage allowed the patient to consume foods and beverages encouraged from earlier or less advanced stages. Diet-stage suggestions are to be modified on an individualized basis to ensure the successful outcome of each bariatric patient. Table 9.3 offers a general diet-progression suggestion for the post-bariatric patient.

Stage I

The first stage (stage I) of the diet progression following weight loss surgery is to initiate a clear-liquid diet within 24 h and to continue this stage for 1–2 days. Initiation of ingestion of clear liquids for post-RYGB or BPD/DS patients should only occur after the patient has successfully passed a swallow study to rule out any surgical complications such as anastomotic leaks or strictures. This initial diet stage typically encourages the patient to consume approximately 30–60 milliliters (ml) (1–2 oz) of clear liquids every hour including ice chips and sips of non-carbonated, sugar-free, calorie-free, non-caffeinated beverages (e.g., water, herbal teas, clear-liquid nutrition supplements), sugar-free gelatin, broth, sugar-free popsicles. Available commercial nutrition supplements providing low calories, low-to-no sugar, and added protein approved for clear-liquid diets should also be encouraged. The purpose of stage I is to provide hydration to the patient, stimulate GI motility, and prevent a gastric ileus from occurring. Oftentimes, patients are discharged to home after only progressing to a clear-liquid diet. However, it may be beneficial for the patient to experiment with the second stage of the diet progression prior to discharge.

Stage II

The second stage (stage II) of the diet progression usually consists of a full-liquid diet. Full-liquid diets are considered nutritive (provides macronutrients and thus calories) and is usually initiated by postoperative day 3 [2]. The duration of the full-liquid diet is usually based on a patient's tolerance; however, some authors recommend that patients adhere to stage II for 10–14 days [13]. The goal of this diet stage is for the patient to work towards his or her specific protein goal per day, typically 60–90 g among LAGB patients or higher for BPD/DS patients [13]. During stage II, patients should consume a minimum of 48–64 fluid ounces of total fluids per day—consisting of ~24–32 oz of clear liquids (as described in the previous paragraph) plus 24–32 oz of any combination of full liquids. These would include high-quality protein sources such as 1 % or skim milk yogurt, nonfat milk, or milk alternatives (e.g., soymilk, almond milk, rice milk), vegetable juice, strained creamed soups, cream cereals, and low-fat or nonfat sugar-free puddings [3, 13]. The use of commercial protein supplements is also encouraged at this stage in order to facilitate the ability for patients to meet their protein intake goals. These include whey/casein, egg, and/or soy protein supplements with 100 % protein digestibility corrected amino acid score (PDCAAS) [13]. Stage II is also an optimal diet stage for post-LAGB patients who have undergone an adjustment or "fill" of their port. Patients post-"fill" should follow a full-liquid diet (emulate Stage II guidelines) for 2 days post-fill and then advance diet as tolerated to stage III or IV [2].

Stage III

The next suggested stage of the diet progression should consist of a blenderized/pureed diet and should be introduced to the patient once stage II is well tolerated. Stage III is generally encouraged for the duration of 10–14 days [13]. The foods most commonly recommended in the puree phase include scrambled eggs and egg substitute, pureed meat, flaked fish and meat alternatives (e.g., tofu, tempeh, textured vegetable protein [TVP]), cooked lentils and beans, pureed fruits and vegetables, soft cheeses (e.g., ricotta, cottage), and hot cereal and other easily digested complex carbohydrates (e.g., easily digested crackers and quinoa).

Stage IV

Stage IV consists of a soft diet, sometimes referred to as "mechanically soft diet," and is usually encouraged for more than 2 weeks in duration [13]. Nutrient dense, low-residue foods are recommended in this stage including eggs, ground or chopped soft meats, flaked fish and meat alternatives, canned fruits, soft fresh fruit, canned or well-cooked vegetables, cooked beans and lentils, hearty bean soups, soft cheeses, and grains as tolerated.

Other eating behaviors that may increase the tolerance and adherence to stage IV include keeping foods moist since oftentimes dry foods are not tolerated, especially those post-gastric banding, as some patients report food "getting stuck." Therefore, added fat-free gravy, bouillon, light mayonnaise, ricotta cheese, cottage cheese, and yogurt can help the patient's tolerance to soft foods, which may be more difficult to swallow. Furthermore, encouraging patients to avoid stringy vegetables and the tough outer peels of fruits can also increase the acceptance and tolerance of the stage III diet progression [13].

Stage V

Stage V is considered the regular bariatric diet stage, usually initiated after 8 weeks for the RYGB and after 6–8 weeks for AGB [13]; however, other practitioners recommend that patients reach stage V at the 3-month postsurgical follow-up visit [3]. This diet stage consists of healthy, balanced meals with calorie needs based on weight loss goals, height, weight, and age. Typically, patients can meet their estimated calorie and nutritional requirements with 1–1.5 cups of food three times daily; however, some may need to obtain 3–6 "mini-meals" depending upon the volume tolerance. Foods of any consistency may be tried carefully one at a time in order to evaluate tolerance and palatability. In stage IV, the dietitian can help the patient with meal planning and eating behaviors, discourage "grazing" or snacking, and educate the patient on how to obtain optimal nutrition from healthy meals.

Nutrition Assessment of Protein Malnutrition

Protein intake is of concern after bariatric surgery because decreased protein intake and/or intolerance of protein-containing foods and beverages exist, and the rearranged anatomy after many weight loss surgeries results in protein malabsorption [3]. Protein malnutrition is the most severe macronutrient complication following bariatric surgery; thus, regular monitoring and assessment of protein intake and status is very important [13]. Prevention of protein malnutrition requires regular assessment of protein intake and counseling regarding assessment of protein intake and counseling regarding ingestion of protein from protein-rich foods and modular protein supplements [6].

The RD should utilize all assessment domains including the biochemical domain (including laboratory assessment of visceral protein status), clinical (including functional status and anthropometrics), and behavioral/environmental (including limited adherence to postsurgical nutrition-related recommendations) in order to detect, treat, and monitor for protein malnutrition [8]. If parenteral nutrition support is required to maintain lean body mass and meet nutrition needs while allowing bowel rest, patients should be fed by utilizing permissive underfeeding nutrition support guidelines by the American Society of Parenteral and Enteral Nutrition (ASPEN) [19]. Parenteral nutrition should be considered in high-risk, critically ill patients unable to tolerate sufficient enteral nutrition for >5–7 days or non-critically ill patients unable to tolerate sufficient enteral nutrition for >7–10 days. Caution must be exercised when initiating nutrition support in the setting of severe malnutrition to avoid refeeding syndrome manifesting with signs and symptoms of volume overload, edema, hypokalemia, hypophosphatemia, and hypomagnesemia [6].

Protein intake, in general, among post-bariatric surgery patients have been recommended as 60–120 g per day [2, 6]. According to ASMBS Allied Health Nutritional Guidelines for the Surgical Weight Loss Patient, however, 60–90 g of protein is recommended for the post-RYGB patient and 90–120 g of protein is recommended for the post-BPD or BPD/DS patient [13]. It can be difficult for patients to meet their protein intake goals after surgery, especially during the early postoperative period. For each 4 oz serving of lean beef, approximately 30 g of high-quality protein can be consumed. However, due to the altered GI anatomy associated with most weight loss surgeries, patients may find consuming a 4 oz serving of beef an impossible task. Patients are encouraged to "work up" to their protein intake goals. Strategies to help patients obtain their protein goal include the addition of commercial protein supplements; small, frequent meals of thoroughly chewed high-quality protein food sources; and eating protein first at any meal. Although no studies have examined the most optimal protein intake to stimulate muscle protein synthesis (MPS) and other metabolic advantages [20] among bariatric patients, Symons et al. [21] demonstrated that the ingestion of more than 30 g of protein in a single meal does not further enhance MPS. Furthermore, Paddon-Jones et al. [22] showed that a dietary plan that includes 25–30 g of high-quality protein per meal, distributed evenly (no more than 5 h apart), had a greater effect on stimulating maximum MPS compared to an uneven distribution of higher grams of protein intake.

Vitamin and Mineral Supplementation

Nutrition assessment and follow-ups should include the evaluation of patient compliance to bariatric surgery nutrition guidelines and vitamin and mineral supplementation adherence. Nutritional labs are recommended to be drawn at regular intervals, such as presurgery and then at 3, 6, 9, and 12 months postsurgery; every 6 months in the second year postsurgery; and then annually [13]. Furthermore, baseline and diagnostic tests can be utilized to determine micro- and macronutrient deficiencies. For example, the use of Dual-Energy X-ray Absorptiometry (DEXA) scans can be a reliable measure of bone mineral density, recommended to be performed presurgery as well as every 2 years postsurgery [2].

Taking daily micronutrient supplements and eating foods high in vitamins and minerals are important aspects of any successful weight loss program. Patients are encouraged to begin supplementation as soon as possible and to continue supplementation for life. Guidelines for nutrition supplementation postsurgery have been published [12]. Routine supplementation after bariatric surgery includes one to two multivitamins daily inclusive of 400 μ(mu)g folic acid and 40–65 mg elemental iron (recommended for menstruating women), 1,200–2,000 mg/day of calcium citrate with added vitamin D (400–800 IU daily), and ≥350 μg vitamin B12 orally (or 1,000 μg per month intramuscularly or 3,000 μg every 6 months intramuscularly or 500 μg per week intranasally) [2]. Due to the risk of micronutrient deficiencies among BPD and BPD/DS patients, suggested prophylactic vitamin/mineral supplements are similar to other types of surgery patients with some exceptions: a fat-soluble vitamin inclusive of 5,000–10,000 IU vitamin A, 600–50,000 IU vitamin D supplement, 400 IU vitamin E, and 1 mg vitamin K.

Suboptimal Weight Loss and Weight Regain

Despite the significant weight loss and dramatic improvements in comorbidities associated with bariatric surgery, a minority of patients appear to experience suboptimal weight loss, either by not meeting their weight loss goals or by experiencing weight regain. Although weight loss surgery has been shown to be a durable treatment for obesity and obesity-related comorbidities [1], it can be expected that 20–25 % of the lost weight will be regained over a period of 10 years [6]. Although the reasons for this are not well understood, suboptimal weight loss and weight regain have been shown to be due to noncompliance with dietary and lifestyle recommendations, physiological factors, and surgical failure [6].

The long-term success of bariatric surgery relies on the patients' ability to make sustained lifestyle changes in the areas of nutrition and physical activity [3]. Suboptimal weight loss is often attributed to preoperative psychosocial characteristics and/or eating behaviors, as well as poor adherence to the recommended postoperative diet. Sarwer et al. [7] reported that baseline cognitive restraint and adherence to the recommended postoperative diet were associated with the percentage of weight loss after gastric bypass surgery. Patients often increase calorie intake after 1–2 years postsurgery and lack adherence with regular, planned, consistent exercise intervention, both contributing to suboptimal weight loss and/or weight regain [6].

Research has shown that up to 20 % of post-gastric bypass patients cannot sustain their weight loss beyond 2–3 years after surgery [23]. Again, although the mechanisms for this weight regain are unclear, weight regain-promoting consequences such as a failure to sustain elevated satiety gut hormones (glucagon-like peptide 1 [GLP-1] [6] and plasma PYY^{3-36} concentrations [23]) may be to blame. Other physiological factors contributing to weight regain after bariatric surgery include several adaptive intestinal mechanisms leading to changes in the absorptive capacity of the small bowel as well as other biologic drivers [6].

Prevention of weight regain is essential to maintain the benefits of bariatric surgery on a long-term basis [6]. Postoperatively, the nutrition professional can play a role in assisting the patient in obtaining and maintaining their weight loss goals as well as monitoring and evaluating the patient's nutritional status. Furthermore, the nutrition professional can help the patient troubleshoot dietary challenges and continue to offer support and education regarding post-surgical bariatric nutrition issues. Patients should also be advised to increase their physical activity and engage in aerobic and strength-training exercise to a minimum of 30 min a day as well as increase physical activity throughout the day as tolerated [2]. Moreover, weight loss appears to be improved by attendance of structured events and motivational forums such as support groups and face-to-face encounters with behavioralists and/or exercise specialists [15, 16]. The nutrition professional can help patients with their physical activity program and goals and refer patients to certified exercise specialists possessing knowledge and training of the bariatric patient.

Conclusion

Due to the continuing trend of obesity and utilization of bariatric surgery for the treatment of obesity, there will undoubtedly be a growing role for the registered dietitian [5]. Both presurgical and postsurgical nutrition assessments are mandatory in order to improve patient outcomes, primarily by assisting patients to meet their weight loss goals while preventing complications such as nutrient deficiencies [3, 6]. The role of nutrition education and medical nutrition therapy in bariatric surgery will continue to grow as tools to enhance surgical outcomes and long-term weight loss maintenance are further identified [13]. By using a systematic nutrition care process and critical thinking skills unique to the registered dietitian and other expert multidisciplinary care providers, the bariatric patient can experience successful patient outcomes.

Question and Answer Section

Questions

1. What component of the nutrition care process is used by practitioners to obtain, verify, and interpret data needed to identify nutrition-related problems, their causes, and significance?
   A. Nutrition diagnosis
   B. Nutrition counseling
   C. Nutrition education
   D. Nutrition assessment
2. Your patient is consuming a full-liquid diet (stage II in the diet-progression stage) after undergoing a Roux-en Y gastric bypass 10 days ago. However, she states that she is only having one "meal" per day because she found a protein supplement providing 60 g protein per serving. You advice that based on the literature, there are metabolic advantages from ingesting___ to ____ grams of protein distributed at least three times throughout the day including maximum stimulation of muscle protein synthesis.
3. Common food intolerances of the bariatric patient include meat, bread, rice, pasta, milk, and _____.
   A. Fruit
   B. Carbonated beverages
   C. Beans
   D. Tofu

Answers

1. Answer: **D**. Nutrition assessment. The purpose of the nutrition assessment is to obtain, verify, and interpret data needed to identify nutrition-related problems, their causes, and significance. Nutrition assessment is an ongoing, nonlinear, dynamic process that involves initial data gathering from five categories: patient medical/surgical, social, health and family history, food/nutrition-related history, anthropometrics, biochemical data/medical tests and procedures, and nutrition-focused physical findings. Continual reassessment and analysis of the patient's status compared to specified criteria is recommended for improved patient outcomes.
2. Answer: 25–30 g.
3. Answer: **B**. Common food intolerances include meat, bread, rice, pasta, milk and carbonated beverages.

References

1. Delling L, Karason K, Olbers T, Sjostrom D, Wahlstrand B, Carlsson B, et al. Feasibility of bariatric surgery as a strategy for secondary prevention in cardiovascular disease: a report from the Swedish obese subjects trial. J Obes. 2010;2010. pii: 102341. doi:10.1155/2010/102341. Epub 2010/09/18.
2. Mechanick JI, Kushner RF, Sugerman HJ, Gonzalez-Campoy JM, Collazo-Clavell ML, Spitz AF, et al. American Association of Clinical Endocrinologists, The Obesity Society, and American Society for Metabolic and Bariatric Surgery medical guidelines for clinical practice for the perioperative nutritional, metabolic, and nonsurgical support of the bariatric surgery patient. Obesity (Silver Spring). 2009;17 Suppl 1:S1–70, v.
3. McMahon MM, Sarr MG, Clark MM, Gall MM, Knoetgen 3rd J, Service FJ, et al. Clinical management after bariatric surgery: value of a multidisciplinary approach. Mayo Clin Proc. 2006;81(10 Suppl):S34–45. Epub 2006/10/14.
4. Kushner RF, Neff LM. Bariatric surgery: a key role for registered dietitians. J Am Diet Assoc. 2010;110(4):524–6.

5. Kulick D, Hark L, Deen D. The bariatric surgery patient: a growing role for registered dietitians. J Am Diet Assoc. 2010;110(4):593–9.
6. Heber D, Greenway FL, Kaplan LM, Livingston E, Salvador J, Still C, et al. Endocrine and nutritional management of the post-bariatric surgery patient: an Endocrine Society Clinical Practice Guideline. J Clin Endocrinol Metab. 2010;95(11):4823–43. Epub 2010/11/06.
7. Sarwer DB, Wadden TA, Moore RH, Baker AW, Gibbons LM, Raper SE, et al. Preoperative eating behavior, postoperative dietary adherence, and weight loss after gastric bypass surgery. Surg Obes Relat Dis. 2008;4(5):640–6. Epub 2008/07/01.
8. [No authors listed]. International Dietetic & Nutrition Terminology [IDNT] reference manual. 3rd ed. Chicago: American Dietetic Association; 2011, 4th edition (August, 2012).
9. Dalle Grave R, Calugi S, Centis E, Marzocchi R, Ghoch ME, Marchesini G. Lifestyle modification in the management of the metabolic syndrome: achievements and challenges. Diabetes Metab Syndr Obes. 2010;3:373–85. Epub 2010/01/01.
10. NIH Conference. Gastrointestinal surgery for severe obesity. Consensus Development Conference Panel. Ann Intern Med. 1991;115(12):956–61.
11. U.S. Food and Drug Administration. FDA expands use of banding system for weight loss. Available at: http://www.fda.gov/NewsEvents/Newsroom/PressAnnouncements/ucm245617.htm.
12. Mechanick, et al. AACE/TOS/ASMBS Bariatric Surgery Clinical Practice Guidelines. SOARD 2013;9:159–191.
13. Aills L, Blankenship J, Buffington C, Furtado M, Parrott J. ASMBS Allied Health Nutritional Guidelines for the surgical weight loss patient. Surg Obes Relat Dis. 2008;4(5 Suppl):S73–108.
14. Shankar P, Boylan M, Sriram K. Micronutrient deficiencies after bariatric surgery. Nutrition. 2010;26(11–12):1031–7.
15. Shen R, Dugay G, Rajaram K, Cabrera I, Siegel N, Ren CJ. Impact of patient follow-up on weight loss after bariatric surgery. Obes Surg. 2004;14(4):514–9. Epub 2004/05/08.
16. Harper J, Madan AK, Ternovits CA, Tichansky DS. What happens to patients who do not follow-up after bariatric surgery? Am Surg. 2007;73(2):181–4. Epub 2007/02/20.
17. Flancbaum L, Belsley S, Drake V, Colarusso T, Tayler E. Preoperative nutritional status of patients undergoing Roux-en-Y gastric bypass for morbid obesity. J Gastrointest Surg. 2006;10(7):1033–7. Epub 2006/07/18.
18. Frank P, Crookes PF. Short- and long-term surgical follow-up of the postbariatric surgery patient. Gastroenterol Clin North Am. 2010;39(1):135–46. Epub 2010/03/06.
19. McClave SA, Martindale RG, Vanek VW, McCarthy M, Roberts P, Taylor B, et al. Guidelines for the provision and assessment of nutrition support Therapy in the adult critically Ill patient: Society of Critical Care Medicine (SCCM) and American Society for Parenteral and Enteral Nutrition (A.S.P.E.N.). JPEN J Parenter Enteral Nutr. 2009;33(3):277–316.
20. Westerterp-Platenga MS, Nieuwenhuizen A, Tomé D, Soenen S, Westerterp KR. Dietary protein, weight loss, and weight maintenance. Annu Rev Nutr. 2009;29:21–41.
21. Symons TB, Sheffield-Moore M, Wolfe RR, Paddon-Jones D. A moderate serving of high-quality protein maximally stimulates skeletal muscle protein synthesis in young and elderly subjects. J Am Diet Assoc. 2009;109(9):1582–6. Epub 2009/08/25.
22. Paddon-Jones D, Rasmussen BB. Dietary protein recommendations and the prevention of sarcopenia. Curr Opin Clin Nutr Metab Care. 2009;12(1):86–90. Epub 2008/12/06.
23. Meguid MM, Glade MJ, Middleton FA. Weight regain after Roux-en-Y: a significant 20% complication related to PYY. Nutrition. 2008;24(9):832–42. Epub 2008/08/30.

Nutrition Education and Counseling of the Bariatric Surgery Patient

Toni Piechota

Chapter Objectives

1. To identify the nutritional and dietary educational needs of the weight loss surgery population both presurgery and postsurgery
2. To identify key factors that affect patient learning
3. To identify key counseling strategies for the weight loss surgery population
4. To describe the application of the Nutrition Care Process to weight loss surgery nutrition education and counseling

Introduction

The success of weight loss maintenance following bariatric surgery has exceeded that of conventional and pharmaceutical treatments. A meta-analysis by Buchwald et al. [1] reported that the mean weight loss as a percentage of excess body weight (EBW) was 61.2 % for all surgery patients (47.5 % for patients who underwent gastric banding; 61.6 %, gastric bypass; and 70.1 %, biliopancreatic diversion or duodenal). However, there is considerable variability in degree of weight loss, and weight regain can be substantial in some patients. Magro et al. [2] reported that a mean weight regain of 8 % of lost weight occurred within 60 months following surgery and that up to 18.8 % of patients lost less than 50 % of their EBW. The cause of this weight regain is typically attributed to either failure to incorporate adequate lifestyle changes to maintain the weight loss or relapse into prior behaviors favoring weight gain as the body adapts to surgery-induced anatomical changes that caused early satiety and restricted food intake, malabsorption, and food intolerances. In an effort to optimize patient safety and outcomes, the American Society of Metabolic and Bariatric Surgery (ASMBS) The American Association of Clinical Endocrinologists, and The Obesity Society have published clinical practice guidelines which include updated recommendations for adequate nutrition and exercise guidelines [3], which updates the 2008 nutrition guidelines [4]. Beyond merely providing information, however, it is incumbent upon the educator to provide education and counseling in a manner that is effective. In this chapter, an overview of the diet and nutritional information needs of the bariatric surgery patient before and after surgery will be reviewed, as will various principles and strategies of education and counseling that may enhance effectiveness of interventions. Finally, the application of the Nutrition Care Process as it applies to education and counseling in this context is discussed.

Educational and Counseling Needs

Although it is generally accepted that gastric bypass, vertical sleeve gastrectomy, and biliopancreatic diversion with or without duodenal switch influence weight loss by mechanisms other than simply restricting gastric capacity (e.g., by reducing levels of ghrelin and increasing levels of PYY and GLP-1), weight loss surgery is also referred to by some as "forced behavior modification." Anatomical changes associated with bariatric surgery, such as the loss of the pylorus following gastric bypass or significantly decreased intestinal capacity following biliopancreatic diversion, necessitate dietary changes that, if not made, cause discomfort, thereby discouraging the causative behaviors. Anticipatory guidance on the necessary changes associated with weight loss surgeries and counseling to assist patients in the implementation of these changes are the responsibilities of the bariatric surgery team. Education and counseling on issues pertaining to all aspects of diet, nutrition, and lifestyle are the responsibility of the registered dietitian (RD) and should be provided by a qualified registered dietitian familiar with the bariatric surgery procedures and specific needs of this patient population.

T. Piechota, MS, MPH, RD (✉)
Department of Food and Nutrition, University of California, Davis, 2315 Stockton Blvd, Sacramento, CA 95817, USA
e-mail: tpiechota@hotmail.com

However, optimal education and counseling occurs when a multidisciplinary team communicates findings and shares expertise to reinforce and optimize conveyance of accurate health messages in a manner best suited to each individual. The registered dietitian, in identifying patient needs and optimal counseling strategies, must work closely with other healthcare providers, including the bariatric surgeon, nursing staff, psychologist, physical therapist, and other practitioners.

Lifestyle changes that are required for safe and effective outcomes will vary according to (1) surgical procedure, (2) individual patient needs, and (3) stage in the surgical process. Topics to be covered range from guidance on weight management and preoperative weight loss to nutritional supplementation and weight regain. The emphasis and guidelines will change as the patient progresses through the process, and education should be adapted accordingly. For convenience, educational needs can be divided into three stages including preoperative education, short-term postoperative education (immediately following surgery to approximately 1 year postoperatively), and long-term postoperative education.

Preoperative Nutrition Education and Counseling

Prior to surgery, patients should receive education on the following topics:
- Principles of weight management and individual guidance on preoperative weight loss and glycemic control as indicated
- Realistic weight loss expectations following surgery
- Postoperative diet stages and allowed foods
- Sources of high-quality liquid protein
- Hydration goals
- Vitamin and mineral supplement needs and suggested schedules
- Timing and composition of meals
- Eating behaviors such as rate of ingestion and awareness of altered experiences of hunger and satiety

Patients may be encouraged to practice some of these behavior changes prior to surgery and should prepare for the postsurgical period by having purchased allowed foods, protein supplements, vitamin and mineral supplements, and other tools that may facilitate the process after surgery.

Preoperative Weight Loss

Preoperative weight loss may be indicated before weight loss surgery as a means of improving surgical outcomes [5]. One of the requirements set in the 1991 National Institutes of Health (NIH) consensus statement on weight loss surgery is that qualified candidates for bariatric surgery will have tried and failed at weight loss [6]. However, it should not be assumed that patients have had guidance by a qualified individual on nutrition or behavior change. Many patients who present for weight loss surgery lack even basic knowledge of weight loss principles. The dietitian serves an important role in educating surgical candidates on accurate principles of weight management, facilitating skill development, and increasing patient awareness of their own behaviors. This is necessary both for preoperative weight management and to encourage behaviors that will prevent early plateau and weight regain. In addition, the dietitian can offer specific guidance for individual weight loss strategies such as appropriate use of meal replacements supplements or structured meal plans.

Realistic Weight Loss with Weight Loss Surgery

It is important that patients be educated prior to surgery on average and realistic weight loss with the surgical procedure they will be having. It has been found that bariatric surgery candidates often overestimate the amount of weight they will lose with surgery as well as the degree to which bariatric surgery will affect their eating behaviors [7]. Because unrealistic weight loss expectations have been linked to poor outcome in conventional weight loss patients [8] and in the spirit of having a well-informed patient, average weight loss achieved with their surgical procedure should be discussed as well as factors that positively and negatively impact those averages.

Diet Stages

Following bariatric surgery, patients typically progress through five diet stages of advancing texture as follows:
1. Low-sugar clear liquid
2. Low-sugar full liquid
3. Mechanical soft
4. Soft and low sugar
5. Low-fat regular

At present there are no specific guidelines recommending specific duration of stages, and diet advancement should be individualized. Patients should, however, be provided with an overview of dietary guidelines and appropriate foods to include a shopping list, suggested meal plans, and recipes that will be texturally appropriate while providing adequate protein.

Hydration

Early after surgery, patients should aim for > 1.5 L of fluid daily, increasing as tolerated from an initial goal of 48 ounces daily. Patients should be instructed to proceed gradually, slowly increasing their rate of sipping to prevent vomiting. The slow rate of drinking requires sipping liquids throughout the day in order to prevent dehydration. Sippy cups, 1 oz (30 ml) medicine cups, sugar-free popsicles, kitchen timers, and fluid tracking sheets are tools that may help the patient adhere to these guidelines.

Protein

Protein needs following weight loss surgery are estimated at 1.0–1.5 g/kg ideal body weight. Patients should be instructed on this goal and how to meet this goal. Food sources of protein are typically inadequate to meet patient needs and supplemental protein drinks are indicated during the early postoperative period. The array of protein powders and drinks can be overwhelming and patients should receive specific guidance on high-quality protein supplements that are adequate to meet their protein needs within their volume restrictions. Low-sugar supplements made from appropriate protein sources such as soy protein isolate and whey protein isolate are advised. However, patients may benefit from specific brand names and products as marketing claims and scientific jargon on labels can confuse and overwhelm patients.

Eating Behaviors

Patients should be educated on the role of the stomach, the pyloric sphincter, and the small intestine on digestion as appropriate. Implications of these changes are that the patient must be diligent about chewing food thoroughly, eating and drinking slowly, separating liquids from solids by 30 min, be alert to altered sensations of hunger and satiety, limit portion size, avoid snacking, emphasize eating protein first to ensure adequate intake, and avoid tough, stringy and doughy foods. Failure to comply with these behaviors may result in dumping syndrome, vomiting, plugging, weight regain, malnutrition, and possibly more serious complications.

Short-Term Postoperative

Although patients have been exposed to information about suggested behaviors and complications prior to surgery, the volume of information can be overwhelming and requires review at follow-up. Additionally, information that may have been dismissed as irrelevant before surgery often becomes more meaningful as patients encounter various situations. Nutrition and diet-related issues encountered in the early postoperative stages provide an opportunity to teach patients problem-solving skills as you work with them to identify causes and solutions. Some common problems encountered during this period include nausea and vomiting, dehydration, difficulty ingesting adequate protein, dumping syndrome, inappropriate vitamin and mineral supplementation, and diarrhea and constipation.

Addressing Common Concerns

- Nausea and vomiting: Advise to sip fluids slowly throughout the day, ensure adequate hydration, drink protein drinks on ice, hydrate with sugar-free popsicles, or try warm herbal tea and ginger, and avoid strong smells. If symptoms do not respond, consult with medical providers regarding indications for medication or possible anatomical complications if severe.
- Dehydration: Review signs and symptoms of dehydration. Early dehydration can cause nausea, which makes it harder to continue drinking. Reinforce fluid goals and sources. Consult with medical providers regarding the need for intravenous rehydration.
- Inadequate protein intake: Obtain a diet recall or review patient tracking sheets. Review their individual goals, and review their protein sources for adequacy and quality of protein. Query patients on food sources of protein and their individual needs to reinforce information, and remind them of consequences of inadequate protein intake.
- Dumping syndrome: Review symptoms and causes of dumping syndrome. Simple sugars including honey, dehydrated cane juice, fructose, and other sugar additives can cause dumping even in small amounts. Additionally, drinking too soon after a meal, eating greasy foods, and drinking alcohol can cause dumping. Review reported symptoms, diet recall, and hidden sources with patients.
- Vitamin and mineral supplements: The follow-up appointment is an opportunity to assess and reeducate on the need for lifelong supplementation and to problem-solve solutions for non-adherence.
- Diarrhea: Rule out lactose intolerance, which may manifest after bariatric surgery; rule out dumping syndrome or inappropriate intake of simple carbohydrates, and if persistent and unresolved with simple dietary changes, coordinate with medical provider to rule out gastrointestinal infection. Probiotics can sometimes help.
- Constipation: Provide instruction on lifestyle factors that prevent constipation including adequate fluid intake, daily physical activity, and fiber intake. Fiber intake may be limited early on due to emphasis on protein foods and limited gastric capacity. Soluble fibers may help.

Short-term postoperative complications typically resolve within a few months. The following few months provide an opportunity to coach patients on healthy diet selection, meal patterns, and exercise goals. As a patient moves beyond the first year, other issues begin to emerge.

Long-Term Postoperative

Concerns encountered after the first year include weight plateaus and even weight regain, non-adherence to nutrient supplements, dumping syndrome, maladaptive eating patterns and unhealthy food choices, and others.

Early Plateau and Weight Regain

Early plateau refers to a cessation of weight loss before optimal weight loss is achieved. When this occurs, assess the duration of the stall and rule out a shift in body composition.

Body composition assessments can be useful if obtained at different points throughout the postoperative period. These patients need reassurance that they are on the right track and that this is typically a temporary stall. On the other hand, when obtaining information about dietary intake, probing is required to assess frequency of eating, liquid calories, deviations from reported "typical" intake, and frequency, duration, and intensity of physical activity. Nutritional adequacy should also be assessed. Patients should be advised to limit the number of snacks and calorie-dense foods and on diet quality and exercise.

Noncompliance with Vitamin and Mineral Supplementation and Nutrient Deficiencies

At each follow-up appointment, adequacy of supplement intake should be assessed and reviewed as indicated. Brands, quantity, frequency of compliance, as well as barriers and solutions should be discussed. Forgetting supplements and lack of perceived importance of ongoing supplementation are frequent barriers that the dietitian can assist with using education and counseling strategies.

Dumping Syndrome

Although many patients are familiar with the distinct symptoms of early-onset dumping syndrome, the less-specific symptoms of delayed dumping syndrome are often overlooked. Educate patients based on symptoms about causes of delayed dumping syndrome, which include ingestion of simple sugar, greasy foods, alcohol, and fluid with meals as well as excessive intake of refined carbohydrates with inadequate protein intake. Also review symptoms of delayed dumping syndrome, which may present as fatigue, shakiness, irritability, and even syncope about 2–3 h after ingestion.

Maladaptive Eating

Eating behaviors that are counterproductive, unhealthy, or lead patients away from their goals are considered maladaptive. Examples include grazing, emotional eating, mindless eating, and eating disorders:
- Grazing: The term grazing refers to a pattern of frequent snacking throughout the day and has been identified as a significant factor in weight regain following bariatric surgery [9]. As diet recall and food records are reviewed, assess frequency of intake, and when greater than 3–6 eating episodes a day, remind patients of the need to plan meals and snacks regularly with protein and complex carbohydrates. Cognitive behavioral principles including self-monitoring, contingency planning, and stimulus control can be helpful.
- Emotional eating: The learned behavior of eating in response to emotions is generally interrupted to some extent by anatomical changes early after surgery, but the inclination to turn to food for comfort remains. Failure to adopt alternative coping strategies can lead to a pattern of grazing and weight regain or to alternative destructive coping strategies, such as drinking alcohol. Self-monitoring of eating behaviors and thoughts and development of alternative coping strategies can help. Psychological intervention may be indicated.
- Mindless eating: Patterns of eating at a desk, in the car, or while watching television can lead to excessive calorie intake. Snack foods tend to be calorie dense, and foods such as crackers and chips pass through the gastric pouch easily allowing for high-volume intake. The result is weight regain and unhealthy diet patterns that can reverse some of the health benefits gained by weight loss surgery. Self-monitoring, contingency planning, and stimulus control can be helpful.
- Eating disorders: Eating disorders can present in several ways and may be different than in patients who have not had bariatric surgery. Anorexia nervosa can be overlooked as patients may demonstrate excessive weight loss while complaining of an inability to eat adequate amounts to sustain weight or inability to eat due to abdominal pain. Bulimia can present as excessive exercise, vomiting for calorie control (which may be attributed by the patient to nausea or plugging), or laxative abuse. Binge eating will more often appear as grazing. Other manifestations may include severely limiting diet choices or preoccupation with food or weight. Persistent inability to eat adequate amounts to maintain a desirable weight should be discussed with the medical team. If an eating disorder is suspected, a psychological consultation is indicated. Nutrition support may also be indicated.

Unhealthy Eating Habits

A pattern of limiting calories to maintain weight loss without regard to diet quality can result in diet-related chronic diseases in addition to eventual weight regain as tolerance for unhealthy foods increases. Patients may also develop malnutrition when diet quality is compromised. Although there may be some food intolerances and volumes of food may be limited, a healthy diet following bariatric surgery is a balanced diet containing low-fat and low-sugar unrefined foods from all food groups.

Inactivity

Regular exercise and physical activity has been shown to correlate with amount of weight loss and increased likelihood of maintaining that loss [10]. Patients who had adopted regular exercise may, for various reasons, become inconsistent or stop exercising altogether. Education on the role of exercise in long-term weight management and overall help should be reviewed as should strategies for adopting exercise such as realistic goal setting and self-monitoring. Problem-solving solutions to barriers can also help.

Although general guidance on all of the above should be reviewed prior to surgery, it must also be reiterated at follow-up appointments as indicted by diet recall and laboratory results. Because of the nature of weight loss surgery as a tool in weight management and as a life-altering intervention that has the potential long-term to cause complications such as ulcers and nutrient deficiencies and because maintenance of desired weight loss and health will hinge on conscious behaviors, lifelong education may be necessary.

Components, Theories, and Approaches to Education and Counseling

Beyond the responsibility to provide patients with information, the goal of optimal patient outcomes requires that approaches be effective so patients can understand and apply recommendations to daily life. Both education and counseling are essential components of effective interventions. Education is the imparting of information but the goal is behavior change. The Academy of Nutrition and Dietetics (formerly the American Dietetic Association) distinguishes between education and counseling as follows:

> Nutrition education is defined as "a formal process to instruct or train a patient or client in a skill or to impart knowledge to help [them] voluntarily manage or modify food choices and eating behavior to maintain or improve health." Nutrition counseling is defined as "a supportive process, characterized by a collaborative counselor-patient relationship, to set priorities, establish goals, and create individualized action plans that acknowledge and foster responsibility for self-care to treat an existing condition or promote health." [11]

As two distinct processes, education and counseling require different practitioner skills. Knowledge of learning and counseling theories helps the practitioner to develop and adapt more effective interventions for a heterogeneous audience. Dietetics practitioners working with bariatric surgery patients require strong skills in both categories of intervention to effectively assist the patients in understanding and applying recommended lifestyle changes associated with bariatric surgery and healthy, lifelong weight management.

The most common educational and counseling theories used in the healthcare setting have some common threads, but each offers additional and unique focus. Although little research has been conducted to demonstrate the superiority or effectiveness of any one educational strategy or behavior change theory or model to bariatric surgery patients, it is reasonable to assume that the counseling theories and strategies that have been successfully applied to health behavior change for other health behaviors also apply to the bariatric surgery population. Components of effective education and counseling theories and models as applied to health behaviors, including those behaviors required for successful bariatric surgery, will be discussed.

Education Components

Prior to intervention, certain patient characteristics and barriers to learning should be considered. These include assessment of patient learning needs (including correction of misconceptions), readiness to learn, preferred learning styles, literacy and numeracy, cognitive capacity, language and cultural factors, and visual and hearing impairment. These are discussed below.

Assessment of Learning Needs

Patient knowledge can be assessed formally through quizzes or questionnaires or informally through queries during face-to-face interactions. Appropriate questions may include "What do you know about weight loss surgery?" or "What do you feel you need to know to be healthy after surgery?" Oral and written assignments can be useful for assessing knowledge base and ability to apply that information. Posttests and questions regarding information provided during instruction allow for assessment of patient understanding and need for further education.

Readiness to Learn

One theory of adult learning states that adults will more readily learn, retain, and apply information they perceive to be important [12]. Information and skills that the patient identifies as valuable and important to learn constitute their perceived learning needs. Patient responses (both verbal and nonverbal) can also allow for assessment of patients' readiness to learn. Questions can include "How do you see yourself applying this information?" When patients do not think the information is important, the educator can identify scenarios in which that knowledge may be useful or research addressing the benefits of a suggested behavior.

Preferred Learning Styles

Learning styles should be considered when developing an educational plan. Three learning styles include auditory, visual, and kinetic. Auditory learners benefit from hearing information and from discussions. Visual learners benefit from having information written and by viewing charts, graphs, pictures, and labels. Kinetic learners learn best by applying information or through active participation in the learning process. They may benefit from role-playing and hands-on experiences such as doing a goal-setting exercise or comparing supplement labels. In teaching a group class or leading a support group, incorporate a variety of teaching strategies to accommodate a variety of learning styles. Handouts, worksheets, discussion, workshops, and lectures can be used.

Literacy, Numeracy, and Cognitive Capacity

Patients may not admit to having difficulty reading or with numbers. Indicators of illiteracy include incomplete forms, frustration, medication non-adherence, or statements such as

"I will go over this when I get home." This may require adapting information to accommodate for deficits, e.g. having pictures or food models and demonstrating behaviors. Written materials should be written at or below the sixth grade level and should include pictures, bullet points, and large easily readable font. Avoid medical jargon and identify a few key messages.

Language and Cultural Factors

Practitioners should be sensitive to cultural issues relevant to diet and nutrition as well as social issues that may affect self-care. Examples include having information available on halal, kosher, or vegetarian supplements and having culturally adapted meal plans. Written materials should be available in the languages when feasible.

Counseling

Various counseling theories have been studied and applied to health-related behaviors such as medication compliance, weight management, healthy eating, and exercise. Some theories and strategies include the health belief model, social learning theory, transtheoretical model, cognitive behavioral therapy, and motivational interviewing.

Health Belief Model

The health belief model is a health behavior theory that attempts to identify those significant variables that affect an individual's decision to engage in health-related behaviors [13]. The model proposes four constructs that impact health behaviors:
1. Perceived susceptibility to a health threat or condition (e.g., possibility or developing osteoporosis)
2. Perceived benefit of a health-altering action (e.g., taking calcium supplements will prevent osteoporosis)
3. Perceived severity of the health threat or condition (e.g., the possibility that a nutrient deficiency could result in immobilization)
4. Perceived barriers or the costs (psychological, social, monetary, and other) to the individual (e.g., the money spent on supplements)

Two additional concepts, self-efficacy and cues to action, are also incorporated into other health behavior models/theories. Self-efficacy refers to an individual's confidence in their ability to comply with a given behavior. Cues to action are those prompts that stimulate an individual to change behavior, such as listening to another bariatric surgery patient in support group discuss their weight regain. While engaging in patient education and counseling, the provider should be mindful of these factors and in communicating the hows and whys of behavior change as they pertain to each patient as well as probing to identify perceived obstacles and solutions and to facilitate improved self-efficacy. This model can serve to prompt healthcare providers to facilitate the individual to explore their personal health concerns.

Social Learning Theory

Social learning theory was introduced in the 1970s by Albert Bandura [13]. It emphasizes the role of external factors, such as social interactions and media, and internal thoughts on behavior. As with the Health Behavior Model, the decision to act is somewhat determined by value placed on the expected outcome and the likelihood of achieving the desired results by taking the action. Reinforcement of information is important, and reinforcement can be achieved through direct information, observation of others, or self-management. Self-efficacy to conduct a behavior and achieve an outcome is an important component of this theory. Self-efficacy is thought to be increased by observing others, achieving mastery of the behavior, and obtaining information on how to behave in situations.

Transtheoretical Model of Change

The transtheoretical model of change states that change is a process and that people go through a series of predictable stages of readiness to change. Although it can be assumed that most patients who seek weight loss surgery are motivated to lose weight, it does not follow that they are motivated to *make changes*. Even when patients are ready to change certain behaviors, they may not be ready to change all behaviors. Interventions should be based on where the patient is in the process of change. The five stages of change are identified as precontemplative, contemplative, preparation, action, and maintenance. Relapse into old behaviors is considered as moving to an earlier stage of readiness. Clinician interventions have been shown to be more effective if the intervention is adjusted based on the patient's state of readiness (Table 10.1) [14].

Cognitive Behavior Therapy

Behavioral therapy has been applied to weight loss and weight loss management with some success since the 1960s and is endorsed by the NIH guidelines on overweight and obesity as an effective strategy in facilitating weight loss [15]. Cognitive behavioral therapy (CBT) as applied to weight management is based on the theory that behaviors are learned and that positive behaviors can be learned to replace destructive behaviors and that addressing destructive thought patterns is part of the change. Adherence to behaviors can be triggered by either internal or external cues. As a result, CBT aims to promote behavior change by increasing awareness of current thought and behavior patterns related to the desired change and utilize various strategies employed in behavior modification [16].

Table 10.1 Stage-appropriate intervention approaches based on the transtheoretical model of behavior change

Stage-appropriate intervention approaches	
Stage of change	Intervention strategies
Precontemplative:	
The patient has no intention to change. He may be in the appointment to fulfill a requirement or may reject certain behavioral recommendations as impertinent	Consciousness raising; education; provide feedback on lab results, weight change
Contemplative:	
The patient acknowledged a problem or potential issue and is thinking about changing	Focus on problem recognition and advantages of change; coach patient in weighing the pros and cons of change
Preparation for action:	
The patient recognizes a problem or potential problem and intends to change behavior within the next month	Offer support, reinforce behavior changes
Action:	
The individual has been engaging in the behavior consistently for 6 months	Reinforce behavior changes, provide support, prepare for high-risk situations (e.g., through visualizations or scenarios), and assist in identifying alternative behaviors
Maintenance:	
The individual has been engaging in the behaviors for 6 months	Continue to support and reinforce changes; contingency planning

Principles of cognitive behavioral therapy can be applied to facilitate any behavior change, including taking supplements, incorporating exercise, and improving dietary compliance. Components of cognitive behavior therapy include goal setting, self-monitoring, problem solving, social support, stress management, cognitive restructuring, relapse prevention, rewards and contingency management, and stimulus control (see Table 10.2).

Motivational Interviewing

One counseling strategy that has received a lot of attention in promoting lifestyle change is motivational interviewing [17]. Motivational interviewing is patient-centered counseling designed to elicit behavior change by helping patients to explore their ambivalence to change and resolve conflicts between where they are and where they want to be. It views the caregiver as a partner in change rather than as an authoritative figure. Some key principles of motivational interviewing are that change is an "inside job" and not something that can be imposed from an outside force; patients must identify and resolve their ambivalence ("If I exercise, I will miss happy hour after work"); the provider does not persuade the patients to change but rather assists in the exploration of sources of ambivalence; and readiness to change is not a fixed state but that it ebbs and flows. The provider should:

- Exhibit empathy for the patient. Try to understand the patient's frame of reference and why they do what they do. This facilitates an important component of behavior change: the therapeutic alliance. Recognize that sometimes the overt behavior is a coping mechanism. An angry reaction or underreporting on food records may be a way of maintaining self-dignity, for example. Empathy helps to get past this.
- Allow the patient to explore and express their motivation to change and their ability to do so. Motivation comes from the difference between where a patient is and where they want to be.
- Acknowledge the patient's autonomy to change or not change and avoid power struggles.
- Support their self-efficacy by focusing on previous successes and identifying their skills regarding diet and exercise or as demonstrated in other areas of their life.

The aforementioned counseling theories and strategies have been incorporated into the language of the Nutrition Care Process and are accepted educational and counseling interventions. The Nutrition Care Process Model and its application to the bariatric surgery population are discussed.

Integrating Education and Counseling with the Nutrition Care Process

The Nutrition Care Process (NCP), developed by the Academy of Nutrition and Dietetics (formerly the American Dietetic Association), is a model for providing nutrition care that promotes improved consistency of quality care and allows for data collection. In addition, standardized terminology including codes has been developed for use with the NCP and is published elsewhere [11]. The NCP divides nutrition care into four distinct steps: assessment, diagnosis, intervention, and monitoring and evaluation. Within each step are specific domains for identifying, prioritizing, and addressing patient nutrition needs and developing and assessing the nutrition care plan. Each step is discussed below (see Table 10.3).

Table 10.2 The application of cognitive behavioral therapy to bariatric surgery patients

Cognitive behavioral therapy for bariatric surgery patients		
Cognitive behavioral therapy strategy	Rationale	Example
Goal setting • Specific • Measurable • Attainable, agreed upon • Realistic, rewarding, relevant • Timely	Setting specific goals increases the likelihood of behavior change	Walk for 1 mile over 20 min for 3 days next week
Self-monitoring	Increases awareness of behaviors and used to identify behaviors that detract from goals	Tracking intake of food, thoughts, feelings, and exercise
Problem solving	Self-correcting problematic behaviors	Working with patient to identify a barrier to a goal-related behavior and developing solutions
Social support	Patients who perceive that they have more social support are more likely to achieve goals	Attend support group; foster relationships with significant others
Stress management	Adoption of stress-reduction techniques and alterations in cognitions provide alternatives to eating in response to stress	Investigating stressors and developing alternative thoughts; breathing exercises
Cognitive restructuring	Cognitions are thought to be important in determining behavior. This can be thought of in the context of the role of self-efficacy in behavior change	Identify destructive thoughts and develop realistic viewpoints: "I've blown it. I'm a failure." Change to "I ate 500 cal above my goal. In the long run, occasional splurges aren't a big deal as long as I get back to my plan"
Relapse prevention	Identify events, situations, and circumstances that may result in a return to old behavior and develop alternatives	In anticipation of holidays during which one typically overeats, develop plans to have low-calorie foods available and to incorporate exercise on busy days
Rewards/contingency management	Tangible rewards enhance behavior changes, particularly when consequences of the behavior are delayed	Buy a new outfit after completing 4 weeks of daily self-monitoring
Stimulus control	Removes cues that trigger undesirable behaviors and places cue that trigger positive behaviors	Keep vitamin supplements in a place to cue intake Shop from a list

Assessment

During the nutrition assessment, the dietitian collects data about the patient in five different categories: client history; food- and nutrition-related history; anthropometrics; biochemical data, medical tests, and procedures; and nutrition-focused physical findings.

Diagnosis

Based on the data from the nutrition assessment, a nutrition diagnosis is made. The nutrition diagnosis is derived from any of three domains: intake, clinical, and knowledge/belief. A patient may be given more than one nutrition diagnosis. Each diagnosis is stated in terms of the nutrition related problem (P), the etiology of the problem (E), and the signs and symptoms (S) on which those determinations were made. This is identified as a PES statement. Examples of PES statements include:

- Inadequate protein intake related to food- and-nutrition-related knowledge deficit as evidenced by taking an incomplete protein supplement
- Altered GI function related to rapid fluid ingestion as evidenced by vomiting with drinking and report of gulping fluids
- Self-monitoring deficit related to unable to determine portion sizes as evidenced by food records without portions and patient report of confusion

The problem is derived from the assessment; the etiology should be something that can be impacted by a dietitian intervention, and the signs and symptoms will provide the basis for monitoring and evaluation.

Intervention

Nutrition intervention will be based on the etiology stated in the nutrition diagnoses. Determining the intervention requires prioritizing issues identified in the nutrition diagnoses and

Table 10.3 The Nutrition Care Process for weight loss surgery

Step	Domain	Common terms used in weight loss surgery
Assessment terminology	Client history	Race/ethnicity, language, literacy, mobility
		Socioeconomic factors (living/housing situations religion, daily stress level)
	Food- and nutrition-related history *(includes knowledge, beliefs, and attitudes* and *behaviors)*	Food and nutrition intake (meal/snack pattern), protein intake, vitamin intake, mineral intake, diet experience
		Previous diet/nutrition counseling, dieting attempts, food- and nutrition-related knowledge, beliefs and attitudes, distorted body image, motivation, preoccupation with food and nutrients, preoccupation with weight, readiness to change nutrition-related behaviors, self-efficacy, self-talk/cognitions, emotions, adherence
		Ability to recall nutrition goals, self-monitoring at agreed upon rate, avoidance behavior, restrictive eating
	Biochemistries and other tests	Vitamin labs, gastrointestinal studies
	Anthropometrics	BMI, excess weight loss, weight gain
	Nutrition-focused physical findings	Appetite, constipation, body language, cognition
Diagnosis terminology	Intake	Excessive energy intake (NI-1.5) inadequate fluid intake (NI-3.1)
	Clinical	Obesity
		Undesired weight gain
	Behavioral/environmental	Food- and nutrition-related knowledge deficit, self-monitoring deficit, disordered eating pattern, limited adherence to nutrition-related recommendations, not ready for diet/lifestyle changes
Intervention	Food and nutrient delivery	Vitamin and mineral supplements, protein supplements
	Nutrition education	
	Nutrition counseling	
	Coordination of nutrition care	
Monitoring and evaluation	Food- and nutrition-related history *(includes knowledge, beliefs, and attitudes* and *behaviors)*	Energy intake, oral fluids, amount of food, meal and snack pattern, types of food eaten, food variety, alcohol intake, macronutrient intake, protein intake (including sources), vitamin/mineral intake, fiber intake, ability to recall goals, self-monitoring
	Biochemistries and other tests	Nutritional anemia profile, vitamin and mineral, metabolic rate
	Anthropometrics	Weight, weight change, body mass index
	Nutrition-focused physical findings	Digestive system, hair or skin quality

establishing goals with the patient. Implementation includes taking action on the plan and may include establishing follow-up care or communicating the care plan with the patient and other providers. The four domains of nutrition intervention (coded "NI") are food and nutrient delivery, nutrition education, nutrition counseling, and coordination of nutrition care. Data from the nutrition assessment, such as literacy and readiness to learn, are important for determining educational approaches and content delivery.

Nutrition education is divided into (1) content and (2) application. Content may include the purpose of the nutrition education, priority modifications, survival information, nutrition relationship between health and disease, and recommended modifications. In the context of weight loss surgery, common educational content will include fluid needs, protein sources, foods to avoid, and other topics discussed previously. Application will commonly refer to training related to skills, such as dietary protein assessment and self-monitoring skills.

Specific theoretical bases or approaches to nutrition counseling that have been identified and for which standardized language and codes have been developed include cognitive behavioral therapy (C-1.1), health belief model (C-1.2), social learning theory (C-1.3), transtheoretical model/stages of changes (C-1.4), and "other" (C-1.5). Specific counseling strategies ("selectively applied evidence-based methods or plans of action to achieve a particular goal") identified include motivational interviewing, goal setting, self-monitoring, problem solving, social support, stress management, stimulus control, cognitive restructuring, relapse prevention, rewards and contingency management, and "other."

Monitoring and Evaluation

The final step in the NCP is to evaluate progress toward the desired outcomes as determined by the nutrition diagnosis. Monitoring involves assessing patient understanding of and compliance with the nutrition care plan, evaluating outcomes parameters such as weight loss, and evaluating outcomes based on previously established goals or criteria, such as excess weight loss [18].

Conclusion

As the popularity of bariatric surgery continues to increase, the need for well-trained practitioners competent in the care of this population will expand. Risks for weight regain, malnutrition, and complications associated with dumping syndrome and other nutrition-related health concerns is a lifelong concern. Patients in need of education and counseling may appear in any healthcare setting many years after surgery presenting and the long-term effectiveness of bariatric surgery as a life-enhancing procedure depends upon the ability to quickly identify and address these needs.

Question and Answer Section

Questions

1. Several years after weight loss surgery, which of the following diet and nutrition concerns may be encountered by a bariatric surgery team?
   A. Weight regain
   B. Vitamin deficiencies
   C. Eating disorders
   D. All of the above
2. List five common strategies used in cognitive behavioral therapy for behavior change.

Answers

1. Answer **D**. Although the success rate for weight loss management following bariatric surgery is encouraging, patients are always at risk for weight regain depending upon the balance between calorie intake and calorie expenditure. In addition, patients who have had malabsorptive procedures remain at risk for vitamin and mineral deficiencies for life. Underlying psychological issues that are present before weight loss surgery can manifest after surgery, though presentation may be somewhat different than in the preoperative patient.

2. Answers: The key behavioral strategies applied with cognitive behavioral therapy include goal setting, self-monitoring, problem solving, social support, stress management, cognitive restructuring, relapse prevention, rewards, and contingency management and stimulus control.

References

1. Buchwald H, Avidor Y, Braunwald E, Jensen MD, Pories W, Fahrbach K, et al. Bariatric surgery. A systematic review and meta-analysis. JAMA. 2004;13:1724–37.
2. Magro DO, Geloneze B, Delfini R, Pareja BC, Callejas F, Pareja JC. Long-term weight regain after gastric bypass: a 5-year prospective study. Obes Surg. 2008;18:648–51.
3. Mechanick JI, Youdin A, Jones DB, Garvey WT, Hurley DL, McMahon MM, Heinberg LJ, Kushner R, Adams TD, Shikora S, Dixon JB and Brehauer S. Clinical practice guidelines for the perioperative nutritional, metabolic and nonsurgical support of the bariatric surgery patient-2013 update: Cosponsored by American Association of Clinical Endocrinologists, The Obesity Society, and the American Society for Metabolic & Bariatric Surgery. Surg Obes Rel Dis. 2013;9:159–91.
4. Aills L, Blankenship J, Buffington C, Furtado M, Parrott J. ASMBS Allied Health Nutritional Guidelines for the surgical weight loss patient. Surg Obes Relat Dis. 2008;4:S73–108.
5. Alami RS, Hsu G, Safadi BY, Sanchez BR, Morton MJ. The impact of preoperative weight loss in patients undergoing laparoscopic Roux-en-Y gastric bypass. Obes Surg. 2005;15:1282–6.
6. Gastrointestinal surgery for severe obesity. NIH Consensus Statement. 1991;9(1):1–20. http://consensus.nih.gov/1991/1991gisurgeryobesity084html.htm. Accessed 16 May 2013.
7. Kaly P, Orellana S, Torrella T, Takagishi C, Saff-Koche L, Murr MM. Unrealistic weight loss expectations in candidates for bariatric surgery. Surg Obes Relat Dis. 2008;4(1):6–10.
8. Foster GD, Wadden TA, Phelan S, Sarwer DB, Sanderson RS. Obese patients' perceptions of treatment outcomes and the factors that influence them. Arch Intern Med. 2001;161:2133–9.
9. Saunders R. "Grazing": a high-risk behavior? Obes Surg. 2004;14: 98–102.
10. Egberts K, Brown WA, Brennan L, O'Brien PE. Does exercise improve weight loss after bariatric surgery? Obes Surg. 2012;22:335–41.
11. [No authors listed] International Dietetics & Nutrition Terminology (IDNT) reference manual: standardized language for the nutrition care process. 3rd ed. Chicago: American Dietetic Association; 2010.
12. Ghorbani E, Khodamoradi M, Bozorgmanesh. Different aspects of adult learning principles. Life Sci J. 2011;8(2):540–6.
13. Rosenstock IM, Strecher VJ, Becker MH. Social learning theory and the health belief model. Health Educ Behav. 1988;15:175.
14. Prochaska JO, Velicer WF. The transtheoretical model of health behavior change. Am J Health Promot. 1997;12(1):38–48.
15. [No authors listed] Clinical guidelines on the identification, evaluation, and treatment of overweight and obesity in adults: the evidence report. National Institutes of Health. Obes Res. 1998;6:51S–209. http://www.nhlbi.nih.gov/guidelines/obesity/ob_gdlns.pdf.
16. Foreyt JP, Poston 2nd WS. What is the role of cognitive-behavior therapy in patient management? Obes Res. 1998;6 Suppl 1:18S–22.
17. Rubak S, Sandbaek A, Lauritzen T and Christensen B. Motivational interviewing: a systematic review and meta-analysis. BJGP. 2005; 55(513): 305–12.
18. [No authors listed] Writing Group of the Nutrition Care Process/Standardized Language Committee. Nutrition care process and model Part II. Nutrition care process part II: using the International Dietetics and Nutrition Terminology to document. J Am Diet Assoc. 2008;108(8):1287–93.

Macronutrient Recommendations: Protein, Carbohydrate, and Fat

Mary Demarest Litchford

Chapter Objectives

1. Explain the role of macronutrients in energy balance and weight management.
2. Describe the weight loss implication of dietary macronutrient distribution.
3. Describe implications of weight loss surgery on macronutrient utilization.
4. Discuss dietary recommendations for weight loss and weight maintenance following weight loss surgery.

Introduction

Metabolic Trajectory of Macronutrients

Macronutrients are not metabolized and utilized equally by the body. A hierarchy exists for the satiating efficacies of the macronutrients with protein being the most satiating and fat the least. This sequence also represents the priority with respect to metabolizing these macronutrients [1]. The metabolic fate of the ingested macronutrients is related to their storage capacity in the body. The storage capacity for protein and carbohydrate is limited and converting these nutrients to a more readily stored form requires energy expenditure. Conversely, the storage capacity for fat is potentially unlimited. The clinical implication of storage capacity is that energy expenditure has a specific order in which it utilizes the macronutrients since it can store an excess intake of fat far more readily than carbohydrate and protein. For example, the postprandial energy expenditure of a mixed meal is mainly oxidation of carbohydrate and protein followed by fat oxidation in the fasted state [2].

M.D. Litchford, PhD, RD, LDN (✉)
Case Software & Books,
5601 Forest Manor Dr, Greensboro, NC 27410, USA
e-mail: MDLPHD@casesoftware.com; MDLPHD@yahoo.com

The metabolic expenditure of utilizing macronutrients follows a similar order. Reported thermic effect of food-induced energy expenditure values for the separate nutrients are 20–30 % for protein, 5–10 % for carbohydrate, and 0–3 % for fat. Protein intake stimulates the largest rise in energy expenditure due to the metabolic cost of protein synthesis, gluconeogenesis, and ureogenesis [3]. Energy expenditure and substrate oxidation measured over 24 h in a respiration chamber shows that protein intake is associated with almost threefold higher diet-induced energy expenditure in comparison with fat intake, without a difference between lean and obese participants [2].

Interplay of Protein and Energy Intake

The interplay between protein intake and energy intake is both complex and noteworthy. Changes in dietary consumption of protein and energy significantly influence human nitrogen metabolism. This arises both from changes in the supply of amino acids that serve as substrates for the formation of polypeptides and from changes in the amounts and sources of chemical energy for the synthesis of ATP and GTP, amino acyl-tRNAs, and peptide bond formation and for the release of amino acids from dietary and endogenous proteins into the tissue-free amino acid pools.

The clinical implication of this construct is that an individual's indispensable amino acid (IAA) requirement and protein requirement are affected by the characteristics of the diet, i.e., the amounts of IAA and dispensable amino acids (DAA), as well as the overall level of dietary protein and energy [4, 5]. The effects of protein on energy metabolism are generally less significant, in the context of requirement estimates, than are the effects of energy on protein metabolism.

The practical application is that a person who has been habitually consuming a low-protein diet will, to a limited degree, adapt to that protein level and be able to maintain nitrogen balance on a lower level of dietary protein.

Moreover, the protein requirement is significantly increased for an individual who is consuming less than his/her energy needs. The converse is true as well. The protein requirement is significantly decreased for an individual who is in positive energy balance. Following weight surgery, the energy intake is greatly reduced and the percentage of calories from protein should be higher to compensate for the very low energy intake. While it is much easier to achieve nitrogen balance if nonprotein energy intake is increased, this may not be an applicable nutrition strategy for weight loss following bariatric surgery.

Protein Quality

In 1991, the Joint World Health Organization (WHO), Food and Agriculture Organization (FAO), and United Nations University (UNU) Expert Consultation on Protein and Amino Acid Requirements in Human Nutrition [6] established a methodology to measure protein value and to make recommendations for individual IAA requirements. Protein digestibility correct amino acid score methodology (PDCAAS) was adopted by WHO/FAO/UUN and later by the Food and Nutrition Board of the Institute of Medicine (FNB IOM) [7] as the preferred method for the measurement of the protein value in human nutrition. PDCAAS replaced traditional biological methods, i.e., protein efficiency ratio (PER) in rats. The principle behind PDCAAS is that utilization of any protein will be first limited by digestibility, which determines the overall available amino acid nitrogen from food. Secondly, the PDCAAS reflects the relative adequacy of its most limiting IAA with a score of zero to 100 %. A score of zero indicates that one or more of the IAAs is missing, while a score of 100 % means that the protein contains a sufficient amount of each of the IAAs. A score of greater than zero but less than 100 denotes insufficient quantity of one or more of the IAAs.

Macronutrient: Protein

Protein is associated with all forms of plant and animal life. Yet, dietary sources of plant and animal protein are not nutritionally equivalent due to differences in amino acid composition. Protein is composed of 20 amino acids or subunits of protein. The amino acids are either synthesized by the body from nonspecific nitrogen substrate (i.e., dispensable amino acids) or must be derived from food (i.e., indispensable amino acids). Amino acids are required to synthesize nitrogen-containing compounds, i.e., enzymes, hormones, antibodies, and DNA. Daily protein intake is the most important dietary determinant of whole-body protein turnover. Furthermore, protein turnover and metabolism is strongly influenced by protein quality, because protein synthesis requires adequate availability of IAA. Nitrogen or protein metabolism takes place through the amino acid pool, which receives amino acids from dietary protein, breakdown of lean body reserves, and is the precursor for nitrogen excretion—predominantly as urea.

The major metabolic cycles involving nitrogen include the protein cycle and the nitrogen cycle. In the protein cycle, amino acids move into and out of protein through the processes of protein synthesis, degradation, and protein turnover. The clinical implication is that the intake of sufficient levels of these IAAs is crucial for preventing negative nitrogen balance and required for tissue accretion [8–10].

In the nitrogen cycle, urea-N moves into the bowel and is salvaged as metabolically useful nitrogen. One adaptation to a very low dietary protein intake is to salvage amino acids from urea through the metabolic activity of the colonic microflora. The rate of salvage is responsive to the dietary protein intake. As the protein intake decreases, there is an increase in the proportion of urea-N produced that is salvaged. The converse is that as the intake falls, the proportion of urea production that is excreted falls. The clinical implication for these findings is that, at least in part, the extent to which the urea produced is excreted is determined by the extent of salvage [5, 10]. The practical application is that through this process, IAA may be salvaged to meet protein requirements when dietary protein intake is poor either in quality, quantity, or both. The extent to which external nitrogen balance is achieved through the internal salvaging of urea nitrogen as an effective source of indispensable amino acids remains to be determined.

Insufficient Protein Intake

During times of inadequate protein and energy intake, the reduced carbon skeleton may be used for energy production. While the body may adapt to a low-protein intake by salvaging amino acids from urea, this is self-limiting process and it is not the preferred source of IAA [10]. Since daily protein intake is the most important dietary determinant of whole-body protein turnover and metabolism is influenced by protein quality, it is vital that WLS patients consume sufficient amounts of high-quality protein. The practical application is that WSL patients may need to consume concentrated forms of high-quality protein, providing sufficient quantities of IAAs, since energy intake is low and total food intake is limited by the surgical procedure.

Surplus Protein Intake

When consumed in surplus of postprandial protein synthesis, amino acids can readily be used as substrate for oxidation. Increasing the amount of dietary protein from 10 to 20 % of

Table 11.1 Protein intake: relative versus absolute

Energy intake/day (kcal)	Protein intake in relative terms	Protein intake in absolute terms
500	WHO 10–15 %	12–18 g/day
	IOM 10–35 %	12–44 g/day
1,000	WHO 10–15 %	25–38 g/day
	IOM 10–35 %	25–88 g/day
1,500	WHO 10–15 %	38–56 g/day
	IOM 10–35 %	38–131 g/day

energy resulted in a 63–95 % increase in protein oxidation, depending on the protein source. However, the body does not utilize all sources of dietary protein equally. The largest (95 %) increase in protein oxidation is observed when the predominant protein source is of animal origin, whereas this increase is only 63 % when soy protein is the predominant protein source in the diet [9]. Differences in digestion rate of the various protein sources may contribute to differences in postprandial protein oxidation as well. The clinical implication of these differences is that the consumption of rapidly digested protein results in a stronger increase in postprandial protein synthesis and amino acid oxidation than slowly digested protein [11–13].

Protein Requirements

The FAO/WHO/UUN recommends that dietary protein should account for around 10–15 % of energy when individuals are in energy balance and weight stable [14]. The FNB IOM recommends that the average person consume between 10 and 35 % of daily calories from protein [7]. Practitioners may recommend protein intake in absolute terms (i.e., total grams of protein per day) or in relative terms (i.e., percentage of total energy intake).

When recommending high-protein diets for weight loss, the difference between absolute and relative measures should be taken into account. Relatively high protein diets for weight loss and subsequent weight maintenance consist of up to 35 % of energy from protein. The clinical implication of this construct is that these diets are relatively high in protein, expressed as percentage energy from protein, but in absolute terms (i.e., grams of protein) they only contain a sufficient absolute amount of protein but less energy in total (Table 11.1). The practical application of this concept is that to ensure that patients are not in a negative nitrogen and protein balance during weight loss and lose their metabolically active fat free mass, the absolute amount of protein is of greater importance than the percentage of protein.

Protein Utilization for Muscle Accretion

The effects of protein ingestion on muscle protein accretion have been largely attributed to the IAA found in the ingested protein. However, researchers found that whey protein results in greater anabolic effect in older adults than its IAA. The clinical application of these findings is that whey protein ingestion improves muscle protein accretion in older adults through mechanisms that are beyond those associated with its EAA content. The practical application of these findings is that high-quality intact protein, either from food or supplements, may stimulate muscle protein accretion to a greater degree than fortified low-quality source protein supplements [15].

Researchers examined the effect of protein dose on muscle protein synthesis using a high-quality, protein-rich food. The data suggests that ingestion of 25–30 g of high-quality protein (PDCAAS = 100 %), which provides about 10 g of IAA, is necessary at a meal to maximally stimulate skeletal muscle protein synthesis. Ingestion of 90 g of protein, distributed evenly over three meals, is more likely to provide a greater 24-h protein anabolic response than an unequal protein distribution. Smaller meals with less protein may not reach the leucine threshold to initiate protein synthesis. Intakes of greater than 30 g of protein per meal do not appear to promote increased muscle accretion but may be used for energy or other purposes [16, 17].

Following WLS, it is unknown if having a minimum of 25–30 g of high-quality protein per meal is needed to achieve an anabolic effect. However, ingestion of 25–30 g of protein at each meal can be achieved by using concentrated high-quality protein supplements.

Lean Body Mass Loss with WLS

Rapid weight loss following bariatric surgery reflects a loss of both lean and fat mass. While loss of protein reserves is undesirable, it appears to be unavoidable [18]. Once glycogen stores are depleted, all body glucose must come from gluconeogenesis, either from glycerol and glucogenic amino acids or lactate and pyruvate. However, if the diet is excessive in carbohydrate-derived calories and deficient in protein, hyperinsulinemia will blunt fat breakdown. Over time, the body will not be able to spare protein reserves, resulting in impaired immunity and hypoalbuminemia due in part to extravascular fluid accumulation and inflammatory response [10].

Very low energy intake and malabsorption due to surgery contributes to depletion of protein reserves.

Individuals undergoing BPD/DS are at greatest risk of developing a protein deficiency. However, all WLS patients who are noncompliant with nutrition instructions regarding adequate protein intake are at risk as well [18].

Role of Protein in Weight Loss

High-protein diets for weight loss have been popular for decades. The high-protein and/or high-fat and very-low-carbohydrate macronutrient distribution induces ketosis. The very-low-carbohydrate content is critical in inducing short-term weight loss in the first 2–4 weeks, which is largely due to fluid mobilization. Ketone bodies tend to be generated with daily dietary carbohydrate intake of under 50 g, and sodium diuresis is forced, causing most of the short-term weight loss. The premise of the diet is that caloric intake as protein is less prone to fat storage than is the equivalent caloric intake as carbohydrate [10].

Numerous studies have been published on the benefits of high-protein diets for weight loss. In randomized trials, weight loss with Atkins-type diets was compared with conventional low-fat or balanced calorie-deficit diets. Although the Atkins-type diet had the greatest initial weight loss, weight loss became similar within 1 year. Adherence to this diet is poor. Similar approaches to weight loss use the high-protein diets that distinguish between what are considered to be "good" and "bad" carbohydrates on the basis of their glycemic index. Although the relevance and importance of the glycemic index is controversial, the diet encourages increased fiber intake, which is associated with lowered weight even when total caloric intake is relatively unchanged. Low glycemic index diets plus a modest increase in protein intake are better at promoting maintenance of weight loss [19].

Dansinger [20] and colleagues compared the Zone, Ornish, and Atkins diets and a typical balanced, calorie-restricted (e.g., Weight Watchers) diet. No significant differences in weight loss based on the diet were observed. Compliance and caloric deficits were more important predictors of weight loss than was specific dietary composition.

Other researchers found low-carbohydrate diet (20 g/day from low glycemic vegetables) with unrestricted consumption of fat and protein and low-fat diets (55 % of calories from carbohydrate, 30 % from fat, and 15 % from protein) to be equally efficacious in inducing weight loss [21]. When types of high-protein diets are compared, low-fat diets are better than low-carbohydrate diets in achieving sustained weight loss. A realistic high-protein weight-reducing diet was associated with greater fat loss and lower blood pressure when compared with a high-carbohydrate, high-fiber diet in overweight and obese women [22].

Table 11.2 Daily protein intake recommendations

Surgical procedure	Protein in gm/kg [Ref.]
RYGB	1.1 g/kg IBW [23]
RYGB	1.0–1.5 g/kg IBW [18]
Gastric banding	1.0–1.5 g/kg IBW
Gastric sleeve	1.0–1.5 g/kg IBW
BPD/DS	90 g (add 30 % more d/t malabsorption) [24]
BPD/DS	1.5–2.0 g/kg IBW
All	60–120 g/day [25, 26]

Protein Needs of WLS Patients

While the exact protein requirements for postoperative WLS patients are undefined, the current clinical practice recommendations for individuals without complications are consistent with those for medically supervised modified protein fasts [18]. Recommendations for protein intake must be based on individualized nutrition assessment and monitored for expected outcomes using nutrition care process (NCP). Common practices are noted in Table 11.2 [18, 23–26].

Protein malnutrition may be observed at 3–6 months after surgery and is largely attributed to the development of food intolerance to protein-rich foods or maladaptive eating behaviors due to pre- or postsurgical eating disorders. Experts have noted that adding 100 g/day of carbohydrate decreases nitrogen loss by 40 % in modified protein fasts [18]. The AND/ASPEN [27] characteristics of malnutrition are tools to quantify adult malnutrition. Laboratory tests such as albumin, prealbumin, and C-reactive protein are markers of inflammation and are not sensitive enough to reflect changes in protein status or predict protein requirements.

Macronutrient: Carbohydrate

Glucose, found in about 80 % of dietary carbohydrates, is the body's preferred carbohydrate energy source. Disaccharides and polysaccharides are the most common forms of dietary carbohydrates found in foods. The most common dietary disaccharides are maltose, lactose, and sucrose. The most common forms of digestible polysaccharides are amylose and amylopectin. Monosaccharides such as free glucose and fructose are found in honey, certain fruits, and in foods with added high-fructose corn syrup.

Digestion and absorption of dietary carbohydrates is so efficient that nearly all monosaccharides are absorbed by the end of the jejunum. The digestion of carbohydrate begins in the mouth where salivary α(alpha)-amylase initiates hydrolysis of disaccharides and polysaccharides. Few monosaccharides are produced due to the short time period that food is in the mouth. The amylose and amylopectin are hydrolyzed by salivary α(alpha)-amylase into dextrins.

The dextrins pass through the stomach unchanged into the duodenum. The pancreas releases pancreatic α(alpha)-amylase, which reduces the dextrins into maltose. Maltose is hydrolyzed by maltase to glucose at the brush border of the small intestine and absorbed as free glucose.

Glucose and galactose are absorbed into the mucosal cells by active transport requiring ATP. Fructose enters the cells at a slower rate than glucose, but entry into cells is independent of glucose concentration. Co-consumption of glucose and fructose accelerates the absorption of fructose and raises the threshold level of fructose ingestions in which malabsorption symptoms occur.

The fate of carbohydrates depends on the energy needs of body cells. Glucose is stored in the body in the form of glycogen in the liver and skeletal muscle. When blood glucose levels fall, glucagon and epinephrine trigger the conversion of glycogen to glucose, i.e., glycogenolysis. When blood glucose levels remain low and glycogen stores are depleted, cortisol, thyroid hormone, epinephrine, glucagon, and hGH trigger gluconeogenesis to synthesize glucose from protein or fat.

A very high carbohydrate diet has been shown to trigger hypertriglyceridemia if such a diet is sustained [28]. Researchers have theorized that hypertriglyceridemia resulted because of a rapid absorption of large amounts of glucose and that the normal pathways for carbohydrate metabolism were overloaded. Moreover, other metabolic pathways (e.g., the hexose monophosphate shunt) were used, which may favor the synthesis of fatty acids. A significant amount of the triacylglycerol-raising effects of sucrose were attributed to its content of fructose [29]. If the carbohydrate content of the high-carbohydrate diet is primarily monosaccharides, particularly fructose, the hypertriglyceridemia is more extreme than if the diet is predominately disaccharides and polysaccharides.

Carbohydrate Requirements

The RDA for carbohydrate is 130 g/day for adults providing between 45 and 65 % of total energy. Carbohydrates are also the source of many vitamins, minerals, and fiber [7].

Carbohydrate Needs of WLS Patients

Carbohydrate needs are determined on an individual basis by the registered dietitian. The majority of carbohydrates should be from disaccharides and polysaccharides. Intake of simple sugars is discouraged to minimize gastrointestinal symptoms associated with dumping. Symptoms of early dumping (i.e., 10–30 min after meals) is usually due to accelerated gastric emptying of hyperosmolar content into the jejunum, followed by fluid shifts from the intravascular compartment into the intestinal lumen. This leads to small bowel distention and increased intestine contractility. Late dumping is thought to be a consequence of reactive hypoglycemia from an exaggerated release of insulin. Dumping may be controlled by (1) eating small, frequent meals; (2) avoiding ingestion of liquids within 30 min of a solid-food meal; (3) avoiding simple sugars and increasing intake of fiber and complex carbohydrates; and (4) increasing protein intake [26].

Role of Carbohydrate in Weight Loss

The relationship between the carbohydrate content of the diet and weight loss has generated mixed results. The Diabetes Excess Weight Loss Trial compared high-protein (30 % calories), low-carbohydrate (40 % calories), low-fat (30 % calories) versus high-carbohydrate (55 % calories), low-protein (15 % calories) low-fat (30 % calories) diets over 2 years in individuals with type 2 diabetes and found no differences between groups in terms of weight loss, reduction of waist circumference, and other measures of diabetes management [30].

The role of carbohydrate in weight loss has been linked to glycemic load. Dietary sources of carbohydrates are grouped by glucose response. Researchers noted that foods with high glycemic index scores were rapidly digested and foods with a low glycemic index scores were digested more slowly and reported to help control appetite. However, the findings of various research studies are mixed in terms of sustained weight loss. The amount of protein in the diet was a stronger predictor of weight loss success than the glycemic index of carbohydrates consumed [20, 31].

Faria [32] examined the effect of grams of carbohydrate and glycemic load and in weight loss on patients who had undergone bariatric surgery and found correlations between weight loss and glycemic load suggesting a role in long-term weight maintenance following gastric bypass. However, long-term weight maintenance may be related to changes in glucose kinetics and glucoregulatory hormone secretion secondary to anatomical rearrangement [33].

Macronutrient: Fat

Fat is the most energy dense of the essential macronutrients, providing more than twice the energy by weight compared to protein or carbohydrate. The terms "fat" and "lipids" are often used interchangeably, but are not the same. The term lipid encompasses not only dietary sources of energy, but also all compounds that dissolve in organic solvents, i.e., fat-soluble vitamins, corticosteroid hormones, and some enzymes such as coenzyme Q.

Fats are hydrophobic, meaning that they do not dissolve in an aqueous environment. In order for fat to be digested, it must be emulsified. Lingual lipase begins the emulsification of lipid in the mouth followed by gastric lipase, activated by low pH in the stomach. The churning of the stomach contents helps to physically separate fats. Digestion begins in the duodenum and jejunum where bile acids and lecithin emulsify fat into smaller particles. Phospholipase breaks the phospholipids into glycerol, fatty acids, phosphoric acid, and choline. Glycerol and free fatty acids (i.e., short-chain and medium-chain fatty acids) are absorbed directly into the bloodstream via intestinal cells. Fatty acids are transported to the mitochondria by carnitine. Pancreatic lipase breaks long-chain fat into monoglycerides and fatty acids. Monoglycerides and fatty acids are absorbed through the villi in the distal duodenum and jejunum via micelles and then are reformed into triglycerides, which are then absorbed by the lacteals. The bile salts are absorbed in the ileum and returned through the portal vein for re-secretion in the bile, i.e., enterohepatic circulation. The reformed triglycerides, with phospholipids and cholesterol, are packaged together to form chylomicrons.

Difficulties with fat absorption and utilization are common following many types of WLS. Reducing the size of the stomach raises the pH by reducing the production of pepsin, thereby limiting the early steps in fat digestion. The surgical bypass of the duodenum and jejunum results in malabsorption of fat since these are the primary sites for fat digestion and absorption [18].

Regulation of Lipolysis and Lipogenesis

The regulation of fatty acid synthesis is closely linked to carbohydrate status. Fatty acids that are not used for synthesis of eicosanoids or incorporated into tissues are oxidized for energy (i.e., lipolysis). Fatty acids yield energy by beta oxidation in the mitochondria of all cells, except those in the brain and kidney. They enter the mitochondria as specific acyl carnitine derivatives. The enzyme carnitine acryl transferase I catalyzes the transfer of fatty acryl groups to carnitine. Saturated short-, medium-, and long-chain fatty acids undergo the first step of beta oxidation with different dehydrogenases. The process yields successive acetyl CoA molecules, which enter the tricarboxylic acid cycle or other metabolic pathways.

The rate of fatty acid synthesis can be influenced by diet. Diets high in simple carbohydrates and low in fats trigger lipogenic enzymes. A low level of insulin accompanied the hypoglycemia would favor lipolysis. Hypoglycemia stimulates the rate of fatty acid oxidation followed by a reduction in TCA cycle activity, which in turn results in inadequate oxaloacetate availability.

Elevated blood glucose levels can affect lipolysis and fatty acid oxidation as well. Hyperglycemia triggers the release of insulin, which promotes glucose transport into the adipose cell and promotes lipogenesis. Malonyl CoA concentration increases whenever a person consumes sufficient amounts of carbohydrate. Carnitine acryl transferase I is inhibited by malonyl CoA. Excess glucose that cannot be oxidized through the glycolytic pathway or stored as glycogen is converted to triacylglycerols for storage using the available malonyl CoA. This pathway requires ATP, biotin, niacin, and pantothenic acid. Excess dietary glycerol and fatty acids undergo lipogenesis to form triglycerides, primarily in the liver. The body has an unlimited capacity to store fat as triglycerides in adipose tissue. The clinical implication of this construct is that high carbohydrate intake will result in increased fat storage. The practical application for the WLS patient on a very low energy diet is that a high carbohydrate intake may blunt the utilization of stored fat for energy and stall weight loss.

Recommendations for Fat Intake

Fat is an essential nutrient providing essential fatty acids and fat-soluble vitamins. Recommended fat intake guidelines have not been published beyond limiting total intake of dietary fat.

Diets very low in fat, especially with significant fat malabsorption, have the potential for essential fatty acid and fat-soluble vitamin deficiencies. Biliopancreatic diversion surgery has been shown to decrease fat absorption by 72 % [18]. Therefore it is reasonable to expect that these individuals have an increased risk for essential fatty acid and fat-soluble vitamin deficiencies.

To assess for essential fatty acid deficiencies, evaluate the triene/tetraene ratio. A ratio of >0.2 indicates deficiency of linoleic and linolenic fatty acids [25]. Nutrition-focused physical assessment may note signs of essential fatty acid deficiency including dry scaly skin, hair loss, decreased immunity, and increased susceptibility to infections, anemia, mood changes, and unexplained cardiac, hepatic, gastrointestinal, and neurological dysfunction.

Dietary sources of linoleic and linolenic fatty acids include polyunsaturated vegetable oils such as soybean, linseed, and canola oils. The recommended intake to prevent or reverse symptoms of linoleic acid deficiency is approximately 3–5 % of energy intake. The recommended intake to prevent or reverse symptoms of linolenic acid deficiency is approximately 0.5–1 % of energy intake [25].

Deficiencies of vitamins A, E, and K have been reported following WLS. Normal absorption of fat-soluble vitamins occurs passively in the upper small intestine. The digestion of dietary fat and subsequent micellation of triglycerides is associated with fat-soluble vitamin absorption. Additionally, the transport of fat-soluble vitamins to tissues is reliant on lipid components such as chylomicrons and lipoproteins. The changes in fat digestion produced by surgical weight loss procedures consequently alter the digestion, absorption, and transport of fat-soluble vitamins [18].

Role of Fat in Weight Loss

Researchers have examined the role of daily fat intake as it relates to excessive weight gain and reported either clinically insignificant findings or inconclusive results. Jeon [34] reported that obese subjects reported eating about 20 % more calories from fat than normal weight individuals even though total energy intake was not significantly different between obese and normal groups. Findings from the Nurses' Health Study [35] reported a weak associated in the overall percent of calories from fat and weight gain. A positive association between intake of dietary fat and weight gain was observed in the Pound of Prevention [36] study, yet several randomized trials have failed to support such an association [37]. Astrup [38] observed that, among post-obese women, consuming a high-fat diet (50 % of energy derived from fat) resulted in preferential fat storage and impaired suppression of carbohydrate oxidation but found no relationship with oxidation among women on low-fat (20 % of energy derived from fat) or moderate-fat (30 % of energy derived from fat) diets. Other researchers did not observe an impact on energy metabolism when subjects were switched from a high-fat (42 % of calories) to an isocaloric low-fat (27 % of calories) diet. The findings suggest that adoption of a moderately low-fat diet will not have a meaningful impact on weight gain for most adults [39].

Few clinical trials have assessed the impact of type of dietary fat. Findings from the Nurses' Health Study [35] note that increases in monounsaturated and polyunsaturated fat were not associated with weight gain, but increases in animal fat, saturated fat, and trans-fat had a positive association with weight change. In addition, there is evidence that trans-fat intake is more predictive than total fat of changes in waist circumference [40]. Primate studies reported that monkeys on a diet with trans-fat gained more weight (7.2 % versus 1.8 %) than monkeys on a diet with an equivalent amount of fat, but as monounsaturated cis fat [41]. More research is needed to better delineate the mechanism through which trans-fat independently promotes weight gain.

Conclusion: Pearls for Practice

Dietary intake is deemed an important modifiable factor in the overweight. The role of macronutrients in obesity has been examined in a variety of populations, but the results of these studies are mixed, depending on the potential confounders and adjustments for other macronutrients. Total energy intake seems to be more important than protein while consuming excess amounts of energy with respect to increases in body fat. Diets that are higher in energy from protein are metabolically different from diets lower in energy for protein. The quality and quantity of protein eaten per meal is associated with protein muscle accretion. Macronutrient distribution following WLS should be individualized by a registered dietitian to address both nutrient needs and to manage common side effects following WLS. More research is needed to examine the role of macronutrient distribution in weight loss and weight maintenance following WLS.

Question and Answer Section

Questions

1. The metabolic fate of the ingested macronutrients is related to their storage capacity in the body. The practical application of this concept is that:
   A. In a mixed meal the carbohydrate and protein will be oxidized before fat.
   B. In a mixed meal the carbohydrate and protein will be oxidized after fat.
   C. In a mixed meal all macronutrients are oxidized simultaneously.
2. Which statement best describes the thermic effect of macronutrient distribution?
   A. High-carbohydrate diets have the greatest thermic effect compared to high-protein diets.
   B. High-protein diets have the greatest thermic effect than either high-fat or high-carbohydrate diets.
   C. High-fat diets have a greater thermic effect than high-protein diets than high-carbohydrate diets.
3. Using the glycemic index to select healthy carbohydrates
   A. Is strongly correlated with successful weight loss and weight maintenance
   B. Is the best strategy to prevent weight regain once weight goals are reached
   C. Is a controversial issue but appears to be a weaker predictor of weight loss success than total protein intake

Answers

1. Answer: **A**. The storage capacity for protein and carbohydrate is limited and converting these nutrients to a more readily stored form requires energy expenditure. Conversely, the storage capacity for fat is potentially unlimited. The clinical implication of storage capacity is

that energy expenditure has a specific order in which it utilizes the macronutrients since it can store an excess intake of fat far more readily than carbohydrate and protein.
2. Answer **B**. Since protein intake stimulates the largest rise in energy expenditure due to the metabolic cost of protein synthesis, gluconeogenesis, and ureogenesis, a high-protein diet has the greatest thermic effect.
3. Answer **C**. Various research studies are mixed in terms of sustained weight loss. The amount of protein in the diet was a stronger predictor of weight loss success than the glycemic index of carbohydrates consumed.

References

1. Paddon-Jones D, Westman E, Mattes RD, Wolfe RR, Astrup A, et al. Protein, weight management and satiety. Am J Clin Nutr. 2008;87(5):1558S–61.
2. Veldhorst M, Smeets A, Soenen S, Hochstenbach-Waelen A, Hursel R, Diepvens K, et al. Protein-induced satiety: effects and mechanisms of different proteins. Physiol Behav. 2008;94:300–7.
3. Bray G, Smith S, de Jonge L, Xie H, Rood J, Martin CK, et al. Effect of dietary protein content on weight gain, energy expenditure, and body composition during overeating. JAMA. 2012;307(1):47–55.
4. Hoffer LJ. Protein and energy provision in critical illness. Am J Clin Nutr. 2003;78:906–11.
5. Young VR, El-Khoury AE, Raguso CA, Forslund AH, Hambraeus L. Rates of urea production and hydrolysis and Leucine oxidation change linearly over widely varying protein intakes in healthy adults. J Nutr. 2000;130(4):761–6.
6. [No authors listed] Protein Quality Evaluation – Report of a Joint FAO/WHO Expert Consultation. Food and Agriculture Organization of the United Nations. FAO Food and Nutrition Paper, No. 51, 1991. FAO, Rome.
7. [No authors listed] Institute of Medicine of the National Academies. Protein and amino acids. In: Dietary reference intakes for energy, carbohydrate, fiber, fat, fatty acids, cholesterol, protein, and amino acids. Food and Nutrition Board. National Academy of Sciences. Washington, DC: National Academy Press; 2005.
8. Garlick PJ. The nature of human hazards associated with excessive intake of amino acids. J Nutr. 2004;134 suppl 6:1633S–9.
9. Pannemans DL, Wagenmakers AJ, Westerterp KR, Schaafsma G, Halliday D. Effect of protein source and quantity on protein metabolism in elderly women. Am J Clin Nutr. 1998;68(6):1228–35.
10. Matthews DE. Proteins and amino acids. In: Shils ME, Olson JA, editors. Modern nutrition in health & disease. 9th ed. Baltimore: Williams & Wilkins; 2006. p. 23–61.
11. Dangin M, Boirie Y, Garcia-Rodenas C, Gachon P, Fauquant J, Callier P, et al. The digestion rate of protein is an independent regulating factor of postprandial protein retention. Am J Physiol Endocrinol Metab. 2001;280:E340–8.
12. Boirie Y, Dangin M, Gachon P, Vasson MP, Maubois JL, Beaufrere B. Slow and fast dietary proteins differently modulate postprandial protein accretion. Proc Natl Acad Sci U S A. 1997;94:14930–5.
13. Boirie Y, Gachon P, Beaufrère B. Splanchnic and whole-body leucine kinetics in young and elderly men. Am J Clin Nutr. 1997;65(2):489–95.
14. [No authors listed] WHO/FAO/UUN Expert Consultation. Protein and amino acid requirements in human nutrition. World Health Organ Tech Rep Ser. 2007;(935):1–265.
15. Katsanos CS, Chinkes DL, Paddon-Jones D, Zhang XJ, Aarsland A, Wolfe RR. Whey protein ingestion in elderly results in greater muscle protein accrual than ingestion of its constituent essential amino acid content. Nutr Res. 2008;28(10):651–8.
16. Katsanos CS, Kobayashi H, Sheffield-Moore M, Aarsland A, Wolfe RR. A high proportion of leucine is required for optimal stimulation of the rate of muscle protein synthesis by essential amino acids in the elderly. Am J Physiol Endocrinol Metab. 2006;291:E381–7.
17. Paddon-Jones D, Rasmussen BB. Dietary protein recommendations and the prevention of sarcopenia. Curr Opin Clin Nutr Metab Care. 2009;12(1):86–90.
18. Allied Health Sciences Section Ad Hoc Nutrition Committee, Aills L, Blankenship J, Buffington C, Furtado M, Parrott J. ASMBS Allied Health Nutritional guidelines for the surgical weight loss patient. Surg Obes Relat Dis. 2008;4(5 Suppl):S73–108.
19. Larsen TM, Dalskov SM, van Baak M, Jebb SA, Papadaki A, Pfeiffer AF, et al. Diets with high or low protein content and glycemic index for weight-loss maintenance. N Engl J Med. 2010;363(22):2102–13.
20. Dansinger ML, Gleason JA, Griffith JL, Selker HP, Schaefer EJ. Comparison of the Atkins, Ornish, Weight Watchers, and Zone diets for weight loss and heart disease risk reduction: a randomized trial. JAMA. 2005;293(1):43–53.
21. Foster GD, Wyatt HR, Hill JO, Makris AP, Rosenbaum DL, Brill C, et al. Weight and metabolic outcomes after 2 years on a low-carbohydrate versus low-fat diet: a randomized trial. Ann Intern Med. 2010;153(3):147–57.
22. Te Morenga LA, Levers MT, Williams SM, Brown RC, Mann J. Comparison of high protein and high fiber weight-loss diets in women with risk factors for the metabolic syndrome: a randomized trial. Nutr J. 2011;10:40.
23. Moize V, Geliebter A, Gluck ME, Yahav E, Lorence M, Colarusso T, et al. Obese patients have inadequate protein intake related to protein intolerance up to 1 year following Roux-en-Y gastric bypass. Obes Surg. 2003;13(1):23–8.
24. Slater GH, Ren CJ, Siegel N, Williams T, Barr D, Wolfe B, et al. Serum fat-soluble vitamin deficiency and abnormal calcium metabolism after malabsorptive bariatric surgery. J Gastrointest Surg. 2004;8:48–55.
25. Mechanick JI, Kushner RF, Sugerman HJ, Gonzalez-Campoy, Collazo-Clavell ML, Guven S, et al. AACE/TOS/ASMBE Guidelines. Surg Obes Relat Dis. 2008;4:S109–84.
26. Heber D, Greenway FL, Kaplan LM, Livingston E, Salvador J, Still C, Endocrine Society. Endocrine and nutritional management of the post-bariatric surgery patient: an Endocrine Society Clinical Practice Guideline Clinical Practice Guideline. J Clin Endocrinol Metab. 2010;95(11):4823–43.
27. White JV, Guenter P, Jensen G, Malone A, Schofield M, Academy Malnutrition Work Group; A.S.P.E.N. Malnutrition Task Force; A.S.P.E.N. Board of Directors. Consensus statement Academy of Nutrition and Dietetics and American Society for Parenteral and Enteral Nutrition: characteristics recommended for the identification and documentation of adult malnutrition. JPEN J Parenter Enteral Nutr. 2012;36(3):275–83.
28. Parks EJ, Hellerstein MK. Carbohydrate-induced hypertriacylglycerolemia: historical perspective and review of biological mechanisms. Am J Clin Nutr. 2000;71(2):412–33.
29. Frayn KN, Kingman SM. Dietary sugars and lipid metabolism in humans. Am J Clin Nutr. 1995;62(1 Suppl):250S–61.
30. Krebs JD, Elley CR, Parry-Strong A, Lunt H, Drury PL, Bell DA, et al. The Diabetes Excess Weight Loss (DEWL) Trial: a randomized controlled trial of high-protein versus high- carbohydrate diets over 2 years in type 2 diabetes. Diabetologia. 2012;55(4):905–14.
31. Vega-López S, Mayol-Kreiser SN. Use of the glycemic index for weight loss and glycemic control: a review of recent evidence. Curr Diab Rep. 2009;9(5):379–88.

32. Faria SL, Faria OP, Lopes TC, Galvão MV, de Oliveira Kelly E, Ito MK. Relation between carbohydrate intake and weight loss after bariatric surgery. Obes Surg. 2009;19(6):708–16.
33. Rodieux F, Giusti V, D'Alessio DA, Suter M, Tappy L. Effects of gastric bypass and gastric banding on glucose kinetics and gut hormone release. Obesity (Silver Spring). 2008;16(2):298–305.
34. Jeon KJ, Lee O, Kim HK, Han SN. Comparison of the dietary intake and clinical characteristics of obese and normal weight adults. Nutr Res Pract. 2011;5(4):329–36.
35. Field AE, Willett WC, Lissner L, Colditz GA. Dietary fat and weight gain among women in the Nurses' Health Study. Obesity (Silver Spring). 2007;15(4):967–76.
36. Sherwood NE, Jeffery RW, French SA, Hannan PJ, Murray DM. Predictors of weight gain in the Pound of Prevention study. Int J Obes Relat Metab Disord. 2000;24(4):395–403.
37. Brehm BJ, Spang SE, Lattin BL, Seeley RJ, Daniels SR, D'Alessio DA. The role of energy expenditure in the differential weight loss in obese women on low-fat and low-carbohydrate diets. J Clin Endocrinol Metab. 2005;90(3):1475–82. Epub 2004 Dec 14.
38. Astrup A, Buemann B, Christensen NJ, Toubro S. Failure to increase lipid oxidation in response to increasing dietary fat content in formerly obese women. Am J Physiol. 1994;266(4 Pt 1): E592–9.
39. Roust LR, Hammel KD, Jensen MD. Effects of isoenergetic, low-fat diets on energy metabolism in lean and obese women. Am J Clin Nutr. 1994;60(4):470–5.
40. Koh-Banerjee P, Chu NF, Spiegelman D, Rosner B, Colditz G, Willett W, et al. Prospective study of the association of changes in dietary intake, physical activity, alcohol consumption, and smoking with 9-y gain in waist circumference among 16,587 US men. Am J Clin Nutr. 2003;78(4):719–27.
41. Kavanagh K, Jones K, Keliy K, Rudel LL, Sawyer J, Wagner JD. Trans fat diet induces insulin resistance in monkeys. Diabetes. 2006;55 Suppl 1:A77.

Identification, Assessment, and Treatment of Vitamin and Mineral Deficiencies After Bariatric Surgery

Margaret M. Furtado

Chapter Objectives

1. Identify and understand potential vitamin/mineral deficiencies seen among preoperative bariatric surgery patients, as well as most common deficiencies s/p weight loss surgery.
2. Recognize appropriate laboratory analyses to assess for vitamin and mineral deficiencies after bariatric surgery.
3. Describe guidelines for effective treatment of vitamin and mineral deficiencies after weight loss surgery.

Introduction

Although much remains to be established regarding the prevalence and etiology of vitamin and mineral deficiencies after bariatric surgery, this chapter serves as a guideline for the identification, assessment, and treatment of potential vitamin/mineral deficiencies after commonly performed bariatric surgery procedures. In 2008, the *ASMBS Allied Health Nutritional Guidelines for the Surgical Weight Loss Patient* was published as a supplement in *Surgery for Obesity and Related Diseases* (*SOARD*) [1]. It included suggestions for preoperative and postoperative nutrition screening, assessment, and treatment of the bariatric patient, including vitamin and mineral deficiencies commonly seen after these procedures. Although gastric bypass, gastric banding, and biliopancreatic diversion (BPD) and BPD with duodenal switch (D/S) were included in this paper, vertical sleeve gastrectomy (VSG) was not included, although plans are underway to add this as a supplement to this paper in the future. In the interim, suggestions for vitamin/mineral assessment and guidelines for the treatment of the VSG patient will be based upon the most recent reports in the literature. Although it is commonly known that bariatric surgery patients may be at risk for particular vitamin/mineral deficiencies associated with surgery, it may not be as clear that there are possible micronutrient deficiencies evidenced *prior* to surgery that bear mentioning. An overview of micronutrients most at risk after bariatric surgery is provided, as well as guidelines for the assessment and treatment of common vitamin/mineral deficiencies seen postoperatively.

Potential Preoperative Micronutrient Deficiencies

Ernst et al. [2] performed a systematic assessment of micronutrient status before bariatric surgery on 232 patients with severe obesity. Parameters studied included calcium, magnesium, zinc, folic acid, phosphorus, vitamin B12, and 25-OH vitamin D. In a subsample of 89 subjects, additional laboratory tests were performed, which included thiamin, niacin, vitamin A, vitamin E, selenium, and copper levels. Deficiencies found included:

- Zinc – 24.6 %
- Vitamin B12 – 18.1 %
- Magnesium – 6.9 %
- Phosphorus – 4.7 %
- Folic acid – 3.4 %

In addition, 25.4 % of patients assessed in this study were deemed to have a severe vitamin D deficiency (defined as 25-OH vitamin D3 level < 25.0 nmol/l), which was accompanied by a secondary hypoparathyroidism in 36.6 % of cases. Also, 48.7 % of subjects were found to have at least one of the most prevalent micronutrient deficiencies (e.g., vitamin B12, zinc, 25-OH vitamin D deficiency). Among the 89 subjects in the subsample, 32.6 % exhibited a selenium deficiency, 5.6 % a niacin deficiency, 2.2 % a vitamin B6 deficiency, and 2.2 % a vitamin E deficiency. Thiamin, copper, and vitamin A deficiencies were not demonstrated among these subjects [2]. Based upon these findings, the

M.M. Furtado, MS, RD, LDN, RYT (✉)
Department of Bariatric Surgery, University of Maryland Medical Center, 22 South Greene St., Baltimore, MD 21201, USA
e-mail: margaretfurtado@hotmail.com;
mfurtado@mail.umaryland.edu

authors strongly recommended a systematic assessment of the micronutrient status in all candidates for bariatric surgery.

Vitamins and minerals serve as essential cofactors in a number of biological processes that may affect body weight regulation, including appetite, metabolic rate, nutrient absorption, thyroid and adrenal gland function, energy storage, glucose homeostasis, and neural activities [1]. Therefore, vitamin/mineral repletion and adherence is imperative for successful long-term weight management.

The majority of B-complex vitamins, significant for proper metabolism of carbohydrates and integral in normal neural functions that regulate appetite, have been determined to be deficient among some preoperative patients with severe obesity [3]. These include iron deficiencies, which may diminish energy use and have been reported in approximately 50 % of preoperative bariatric patients with severe obesity. Additionally, zinc and selenium deficiencies have been reported, as well as suboptimal levels of vitamins A, C, and E – all imperative for regulation of energy production and many other processes in the body related to body weight regulation [3–5].

Overview of General Vitamin/Mineral Deficiency Risk After Bariatric Surgery

Overall, the risk of vitamin/mineral deficiencies after bariatric surgery continues to be relatively high, particularly after surgical procedures that impact the digestion and absorption of micronutrients, such as Roux-en-Y gastric bypass surgery (RYGB) and biliopancreatic diversion with or without duodenal switch (BPD/DS) [1]. RYGBP may result in significantly higher risks of vitamin B12 deficiency, as well as other B vitamins, as well as calcium and iron [1]. BPD/DS patients are at high risk for these same deficits, as well as significantly higher rates of deficiencies of fat-soluble vitamins A, D, E, and K (due to estimated fat malabsorption of ~72 % postoperative BPD/DS). These vitamins are imperative for the functioning of many biological processes that involve healthy weight body regulation [6, 7]. Additionally, as nonadherence with prophylactic vitamin/mineral regimens rises, the risk of postoperative deficiency may double [8]. Purely restrictive procedures, such as gastric banding, may still pose risks for micronutrient deficiencies related to decreases in dietary intake and/or nonadherence to the suggested vitamin/mineral regimen [1].

Vertical sleeve gastrectomy (VSG) is a newer bariatric procedure, particularly in the United States, so more research is needed to evaluate long-term vitamin/mineral recommendations and risks. However, one study that compared RYGB to VSG [9] with $n=86$ RYGB patients and $n=50$ VSG patients determined that RYGB patients displayed significantly higher vitamin B12 deficiency rates (58 % versus 18 %), vitamin D deficiency (52 % versus 32 %), and secondary hyperparathyroidism (33 % versus 14 %) than those in the VSG group.

Thiamin deficiency has been reported to be common among patients of varying bariatric procedures, including gastric banding, if there is frequent and/or intractable vomiting. Also, since a great number of micronutrient deficiencies progress with time, patients across all bariatric surgery procedures should be monitored frequently and regularly in order to screen and help prevent and/or treat micronutrient deficiencies in a timely manner [1]. Of course, the exact timetable that is necessary may vary significantly among procedures, and if there were a deemed "ideal lab monitoring schedule" postoperatively, it may not necessarily be feasible for all surgical practices or bariatric patients. The following section provides an overview of the most common vitamin/mineral deficiencies seen after bariatric surgery (Tables 12.1 and 12.2) and suggested guidelines for assessment and treatment.

Most Common Vitamin/Mineral Deficiencies S/P Bariatric Surgery: Assessment and Treatment

While thiamin is not necessarily the most common deficiency after bariatric surgery, given the risk among all of the bariatric procedures, particularly with intractable vomiting, it will be the first micronutrient discussed.

Thiamin

Thiamin (vitamin B1), which is absorbed in the proximal small intestine, may be the micronutrient deficiency evidenced across all bariatric procedures due to a combination of factors, including its short half-life (9–18 days), necessity for metabolism of carbohydrates, higher prevalence of preoperative deficiency, and rapid depletion with intractable vomiting [1]. Thiamin deficiency may be complicated by poor oral intake and prolonged vomiting and may result in anemia that is dilutional in nature when linked with the edematous high-output cardiac failure state, beriberi. Thiamin deficiency has (rarely) been reported to result in macrocytic anemia and myelodysplastic changes in bone marrow precursors, although the significance among bariatric patients has yet to be elucidated. Regardless, weight loss surgery patients whose postoperative course has been complicated by prolonged vomiting have developed Wernicke's encephalopathy, with risks of visual disturbances (including nystagmus and ptosis), ataxia, peripheral neuropathy, memory loss, confusion, apathy, disorientation, and, in some cases, even death; therefore, IV thiamin administration has been deemed appropriate in these instances [13].

Table 12.1 Guidelines for micronutrient assessment and monitoring after bariatric surgery

Micronutrient	Screening	Normal range	Additional labs	Critical range	Notes
Thiamin (B1)	Serum thiamin	10–64 ng/mL	RBC transketolase, pyruvate	Transketolase >20 %; pyruvate >1 mg/dL	Serum thiamin is a poor indicator of total body stores
Pyridoxine (B6)	PLP	5–24 ng/mL	RBC glutamic pyruvate; oxaloacetic transaminase	PLP <3 ng/mL	Consider with unresolved anemia; diabetes may influence values
Cobalamin (B12)	Serum B12	200–1,000 pm/mL	Serum and urinary methylmalonic acid (MMA) Serum homocysteine (tHcy)	Serum B12: <200 pg/mL, deficiency <400 pg/mL, suboptimal sMMA >0.376 mmol/L uMMA >3.6 mmol/mmol CRT tHcy >13.2 mmol/L	Consider MMA and tHcy when symptoms present and serum B12 200–250 pg/mL; serum b12 may miss 25–30 % of deficiency cases
Folic Acid	RBC folate	280–791 ng/mL	Urinary FIGLU; normal serum and urinary MMA; serum tHcy	RBC folate <305 nmol/L, deficiency; <227 nmol/L, anemia	Serum folate reflects recent dietary intake versus folate status; RBC folate more sensitive marker; excessive supplementation may mask B_{12} deficiency in CBC; neurological symptoms will persist
Iron	Ferritin	Males, 15–200 ng/mL; females, 12–150 ng/mL	Serum iron; TIBC	Ferritin <20 ng/mL; serum iron <50 mcg/dL; TIBC >450 mcg/dL	Low Hgb/Hct consistent with iron deficiency anemia, stage 3–4; ferritin also an acute-phase reactant, so elevated with illness and/or inflammation
Vitamin A	Plasma retinol	20–80 mcg/dL	RBP	Plasma retinol <10 mcg/dL	Ocular findings may suggest diagnosis
Vitamin D	25-OH vitamin D	25–40 ng/mL	Serum phosphorus; alkaline phosphatase; serum PTH; urinary calcium	Serum 25-OH vitamin D <20 ng/mL suggests deficiency; 20–30 ng/mL suggests insufficiency	With deficiency, PTH elevated, serum calcium may be low or WNL, serum phosphorus may decrease, and serum alkaline phosphatase increases
Vitamin E	Plasma alpha tocopherol	5–20 mcg/mL	Plasma lipids	<5 mcg/mL	With hyperlipidemia, use low plasma alpha tocopherol to plasma lipids (0.8 mg/g total lipid)
Vitamin K	PT	10–13 s	DCP; plasma phylloquinone	Variable	PT is not a sensitive measure of vitamin K status
Zinc	Plasma zinc	60–130 mcg/dL	RBC zinc	Plasma zinc <70 mcg/dL	Albumin is the primary binding protein for zinc, so monitor albumin levels and interpret zinc accordingly; no reliable method of determining zinc status available, but plasma zinc is the method generally used

Adapted from [1]

Table 12.2 Suggested postoperative vitamin/mineral supplementation

Supplement	Gastric band	RYGB	BPD/DS	Gastric sleeve
MVI/mineral supplement	100 % daily value	200 % daily value	200 % daily value	100 % daily value
Vitamin B12	–	350–500 mcg sublingual daily OR 1,000 mcg/month IM	–	350–500 mcg sublingual daily OR 1,000 mcg/month IM
Additional elemental calcium	1,500 mg/day, in 3 divided doses of 500–600 mg	1,500–2,000 mg/day, in 3–4 divided doses of 500–600 mg	1,800–2,400 mg/day in 3–4 divided doses of 500–600 mg	1,500 mg/day, in 3 divided doses of 500–600 mg
Additional elemental iron	–	Minimum 18–27 mg for a total of 54–65 mg elemental Fe++/day	Minimum 18–27 mg for a total of 54–65 mg elemental Fe++/day	

Adapted from [1, 10–12]

Identifying Thiamin Deficiency

- Paresthesias in lower extremities, which spread upward as it progresses
- Red, burning feet
- Memory loss
- Confusion
- Disorientation
- Ataxia [1]

Rx for Thiamin Deficiency

- B-complex, together with thiamin and magnesium supplementation, for maximal thiamin absorption and optimal neurological function
- Early symptoms of neuropathy often resolved with oral thiamin doses of 20–30 mg/day until symptoms disappear
- 50–100 mg if IV or intramuscular thiamin may be necessary for more advanced signs of neuropathy or protracted vomiting [1]

Vitamin B12

Cobalamin stores are believed to provide for a 3–5-year supply in the body and are dependent on dietary repletion and daily needs. However, RYGB patients exhibit both incomplete digestion and release of vitamin B12 from protein foods. Therefore, they are at highest risk for this deficiency, as compared to other bariatric procedures, including BPD/DS, since RYGB patients exhibit reduced gastric acidity and a decrease in HCl-producing parietal cells [1].

In terms of gastric sleeve and banding patients, one prospective, randomized trial looking at these two procedures comparatively regarding vitamin B12 deficiency risk at 1 and 3 years postoperatively discovered a 10–26 % prevalence of vitamin B12 deficiency among the VSG patients that was not evidenced among the gastric banding patients [10].

Other factors that may increase the risk of vitamin B12 deficiency include:

- Long-term vegan diet
- Malabsorption due to inadequate intrinsic factor (IF) in pernicious anemia
- Inability to release protein-bound vitamin B12 from food, particularly in hypochlorhydria and atrophic gastritis
- Resection or disease of the terminal ileum
- Medications, such as metformin, neomycin, colchicines; medications used in the treatment of inflammatory bowel disease, gastroesophageal reflux disease (GERD), and ulcers (e.g., proton pump inhibitors [PPIs]); and anticonvulsive agents [14]

Identifying Vitamin B12 Deficiency

- Paresthesias to fingers and hands.
- Macrocytic anemia (although may see a false-negative CBC with normalized MCV, MCHC, and RDW in concomitant microcytic anemia).
- Deficiency typically defined at serum vitamin B12 levels <200 pg/mL. However, up to 30 % of patients with obvious signs and symptoms of vitamin B12 deficiency may have normal serum vitamin B12 levels [15].
- Methylmalonic acid (MMA), an important intermediate in vitamin B12 metabolism, is a more accurate test for vitamin B12 screening [15].

Rx for Vitamin B12 Deficiency

- Deficiency usually resolves after several weeks of treatment with 700–2,000 mcg of vitamin B12 per week [16].

Folic Acid

Although folate absorption occurs preferentially in the proximal small bowel, it may occur along the entire length of the small intestines with postoperative adaptation [1].

Therefore, the general consensus is that folate deficiency may be corrected with 1,000 mg of folic acid per day [15].

Etiology of Potential Deficiency
- Inadequate dietary intake.
- Nonadherence with MVI (multivitamin infusion).
- Malabsorption.
- Folic acid stores can be depleted within a few months postoperatively unless replenished by MVI and dietary sources [13].
- Medications, such as anticonvulsants, oral contraceptives, and cancer-treating agents, may increase the risk of folate deficiency [14].

The gastric sleeve, although less invasive than RYGBP or BPD procedures, may result in higher risk for folate deficiency. Gehrer found 22 % of 50 postoperative sleeve patients low in folic acid. Repletion was accomplished with 1 mg po folic acid daily [9].

Identifying Folic Acid Deficiency
- Very GENERAL symptoms initially:
- Fatigue and weakness.
- Headaches.
- Difficulty concentrating.
- Palpitations.
- Diarrhea.
- In the early stages, the tongue may be red and painful leading to a smooth shiny surface in the chronic stages of deficiency.

RBC levels are more accurate in predicting tissue levels than serum folate levels, megaloblastic anemia stage 3 of folic acid deficiency [1].

Rx Folate Deficiency
- Generally agreed that folate deficiency should be corrected with 1 mg/day folic acid [15].
- Preventable with amount typically found in MVI providing 200 % of daily value (800 mcg) [15].
- Folate supplementation >1 mg/day is *not* recommended due to the potential for masking of vitamin B12 deficiency [1].
- Homocysteine is the most sensitive marker of folic acid status, in conjunction with erythrocyte folate level [15].

Iron
- RYGBP: decreased absorption coupled with reduced dietary intake of iron-rich foods (e.g., meat). Vitamin C can enhance absorption in both dietary and supplemental sources of iron.
- Cast-iron skillet may help increase absorption [1].
- Some evidence iron absorption may be an issue after sleeve gastrectomy given 10 % incidence 3 years postoperative gastric sleeve in one study [10].

Identifying Iron Deficiency
- Chronic, incessant cravings for ice (pagophagia), often accompanied by significant ingestion of ice, and/or pica (including cravings for dirt, paper, or other nonfood items)
- Pallor and increased shortness of breath, new onset, with unknown etiology
- Cravings for red meat and/or other significant sources of dietary iron
- Extreme lethargy
- Spoon-shaped nails (koilonychia) [15]

Rx Iron Deficiency
- In addition to iron found in two MVIs, menstruating women s/p GBP and adolescents of both sexes might require additional supplementation to a total of 50–100 mg elemental iron/day; long-term efficacy of this Rx is unknown [1].
- Use of two complete multivitamins with minerals (18 mg each dose or serving) providing a total of 36 mg of Fe++ customary for low-risk (non-anemic men; non-menstruating women) patients after GBP [1].
- History of anemia or change in labs may indicate need for additional supplementation [1] (Table 12.3).
- Recent research among patients status post vertical sleeve gastrectomy determined that the development of iron deficiency 1 year postoperatively was insignificant [11].

Calcium and Vitamin D

- Absorption of calcium facilitated by vitamin D in an acidic environment.
- Low vitamin D levels associated with decrease in dietary calcium absorption [15].
- PTH is considered a better calcium measure than serum calcium, with an elevated PTH level suggestive of suboptimal calcium adherence and/or absorption [15].
- Increased prevalence of low vitamin D with severe obesity and negative correlation between BMI and vitamin D levels [15].
- An inverse correlation was seen between weight loss and vitamin D status 3 months postoperatively among gastric sleeve patients [12].

Calcium Citrate Versus Calcium Carbonate
- Given the low acid in GBP, absorption of calcium carbonate is estimated to be poor.

Table 12.3 Etiologies of postoperative anemia following Roux-en-Y gastric bypass

Early-onset anemia s/p RYGB	Late-onset anemia s/p RYGB
Surgical blood loss	Iron deficiency – malabsorption, poor intake, anastomotic ulceration, gastritis, esophagitis, menorrhagia
Stress gastritis/esophagitis	Vitamin B12 deficiency
Anastomotic ulceration	Folate deficiency
Hemolysis (drug-induced, transfusion therapy, hypophosphatemia)	Thiamin deficiency
Disseminated intravascular coagulation	Riboflavin deficiency
Sepsis-induced bone marrow suppression	Niacin deficiency
Retroperitoneal/intra-abdominal hematoma	Pyridoxine deficiency
Nitrous oxide anesthesia-induced B12 depletion	Vitamin C deficiency
Acute folate deficiency	Copper deficiency
Perioperative thrombotic thrombocytopenic purpura	

Adapted from [13]

- Calcium citrate is better absorbed versus calcium carbonate 22–27 % even among non-bariatric surgery patients, regardless of empty stomach versus meals [15].

Vitamins A, E, K and Zinc

- BPD/DS: decreased intestinal dietary fat absorption r/t delay in mixing of gastric and pancreatic enzymes with bile until the final 50–100 cm of the ileum.
- BPD shown to decrease fat absorption by as much as 72 %, which may significantly increase the risks for deficiencies such as vitamins A, D, E, and K [15].
- Zinc absorption has been found to be significantly decreased (from 32.3 % to 13.6 % in one study [17] at 6 months postoperative RYGB, and no effect of supplement type was observed).
- Gastric sleeve patients may be at risk for zinc deficiency, as one study on sleeve gastrectomy patients cited 34 % postoperative deficiency [9].

Copper

- Absorbed by the stomach and proximal gut, but rarely measured in RYGBP or BPD/DS patients [13].
- Deficiency can cause anemia and myelopathy, similar to that found in deficiency of vitamin B12 [13].
- Two cases of copper deficiency reported in RYGBP, both presenting with ataxia and paresthesias [18, 19].
- Copper status needs to be examined in RYGBP and BPD/DS patients presenting with s/s of neuropathy and normal vitamin B12 levels [19].

Identifying Copper Deficiency
- Numbness and tingling of hands and/or fingers (paresthesias).
- Ataxia and/or difficulty walking or clumsy gait.
- Caution is advised when patients are taking zinc hair/nail formulas without copper [1].

Rx Copper Deficiency
May include 2–4 mg of elemental copper/day, depending on the level of deficiency [1]

Selenium

- Micronutrient deficiencies have been associated with reversible and irreversible cardiomyopathic processes. Recently, a report was cited of selenium deficiency secondary to bariatric surgery, which was associated with life-threatening cardiomyopathy [20].
- Since 1981, ten cases of cardiomyopathy (six fatal) in humans have been linked to non-endemic acquired selenium deficiency [20]. All of the patients were on total parenteral nutrition (TPN), and the patients who survived were able to experience reversal of cardiomyopathic symptoms after a selenium compound was administered via their TPN solutions. Of note, cases that resulted in death have included patients on TPN for 2–16 years due to extensive gastrointestinal disease with glutathione peroxidase levels <10–20 % of normal values, suggestive of severe selenium deficiency [20].

Conclusion

Although there are many significant benefits typically attributed to bariatric surgery, including amelioration of severe obesity and its many accompanying comorbidities, it is imperative to recognize the risk for micronutrient deficiencies, even among patients who have had purely restrictive procedures, such as gastric banding. What is more, with increasing potential for malabsorption of micronutrients seen with procedures such as Roux-en-Y gastric bypass surgery, BPD/DS, and, to a certain extent, vertical sleeve gastrectomy, diligent screening, assessment, and treatment of micronutrient deficiencies may not only be prudent but may also help prevent potentially severe consequences, including, in some cases, death. Therefore, it is imperative that bariatric surgery centers worldwide adopt guidelines for regular screening, assessment, and treatment of vitamin/mineral deficiencies, both pre- and postoperatively.

Question and Answer Section

Questions

1. Appropriate management for prevention of vitamin/mineral deficiencies after Roux-en-Y gastric bypass includes all of the following EXCEPT:
   A. 200 % RDA vitamins/minerals daily
   B. 500 mg elemental calcium as calcium carbonate
   C. 500 mcg sublingual vitamin B12 daily
   D. Total of 50–100 mg elemental iron daily for menstruating women and/or patients with anemia
2. Thiamin deficiency may occur due to all of the following EXCEPT:
   A. Increased carbohydrate consumption in the diet
   B. IV dextrose administration without supplemented thiamin in bag
   C. Excessive protein intake
   D. Chronic alcohol ingestion
3. Which of the following is NOT a common warning sign of iron deficiency?
   A. Intense craving and/or ingestion of ice and sometimes items such as dirt and paper
   B. Extreme lethargy
   C. Sudden and intense craving for red meat
   D. Spoon-shaped nails
   E. Metallic taste

Answers

1. Answer is **B**. Since calcium citrate is believed to be better absorbed than calcium carbonate so the latter would not be recommended for postoperative RYGBP.
2. Answer is **C**. Since thiamin is not involved in protein metabolism but IS involved in the metabolism of carbohydrates and alcohol.
3. Answer is **E**. Since metallic taste may be indicative of zinc deficiency but typically not seen with iron deficiency. All of the other selections are suggestive of iron deficiency.

References

1. Allied Health Sciences Section Ad Hoc Nutrition Committee, Aills L, Blankenship J, Buffington C, Furtado M, Parrott J. ASMBS Allied Health Nutritional guidelines for the surgical weight loss patient. Surg Obes Relat Dis. 2008;4(5 Suppl):S73–108.
2. Ernst B, Thurnheer M, Schmid SM, Schultes B. Evidence for the necessity to systematically assess micronutrient status prior to bariatric surgery. Obes Surg. 2009;19(1):66–73.
3. Flancbaum L, Belsley S, Drake V, Colarusso T, Tayler E. Preoperative nutritional status of patients undergoing Roux-en-Y gastric bypass for morbid obesity. J Gastrointest Surg. 2006;10(7):1033–7.
4. Madan AK, Orth WS, Tichansky DS, Ternovits CA. Vitamin and trace mineral levels after laparoscopic gastric bypass. Obes Surg. 2006;16(5):603–6.
5. Reitman A, Friedrich I, Ben-Amotz L, Levy Y. Low plasma antioxidants and normal plasma B vitamins and homocysteine in patients with severe obesity. Isr Med Assoc J. 2002;4(8):590–3.
6. Alvarez-Leite JI. Nutrient deficiencies secondary to bariatric surgery. Curr Opin Clin Nutr Metab Care. 2004;7:569–75.
7. Bloomberg RD, Fleishman A, Nalle JE, Herron DM, Kini S. Nutritional deficiencies following bariatric surgery: what have we learned? Obes Surg. 2005;15(2):145–54. Review.
8. Brolin RE, Gorman RC, Milgrim LM, Kenler HA. Multivitamin prophylaxis in prevention of post-gastric bypass vitamin and mineral deficiencies. Int J Obes. 1991;15(10):661–7.
9. Gehrer S, Kern B, Peters T, Christoffel-Courtin C, Peterli R. Fewer nutrient deficiencies after Laparoscopic Sleeve Gastrectomy (LSG) than after Laparoscopic Roux-en-Y-Gastric Bypass (LRYGB)- a prospective study. Obes Surg. 2010;20(4):447–53.
10. Himpens J, Dapri G, Cadière GB. A prospective, randomized study between laparoscopic gastric banding and laparoscopic isolated sleeve gastrectomy: results after 1 and 3 years. Obes Surg. 2006;16(11):1450–6.
11. Hakeam HA, O'Regan PJ, Salem AM, Bamehriz FY, Eldali AM. Impact of laparoscopic sleeve gastrectomy on iron indices: 1 year follow-up. Obes Surg. 2009;19(11):1491–6.
12. Ruiz-Tovar J, Oller I, Tomas A, Llavero C, Arroyo A, Calero A, et al. Mid-term effects of sleeve gastrectomy on calcium metabolism parameters, vitamin D and Parathyroid Hormone (PTH) in morbidly obese women. Obes Surg. 2012;22(5):797–801.
13. Marinella MA. Anemia following Roux-en-Y surgery for morbid obesity: a review. South Med J. 2008;10(101):1024–31.
14. Charney P, Malone A, editors. ADA pocket guide to nutrition assessment. Chicago: American Dietetic Association; 2004.
15. Malinowski SS. Nutritional and metabolic complications of bariatric surgery. Am J Med Sci. 2006;331:219–25.
16. Kaplan LM. Pharmacological therapies for obesity. Gastroenterol Clin North Am. 2005;34:91–104.
17. Ruz M, Carrasco F, Rojas P, Codoceo J, Inostroza J, Basfi-fer K, et al. Zinc absorption and zinc status are reduced after Roux-en-Y gastric bypass: a randomized study using 2 supplements. Am J Clin Nutr. 2011;94(4):1004–11.
18. Kumar N, McEvoy KM, Ahlskog JE. Myelopathy due to copper deficiency following gastrointestinal surgery. Arch Neurol. 2003;60(12):1782–5.
19. Kumar N, Ahlskog JE, Gross Jr JB. Acquired hypocupremia after gastric surgery. Clin Gastroenterol Hepatol. 2004;2(12):1074–9.
20. Boldery R, Fielding G, Rafter T, Pascoe AL, Scalia GM. Deficiency of selenium secondary to weight loss (Bariatric) surgery associated with life-threatening cardiomyopathy. Heart Lung Circ. 2007; 16(2):123–6.

Managing Common Nutrition Problems After Bariatric Surgery

13

Claire M. LeBrun

Chapter Objectives

1. To be able to identify nutrition complications in the bariatric surgery patient
2. To learn how to effectively treat common nutrition problems in bariatric surgery patients
3. To be able to assess and correctly treat common vitamin and mineral deficiencies
4. To ensure that you relay the importance of taking advised vitamin and mineral supplements to your bariatric surgery patients daily for the rest of their lives

Introduction

Managing common nutrition problems after bariatric surgery requires clear understanding of the anatomical changes that occur with each type of bariatric surgery, the nutritional implications of these changes after surgery, when to expect these complications to arise, and how to address them. The chapter begins by briefly describing the types of bariatric surgery, changes that may contribute to nutrition problems after surgery, and, finally, how to recognize and treat potential nutrition issues that arise after the surgery.

Types of Bariatric Surgeries

Restrictive Procedures

Surgical options for the morbidly obese reduce body weight by any of the three following mechanisms: restriction of dietary intake, malabsorption of nutrients, and alteration of hormonal metabolism (e.g., decreased ghrelin, pancreatic polypeptide gene PPY, increased leptin, etc.) [1].

The adjustable gastric band (AGB), a purely restrictive procedure, creates a small gastric pouch of 15–30 cm by placing a saline-filled band around the upper curvature of the stomach, just below the gastroesophageal junction. This band is attached to a port that is subcutaneously placed just under the patient's rib cage. The saline fills are deferred until about 6–8 weeks after surgery to give time for gastric swelling to decrease. There are no apparent changes of gut hormones in this procedure [2]. The sleeve gastrectomy (SG), another restrictive procedure, involves removing approximately 60–80 % of the proximal stomach, along with the fundus and greater curvature, but leaving the pylorus and part of the atrium intact [3]. This surgery was originally designed to be the safer, first stage of the biliopancreatic diversion with duodenal switch (BPD/DS) or the Roux-en Y gastric bypass (RNYGB), to help the extremely obese patient (>60 BMI) lose some weight and reduce their comorbidities before completing the second part of the surgery or the malabsorptive stage. It has been successful enough to serve as a stand-alone procedure. The removal of the fundus contributes to this surgery's success, as this is where the appetite-stimulating hormone ghrelin is produced and, therefore, its presence is greatly diminished after the procedure, aiding to the patient's weight loss ability. However, because the SG removes the parietal cells, patients also have reduced gastric acid production and thereby a decreased absorption of B12, iron, and calcium [4].

Combined Restrictive and Malabsorptive Procedures

The biliopancreatic diversion (BPD) is a procedure that produces a minor restriction (200–300 ml) with a considerable intestinal bypass (60 % of the small intestine), making it more malabsorptive than restrictive. A later modification to this procedure is the duodenal switch (BPD/DS), which

C.M. LeBrun, MPH, RD, LD (✉)
Department of Surgery, George Washington Medical Faculty Associates, 2150 Pennsylvania Avenue, NW Suite 6B-412, Washington, DC 20037, USA
e-mail: clebrun@mfa.gwu.edu; cmlebrun@gmail.com

preserves the distal stomach and pylorus (similar to the SG) while maintaining the common channel or degree of malabsorption. Since dietary fats are absorbed in the proximal two-thirds of the jejunum, fat malabsorption and essential fatty acid deficiencies are more likely to occur in this procedure, since the common channel is shorter. Both procedures are less commonly done now due to their high incidence of postoperative complications, most notably protein, calorie, and vitamin-mineral deficiencies due to the increased malabsorption resulting from the shorter common channel.

The Roux-en-Y gastric bypass (RNYGB) procedure, which now comprises 70–75 % of all bariatric procedures done, is both restrictive and malabsorptive. In the RYNGB, a small pouch (usually 30 ml) is created and separated from the distal stomach and then anastomosed (10–13 mm diameter) to the proximal jejunum, essentially bypassing the duodenum and the proximal part of the jejunum [5]. This new channel, which is connected to the gastric pouch, is called the Roux limb, or alimentary limb, as it works by transporting nutrients from the pouch to the small intestine. Roux limbs vary in length but are usually 75–150 cm [6].

There is a second entero-enteric anastomosis made by connecting the duodenum to the distal end of the jejunum. The pancreatic and biliary enzymes enter just below this second anastomosis, into what is known as the common channel. As previously noted, the shorter the common channel (and the longer the Roux limb), the higher the risk for nutrient deficiencies since less nutrient absorption will occur. Most common channels are 50–100 cm long [7]. The combination of gastric restriction and malabsorption, along with gut hormone changes reducing hunger and the reduction of complications as compared to the BPD and DS, makes this surgery considered the "gold standard" of all the bariatric procedures [6].

Preoperative Nutrition

It is not uncommon to see micronutrient deficiencies prior to surgery, as stated in a previous chapter on preoperative assessment (see Chap. 9). Micronutrient deficiencies most prevalent prior to bariatric surgery in order of occurrence are vitamin D (55–80 %) and iron (25–50 %), with a smaller number of B12 and thiamine deficiencies also found [8]. Surgeons should routinely test their surgical candidates for micronutrient deficiencies prior to surgery, given that there is a known association between micronutrient deficiency and postoperative complications in animal studies [9]. Deficiencies are much easier to correct prior to surgery than after surgery; they are especially more difficult to manage after malabsorptive procedures.

Research has shown that a 10 % excess body weight (EBW) loss prior to surgery helps to shrink the liver, thereby reducing surgical complications, operating time, blood loss, and hospital stay. These factors, in turn, improve mortality and also help the patient recover more quickly [4]. One recent study of 150 gastric bypass patients showed that a higher preoperative excess body weight (EBW) loss correlated with a higher EBW loss 3 and 4 years after surgery and therefore greater success with the surgery [10].

Postoperative Nutrition Issues

Most nutritional complications after weight loss surgery are due to inadequate food intake (secondary to reduced stomach size and appetite, malabsorption, and/or incomplete digestion, or often all of the above, in the case of the combined restrictive and malabsorptive procedures. With all bariatric surgeries, there is a reduced intake of food, and less gastric acid and pepsin available, which limits the gut's ability to break down and absorb macro- and micronutrients. The bypass of the first one-third of the small intestine, in the case of the RYNGB procedure, and closer to the first two-thirds of the small intestine in the BPD and BPD/DS procedures contributes to the malabsorption of several macro- and micronutrients, namely, protein, iron, calcium, vitamin D, folate, and B12 with RYNGB surgery and, in addition, the fat-soluble vitamins (A, D, E, and K) with BPD and BPD/DS [11]. Also the prophylactic use of histamine-2 receptor antagonists (H2 blockers), or proton pump inhibitors (PPIs) prescribed by the surgeon to the patient, further reduces the gastric acid secretion and therefore the absorption of iron, calcium, and B12.

The patient's possible nonadherence to dietary and vitamin-mineral supplement guidelines plays into the frequency of nutritional complications.

Early Nutrition Concerns

The main concerns for the first couple of weeks after surgery are ensuring that the patient gets adequate fluids and sufficient protein, in this order. Due to the lack of evidence-based recommendations for diet advancement, facilities and surgeons vary their postoperative diet progression recommendations. However, to help patients adjust slowly to their new anatomy, heal from their surgery faster by enhancing their protein intake, maximize their weight loss, and avoid gastrointestinal complications such as rupture of staple lines, chronic vomiting, and strictures, patients are normally placed on a diet progression usually starting with the liquid phase. To preserve healing of the new gastric anatomy and prevent ulcers, all patients should be instructed to avoid caffeine and alcohol for the first 4–8 weeks, which are known gastric irritants. Usually, the patient is placed on low-sugar clear liquids for the first 1–2 days; then advances to low-fat, low-sugar full liquids for the next 1–2 weeks; then puree/soft foods for 1–2 more weeks; and then eventually to a regular solid food diet by 6–8 weeks after surgery. As they progress to more solid foods, it is helpful to remind patients that they no longer have the ability to digest chunks of food and that all food should be chewed to a pureed consistency before swallowed. In general, moist, soft foods in the forms of stews, casseroles, and soups; well-chopped, ground, moist meats; crunchy or crisp, in the case of grains; and canned products will be easier to tolerate than dry, tough, or stringy foods such as well-done red meat, overcooked chicken or fish, celery, pea pods, fresh pineapple, broccoli and asparagus stems, citrus membranes, popcorn or soft grains such as bread, undercooked rice, and pasta [11]. After AGB fills, patients are usually counseled to revert back to a liquid protein diet for 2–3 days and then slowly resume regular solid foods. Gastric sleeve patients should advance their diet slowly due to their long surgical staple line [4].

Dehydration is one of the most common reasons bariatric patients need to return to the hospital after discharge from surgery [12]. During the first week or two after surgery, patients often struggle to drink enough fluids. The smaller pouch (no matter what size the pouch they were given), which is also edematous from the recent surgery, usually makes it difficult for the patient to drink more than about an ounce at a time. In addition, the patients who have had RYNGB or GS often experience an altered sense of taste and smell, usually described as a heightened sensitivity to sweets and/or an "off taste to water or other fluids" [13]. Patients find that liquids are uncomfortable to swallow or may taste badly; thus, they may avoid drinking and become dehydrated. A possible cause of the patient's dysgeusia and dysosmia is thought to be related to the decrease of ghrelin production, which is an appetite-stimulating hormone significantly reduced after RYNGB and GS [14]. With confirmation of the Tong study in 2011, reduced ghrelin levels inhibit a feeling of satiety, which lessens the olfactory response to the usual pleasurable taste and smell of food [15].

It is important to prepare the patient for this and work with them to find individual solutions of tolerable liquids, ideally one with protein to help them work on building up their protein intake. Sometimes referring them to salty, sour, or bitter foods is preferred and more tolerable, as they are able to advance into these foods. Some examples might be to try adding unflavored protein to a salty soup or bitter herbal tea or eating plain yogurt rather than fruit-flavored yogurts.

To prevent dehydration, it is helpful to counsel patients to drink one ounce of fluid every 15 min. Their initial goal should be a minimum of 40 oz per day, gaining up to an optimal level of 64 oz of fluids per day, as soon as they are able. Since sugary liquids may cause dumping syndrome (explained below), low-calorie beverages are optimal, besides protein supplements, which should also be low in sugar. Drinks are often better tolerated when they are as cold as possible and perhaps covered with a lid to inhibit odors from wafting up to their noses. Some patients find drinking cold beverages painful to their new pouch and therefore tend to tolerate warmer beverages best. This usually resolves within the first couple weeks. As sometimes best described, they should be sipping on some type of fluid continuously throughout the day.

Symptoms of dehydration are dark and strong smelling urine, dry mouth, headache, nausea, fatigue, and muscle aches.

Nausea and vomiting may be caused by overeating or eating too quickly (chunks of food cannot be fully digested), drinking with meals, eating foods that are too spicy or too high in fat or sugar, or not taking their PPIs or H2 blockers. To prevent nausea, it is important to advise patients to eat slowly, to chew food to a pureed consistency, and to stop eating as soon as they feel full. They should be reminded to drink liquids only between meals and to follow the 30:30 rule of not drinking within 30 min before or after a meal. This rule does not really need to be emphasized until the solid food stage, as most of their meals are of the liquid type and their new anatomy will usually be resistant to combining the two. H2 blockers or PPIs are usually prescribed to patients after surgery to help reduce nausea and gastroesophageal reflux disease (GERD). If a patient complains of chronic vomiting and nausea, it is best for them to go back to clear liquids for 1–2 days to rest their gut. If vomiting still persists, they should contact their health-care practitioner to rule out other medical issues such as stenosis, ulcer, strictures, etc.

Gastroesophageal reflux disease or GERD is one of the most common comorbidities of morbid obesity, with an incidence as high as 50–70 % of patients seeking bariatric procedures. RYNGB has been considered as one of the most effective bariatric procedures to eradicate GERD due to the success of the weight loss combined with the absence of gastric and bile acid in the pouch [16]. The AGB procedure normally helps reduce incidence of GERD in the average patient, unless they present with weak esophageal body motility preoperatively – diagnosed by manometry. The RYNGB appears to be the most promising procedure of the three for those patients with chronic GERD issues as it reduces both gastric and bile acids from the stomach and therefore the distal esophagus, along with an increase in gastric motility and weight loss [17].

GERD occurs most commonly after LGS, where it affects an average of 67 % of patients 1 month after surgery. This usually resolves completely within 2 years status post [4]. The increased incidence of GERD comes from removing the angle of His, which impairs the cardia's anti-reflux action

[17]. It may be due to the resection of the natural gastric pacemaker and lack of gastric fundus tone, which may adjust over time. In the meantime, continue to counsel the patient to eat small but frequent meals and low-acid and minimal spicy foods and to avoid drinking fluids with meals. Refer the chronic GERD patient back to the medical team for reevaluation for a possible increase in their PPIs. Because of their heightened risk of GERD after GS surgery, patients with prior history of chronic GERD, weak esophageal body motility, and/or hiatal hernias are not considered good candidates for GS and are often encouraged to consider alternate procedures such as RYNGB.

Flatulence – Many patients complain of gas and bloating immediately after surgery. In part, this is residual from the surgery, as in order to do it laparoscopically, a large amount of air is pumped into the patient's abdomen to provide the surgeon room to operate. There is also an air-gas test just after surgery to look for possible leaks, which contributes to increased flatulence after surgery. In the case of malabsorptive procedures, there is also an increase in transient time with any bypass of the small intestine. Increased flatulence may also be a sign of temporary lactose intolerance (see later), especially if combined with abdominal pain and diarrhea. To help counsel patients who complain of gas, it may be helpful to recommend not to use straws, reduction in gum chewing, and less gas-forming foods (broccoli, onions, garlic, legumes, cauliflower, lactose-containing foods, etc.). Over the counter products like Gas-X and Devrom (flatulence deodorizer) are sometimes helpful for these patients.

Lactose intolerance may occur temporarily after RYNGB and BPD surgery, even if the patient had no history or knowledge of intolerance prior to surgery [11].

Symptoms of lactose intolerance are gas, bloating, cramping, and diarrhea after drinking milk or eating soft dairy products such as cottage cheese, ice cream, and soft cheeses. Lactose-free milk, lite yogurts, and hard cheeses are usually tolerated, unless the patient's intolerance is severe. Milk or milk-like products are often initially not appealing or desired by patients, due to their creaminess, richness, or perceived inability to digest. As alternatives to these types of protein drinks, you may encourage patients to try thin, fruit-juice-like protein drinks or to mix unflavored protein powder with a sugar-free fruit-juice-like beverage. Sometimes the patient will no longer like the sweetness of protein drinks, in which case, you may suggest that they use an unflavored protein powder mixed into a broth, pureed bean or cream soup, or hot cereal. There are also some high-protein savory soups that could be recommended.

If the patient is willing to use milk but intolerant to lactose, unsweetened or original-flavored soymilks may be used since they are complete proteins. Early out from surgery, using almond, rice, hemp, or coconut milks are discouraged, due to their low protein and sometimes high sugar content.

Protein energy malnutrition (PEM) – Protein is primarily absorbed in the jejunum and mid-ileum; therefore, malabsorptive procedures that bypass these gut areas have an increased risk for protein malnutrition. Since the most common procedures do not bypass these areas, PEM is mostly due to the reduced intake of calories. The reduced level of hydrochloric acid and pepsinogen in the malabsorptive procedures also contributes to a reduce level of protein digestion and absorption. The restrictive space of the pouch, anorexia or decreased appetite, heightened sense of taste and smell (which tends to be toward protein-rich supplements in particular), and the limited choices of tolerable protein sources contribute to this dilemma. Also, other postoperative circumstances such as chronic vomiting, diarrhea, depression, and alcohol consumption may exacerbate PEM. The patient's reduction in appetite lasts anywhere from 1 to 3 months for most bariatric patients (except for AGB, which seems to dissipate much sooner due to lack of early restriction), and the patient's sense of fullness comes on very quickly, especially in the first 8 weeks after surgery. Usually, the amount of food they can ingest starts off very small, about one to two teaspoons and then will increase by about an ounce per week from the date of surgery, with liquids progressing about twice as fast as solids (i.e., at week 2, they may be able to eat 2 oz of pureed foods and possibly drink up to 4 oz of fluids at one time).

Recommended levels of protein after bariatric surgery to maintain muscle tissue or fat-free mass vary from 60–120 g per day, with the higher amounts needed for the more malabsorptive procedures. A more accurate method would be to suggest a protein level of 1.5–2.1 g/kg of ideal body weight [18].

The quality of protein is also an important factor with complete protein sources usually coming from animal products. Whey protein, which comes from cows, has been shown to be easy to digest and has been shown to promote satiety better than casein, another milk protein [19]. Liquid protein supplements are a great way to increase protein intake as they are easier to ingest as well as being convenient. Aside from whey protein, other sources of complete protein are casein, egg albumin, soy, and any collagen blends that are enhanced with the missing amino acids to create complete proteins. For those patients with lactose intolerance, ensure that they use lactose-free protein sources such as whey protein isolate (whey protein concentrate may have traces of lactose), soy, egg, and pea, rice collagen protein blends with a protein digestibility corrected amino acid (PDCAA) score closest to 100, meaning that the protein source contains all the correct proportions of the nine essential amino acids [20].

Clinical signs of protein malnutrition are edema, alopecia, low serum albumin levels (<3.5 g/dL), nausea, and reduced weight loss [21]. Serum albumin levels may or may not reflect PEM due to their longer half-life [22]. Prealbumin is a better short-term marker of protein deficiency as it has a half-life of only 1–2 days [11]. While rare in strictly malabsorptive procedures (0–2 %), protein inadequacy has been recorded in 13 % of patients after RYGB [23] and 7–21 % after BPD [11].

It is generally recommended for post-bariatric patients to aim for 60–80 g of protein or 1.0–1.5 g per kg of ideal body weight (IBW) per day. In the initial weeks after surgery, due to healing of the new pouch and the patient's reluctance to eat or drink, it may be more realistic to suggest that the patient strive to reach 40 g of protein per day and then adapt to 50 g per day within 2 weeks status post, aiming for the 60–80 g as soon as they are able (ideally by 3–4 weeks status post). Usually, two to three protein drinks per day, during the liquid through pureed phase, will cover their protein needs. As they are able to achieve their protein goals through protein-rich foods, they may phase out their liquid protein supplement intake.

Dumping syndrome usually occurs only with RNYGB but may also occur sometimes with GS. There are two types of dumping: "early" and "late." After RNYGB, as many as 70 % of patients may experience early dumping syndrome and 5 % may experience severe symptoms [24]. With the lack of a pyloric sphincter after the RYNGB, the undigested carbohydrates in the new gastric pouch may drop through the anastomosis into the small intestine too quickly and therefore cause an osmotic effect of pulling extracellular fluid into the bowel to restore isotonicity. This in turn causes the patient to have an array of simultaneous side effects such as diarrhea, nausea, hypotension, bloating, cold sweats, tachycardia, emesis, and dizziness. These symptoms usually occur within 10–30 min after eating and resolve within 1–2 h. While no anatomical damage occurs, the patient usually feels fairly drained afterward.

Fortunately, most of the time, dumping syndrome may be reduced or eliminated by ensuring that the patient eats small, frequent meals, containing low glycemic index and high-protein foods, and avoids drinking fluids while eating. Highly refined carbohydrates and sweets, especially in the absence of protein, also cause a quick emptying of the new pouch or "early dumping."

RYNGB patients may also experience what is known as "late dumping," or *reactive hypoglycemia* or *hyperinsulinemic hypoglycemia*, which generally occurs 1–4 h after eating and is usually caused by infrequent eating or consuming a meal of simple sugars or refined carbohydrates in absence of protein. Late dumping occurs in 25 % of patients who have early dumping [25]. Most types of dumping improve as the patient modifies their way of eating to include less simple sugars, more protein, and adequate meal frequency.

Halitosis often occurs during the low-calorie, liquid-to-soft food diet phase. In part, malodorous breath is a result of ketone breakdown for energy, in the absence of stored glycogen or blood sugar in the body. This sometimes fruity odor of burning ketones is released in the breath and urine. In addition, during the early months postsurgery, there is a lack of hard, crunchy foods that normally scrape off natural bacterial buildup in the mouth. Encouraging patients to thoroughly brush the interior of their mouths helps treat this issue.

Many patients will complain of *fatigue* early out from surgery. In part, this is due to having just had major abdominal surgery, but their low intake of protein and calories is an obvious factor. It is not unusual for patients to be consuming only around 300–600 cal for the first 2–4 weeks out from surgery. Dehydration or iron deficiency anemia may also be a factors to consider.

"Postsurgery fatigue" could last for the first 3 months after surgery for some. Age is certainly a factor, with older patients often taking longer to recover than younger ones.

If the patient is a premenopausal female and experiencing fatigue or morning nausea, especially if it is beyond 2 months after surgery and they are getting adequate protein, you may encourage them to consider checking for pregnancy.

Constipation may occur in the first couple weeks postoperatively, due to the lack of residue during the liquid phase. It is not unusual for a patient to go without a bowel movement for the first 3–5 days after surgery. Constipation is also due to the low intake of solid foods and lack of fiber early out from surgery. It is preferable that the patient is consuming a low-fiber diet the first 2–3 weeks after surgery while the pouch is healing and the patient is adjusting to his/her decreased ability to break down food. The patients are encouraged to take one to two stool softeners after surgery to help promote and soften their stool, especially while they are still using narcotics, which are a main contributor to early constipation. When counseling patients with diet solutions, applesauce, hot cereals such as oatmeal, berries, and peas or legumes are usually well-tolerated, high-fiber options. As always, ensure that they are staying hydrated and that they start slowly increasing their physical activity, which is of primary importance in increasing bowel motility.

They may need to add a fiber supplement (consider methylcellulose, polycarbophil, or wheat dextrin, which are best tolerated); make sure to recommend sugar-free products to avoid excess calories and dumping syndrome.

Sometimes patients complain of *diarrhea* or *steatorrhea* after surgery, although this happens more commonly with malabsorptive procedures such as RYNGB and BPD. The cause may be due to ingestion of high-fiber or high-fat foods, but sometimes it is a sign of temporary lactose intolerance, too much malabsorption (in the case of a shorter common limb), or small bacteria overgrowth.

If your patient complains of diarrhea, have them avoid dairy, high-fiber (whole grains, fruits, and vegetables with skins), and high-fat foods, as well as caffeine and alcohol.

Ensure that they are getting adequate sugar-free or low-sugar fluids (64 oz per day).

Despite these changes, if their diarrhea persists for more than several days, have them come in to see a member of the healthcare team.

Hair loss, alopecia, or *telogen effluvium* is one of the most feared side effects of many bariatric patients prior to surgery and can be very frustrating to most when it occurs. Interestingly, our hair is always in one of two states: anagen (growth stage) and telogen (dormant or resting stage, which lasts 100–120 days before it falls out). Normally, 90 % of our hair is growing and only 10 % is dormant, which means we have a small and somewhat tolerating amount of hair shedding at any one time. However, whenever our bodies are put into an extremely stressful state (such as surgery or rapid weight loss), for self-preservation purposes, we stop putting energy into things that are not necessary to live, like hair growth. During stressful states, more of our hair is shifted into the telogen stage, which is also called "telogen effluvium." Once the hair is shifted into this stage, there is no possibility of reverting it back to the anagen growth stage, and therefore, it will stay in this stage until it falls out, which may take up to six full months. Some other causes of alopecia are high fevers, severe infection, acute physical trauma, chronic debilitating illness (such as cancer), hormonal disruption (like pregnancy, childbirth, or stopping hormone therapy), anorexia, thyroid or autoimmune disease heavy metal toxicity, and certain medications like beta-blockers, anticoagulants, retinoids, and immunizations. It is important to have a medical professional rule these possibilities out, especially if there is no nutritional cause detected.

When alopecia occurs between 3 and 6 months after surgery, it is most likely a result of the stress of major surgery and low calorie intake. However, there is a possibility that it is due to deficiencies in any of the following: protein, iron, essential fatty acids, biotin, or zinc – especially if the alopecia starts 6 months or later after surgery.

To prevent hair shedding, ensure that your patients consume at least 60–80 g of protein/day, a multivitamin/mineral that provides 15–40 mg zinc, and 18–36 mg of iron. Additional intake of essential fatty acids (fish or flaxseed oils), l-lysine, and 2,500–3,000 mcg of biotin have been shown to be helpful [26].

Obesity and weight loss are known risk factors for gallstone formation. Therefore, *cholelithiasis* or *cholesterol gallstone formation* is very common after bariatric surgery. Within 1 year after surgery, 30–50 % of bariatric patients have cholelithiasis due to their rapid weight loss [27]. Any patient who complains of right upper quadrant pain and nausea should be evaluated for gallstones. It is prudent to put all patients on a gallstone-solubilizing agent such as Actigall for the first 6 months after bariatric surgery. Alternately, a minimum of 10 g of fish oil per day has been found to reduce gallstone formation [28].

Pregnancy

Women often have had fertility issues with central obesity and may be accustomed to not using birth control. After the surgery and with weight loss, there is an increased likelihood of premenopausal women being more fertile and therefore an increased chance of pregnancy [29].

Late Nutrition Issues

Eating disorders after weight loss surgery are not common but do occur. Despite a decreased drive for thinness, less bulimia, plus improved body satisfaction and quality of life, more than half (51 %) of RNYGB patients, 8 years out from surgery, reported either engaging in binge eating or night eating syndrome during the previous month [1].

In an analysis conducted on 59 patients 18–35 months post-RNYGB by de Zwaan et al., bulimic episodes were reported by 25 % of the participants. Also, vomiting for weight and shape reasons was reported by 12 % of the participants, 2 years after surgery. The bulimic episodes were significantly associated with a preoperative binge eating disorder (BED), with more eating-related and general psychopathology after surgery and with less weight loss [30].

Another study by Gorin et al. looked at the effect of mood and eating disorders 6 months out from RYNGB surgery. They analyzed 196 patients and compared those with history of mood and eating disorders (10.2 %) to those of just a mood disorder (24 %) and to those with just an eating disorder (36.7 %) to those with neither (29 %) 6 months after surgery. This study found that the patients with history of both mood and eating disorders were more prone to noncompliance, which included more readmissions to the hospital, dietary violations, and less or no structured exercise. Despite this difference, they ended up losing the same amount of weight as the other participants and reported an improvement in their quality of life [31]. The limitation of this latter study was that they looked at the patients 6 months postoperatively, which is relatively early for eating disorders to start, or to reoccur, considering they should still be actively losing weight.

Anorexia may occur if a patient waits too long to advance with their diet progression [32] and may be exacerbated by inadequate protein intake or a zinc deficiency, both of which can increase nausea. The restrictive and malabsorptive features of RYGB, BPD, and BPD/DS help the patient lose weight fairly quickly after surgery, reaching a nadir usually by 12–18 months after surgery. With the purely restrictive AGB, weight loss is slower, in part due to the lack of restriction within the first 6 months and in part due to the fact that the patients can override volume limitations by snacking on high-calorie liquids or solids throughout the day.

Some research has shown the reoccurrence of eating disorders during the later stages after surgery and may be associated with inadequate weight loss or regaining of weight. Segal and colleagues have proposed a new diagnosis for these patients called "postsurgical eating avoidance disorder (PSEAD)" [33]. It seems appropriate to advise that patients with history of eating disorders should have more intense follow-up with the bariatric team after surgery.

A *weight gain or weight plateau*, which may or may not coincide with the return of hunger for the patient, is always distressing for the patient and a possible red flag for the practitioner. Weight plateaus happen throughout the course of any type of weight loss; however, it is common for the patient to assume it is due to something they did wrong. As a practitioner, it is important to inquire about their protein and calorie intake. Often, their weight loss slows down when they are not getting enough protein or ingesting too many calories. Ensuring that they are getting regular exercise is also important and may be a cause of stalled weight loss. However, if they are engaging in muscle-building exercise, this may also cause a temporary fluid retention, which could also slow down actual weight loss on the scale. It may be helpful to remind them that with any weight loss regime, there are normal periods of weight plateaus and possible slight gains with fluid retention. If your patient is a premenopausal female, you may consider checking for pregnancy.

Permanent weight plateaus are likely to occur after about 1–1.5 years from RYNGB and GS surgeries and about 2–3 years after AGB surgery. By this time, the patient often states that they feel increased hunger and reduced ability to keep continued focus on their calorie and protein intake.

Changes in Bone Metabolism

Due to low stomach acid (gastric acid is normally developed in the distal area of the stomach) and the bypass of the duodenum in malabsorptive procedures, calcium absorption is decreased. Within 3–9 months of a RNYGB surgery, patients display an increase in bone reabsorption, which corresponds to a decrease in bone density; therefore, their calcium need increases during this rapid weight loss stage [34]. Calcium supplements need to be taken in the form of calcium citrate, instead of the more commonly available calcium carbonate, to enhance absorption. Citrate, unlike carbonate, provides an acidic environment, ideal for calcium absorption in the new low-acid pouch. Suggested calcium intake after bariatric surgery increases from the RDA of 1,000–1,200 mg per day to 1,500–2,000 mg per day, to counteract a decreased ability to absorb calcium. Since only 600 mg of calcium can be absorbed at any one time, two to three doses of 500–600 mg of calcium should be taken per day [11].

The reduced intake and absorption of vitamin D and calcium are not the only factors that contribute to bone loss after bariatric surgery. A recent study looking at patients at both 6 and 18 months after RNYGB surgery found that the bone turnover markers of serum osteocalcin, bone alkaline phosphatase, and N-telopeptide (NTX) plus vitamin D levels were all increased while leptin levels were reduced. After regression analysis was complete for this study, the increase in specifically NTX was found to correlate with the decrease in leptin, suggesting that the hormonal changes after bariatric surgery may also contribute to bone loss [35].

Fat-soluble vitamins – Outside of vitamin D deficiency, which is common with all bariatric surgeries, the deficiencies of fat-soluble vitamins A, D, E, and K are more common with the malabsorptive surgeries, especially BPD where only about 32 % of the dietary fat is absorbed [7, 36].

Vitamin D deficiency – The most common deficiency both pre- and postsurgery. The principal site of dietary vitamin D absorption is the jejunum and the ileum; vitamin D is a fat-soluble hormone that is synthesized by the human skin upon exposure to cholecalcifrol (ultraviolet-B radiation) from the sun, as well as a dietary form of vitamin D called ergosterol, found naturally in fatty fish and eggs and fortified in US milk, infant formula, some orange juice, cereals, and soy products. Vitamin D is essential for calcium absorption and has been shown to decrease the incidence of inflammatory diseases such as some cancers, heart disease, and osteoporosis [37–39]. Vitamin D deficiency is also common 1 year after DS and BPD surgeries and detected by testing OH-hydroxy D levels.

Postoperative requirements of intake are 2,000 IU vitamin D3 to prevent deficiency. Unfortunately, 66–80 % preoperative bariatric patients have 25-OH vitamin D levels below 32, causing an automatic deficiency after surgery, with a lessened ability to ingest and absorb this hormone. Postoperative data show that 45 % of these patients continue being vitamin D insufficient despite being supplemented with vitamin D3 [40]. However, the decrease in BMI seems to correlate with an increase in vitamin D levels.

Hyperoxaluria – Gallstones can develop in up to 30 % of patients who experience considerable weight loss. The administration of ursodiol (300 mg four times a day) increases the solubility of bile salts and reduces the risk of developing gallstones to approximately 2 % [41–43].

Ursodiol is given as long as the patient continues to lose considerable weight (3 % of body weight per month) or for the first 6 months after an operation [41].

Question and Answer Section

Questions

1. Your patient is 4 weeks s/p RYNGB and complains about chronic fatigue. Which of the following choices is *least* likely to be the cause of his/her fatigue?
   A. Inadequate protein
   B. Dehydration
   C. Inadequate calories
   D. Iron deficiency
2. Your female patient is 7 months s/p GS surgery and is complaining of hair shedding; which of the following is *least* likely to be the cause?
   A. Iron deficiency
   B. Stress of the surgery
   C. Inadequate protein
   D. EFA deficiency
3. Your patient is 1 year and 3 months out from surgery and states that he is struggling with increased hunger, both with and between meals. His weight loss has stabilized. What would be the most important strategies for him to be doing to prevent weight regain (select all that apply)?
   A. Keeping food records and ensuring that he keeps his calories between 1,200 and 1,400 per day
   B. Ensuring that his protein levels are between 60 and 80 g per day
   C. Exercising at least 30 min per day
   D. Not drinking liquids with meals
   E. Nothing as he has achieved his goal
4. Your patient is 17 months out from surgery and complains of dizziness, irritability, and lightheadedness in the late afternoon. Your patient has no history of diabetes and blood pressure is WNL. What is the most likely cause of these symptoms and the best course of action?
   A. Low blood sugar – assess diet for protein and frequency of eating; ensure protein at each meal and snack.
   B. Low blood sugar – increase calories and frequency of eating.
   C. Insulinoma – refer to endocrinology.
   D. Dehydration – assess and increase fluid intake.
5. Your patient is 5 weeks out from gastric bypass surgery and complains of low energy and frequent vomiting. Her vomiting happens every 2–3 days and is not necessarily associated with any one food. Her fluid intake consists of two protein drinks of 14 oz and 25 g of protein each and one half of a 16.9 oz water bottle. She claims she can tolerate chicken breast, mashed potatoes, raw or cooked spinach, and frozen yogurt but is avoiding most others foods for fear of getting sick. She takes 40 mg of Prevacid daily. What is most likely her issue?
   A. Protein deficiency
   B. Dehydration
   C. Ulcer
   D. Bowel obstruction
6. You have a 33-year-old female patient who is s/p 3 months RYNGB and complains of frequent nausea and vomiting after meals. Below are the possible explanations of her N/V, except for which one?
   A. Pregnancy
   B. Not chewing thoroughly enough
   C. Stricture or ulcer
   D. Drinking and eating at the same time

Answers

1. Answer: **C**. As long as they are getting enough protein, fluids, and iron, their low calorie intake should not be as much of a factor to their fatigue.
2. Answer: **B**. Most hair shedding after 6 months from surgery has more to do with a nutrient deficiency rather than stress from the surgery, which normally shows up prior to 6 months s/p surgery.
3. Answer: **A, B, C, and D** are all important for the patient to be doing – especially if/when hunger cues are increasing – to prevent weight regain.
4. Answer: **A**. Low blood sugar is most likely the cause of her symptoms. Low blood sugar or "late dumping" may occur if the patient is not eating frequently enough and/or if they are eating meals that are low in protein. It is important to increase both the frequency of eating and to ensure protein-rich foods at meal or snack.
5. Answer: **B**. Dehydration. The fact that she can tolerate certain foods rules out ulcer and bowel obstruction. She is getting more than 50 g of protein but only about 36–38 oz of fluid per day, and she confirms that her urine is often dark yellow. She is counseled to increase her fluids up to at least 50 oz per day.
6. Answer: **A**. Pregnancy. Normally with pregnancy, the nausea is more chronic and heightened in the morning, not just after eating.

References

1. Kruseman M, Leimgruber A, Zumbach F, Golay A. Dietary, weight, and psychological changes among patients with obesity, 8 years after gastric bypass. J Am Diet Assoc. 2010;110(4):527–34.
2. Langer FB, Reza Hoda MA, Bohdjalian A, Felberbauer FX, Zacherl J, Wenzl E, et al. Sleeve gastrectomy and gastric banding: effects on plasma ghrelin levels. Obes Surg. 2005;15(7):1024–9.

3. Koch TR, Finelli FC. Postoperative metabolic and nutritional complications of bariatric surgery. Gastroenterol Clin North Am. 2010;39(1):109–24.
4. Snyder-Marlow G, Taylor D, Lenhard MJ. Nutrition care for patients undergoing laparoscopic sleeve gastrectomy for weight loss. J Am Diet Assoc. 2010;110(4):600–7.
5. Smith BR, Schauer P, Nguyen NT. Surgical approaches to the treatment of obesity: bariatric surgery. Med Clin North Am. 2011;95(5):1009–30.
6. Beckman LM, Beckman TR, Earthman CP. Changes in gastrointestinal hormones and leptin after Roux-en-Y gastric bypass procedure: a review. J Am Diet Assoc. 2010;110(4):571–84.
7. Alvarez-Leite JI. Nutrient deficiencies secondary to bariatric surgery. Curr Opin Clin Nutr Metab Care. 2004;7(5):569–75. Review.
8. Manchester S, Roye GD. Bariatric surgery: an overview for dietetics professionals. Nutr Today. 2011;46(6):264–73.
9. Valentino D, Sriram K, Shankar P. Update on micronutrients in bariatric surgery. Curr Opin Clin Nutr Metab Care. 2011;14(6):635–41.
10. Alger-Mayer S, Polimeni JM, Malone M. Preoperative weight loss as a predictor of long-term success following Roux-en-Y gastric bypass. Obes Surg. 2008;18(7):772–5. Epub 2008 Apr 8.
11. Allied Health Sciences Section Ad Hoc Nutrition Committee, Aills L, Blankenship J, Buffington C, Furtado M, Parrott J. ASMBS allied health nutritional guidelines for the surgical weight loss patient. Surg Obes Relat Dis. 2008;4(5 Suppl):S73–108. Epub 2008 May 19.
12. Weller WE, Rosati C, Hannan EL. Relationship between surgeon and hospital volume and readmission after bariatric operation. J Am Coll Surg. 2007;204(3):383–91.
13. Burge JC, Schaumburg JZ, Choban PS, DiSilvestro RA, Flancbaum L. Changes in patients' taste acuity after Roux-en-Y gastric bypass for clinically severe obesity. J Am Diet Assoc. 1995;95:666–70.
14. Cummings D, Shannon M. Ghrelin and gastric bypass: is there a hormonal contribution to surgical weight loss? J Clin Endocrinol Metab. 2003;88(7):2999–3002.
15. Tong J, Mannea E, Aimé P, Pfluger PT, Yi CX, Castaneda TR, et al. Ghrelin enhances olfactory sensitivity and exploratory sniffing in rodents and humans. J Neurosci. 2011;31(15):5841–6.
16. Frezza EE, Ikramuddin S, Gourash W, Rakitt T, Kingston A, Luketich J, et al. Symptomatic improvement in gastroesophageal reflux disease (GERD) following laparoscopic Roux-en-Y gastric bypass. Surg Endosc. 2002;16(7):1027–31. Epub 2002 May 3.
17. Klaus A, Weiss H. Is preoperative manometry in restrictive bariatric procedures necessary? Obes Surg. 2008;18(8):1039–42. Epub 2008 Apr 2. Review.
18. Faria SL, Faria OP, Buffington C, de Almeida Cardeal M, Ito MK. Dietary protein intake and bariatric surgery patients: a review. Obes Surg. 2011;21(11):1798–805.
19. Hall WL, Millward DJ, Long SJ, Morgan LM. Casein and whey exert different effects on plasma amino acid profiles, gastrointestinal hormone secretion and appetite. Br J Nutr. 2003;89(2):239–48.
20. [no authors listed] Food and Nutrition Board. Dietary reference intakes for energy, carbohydrate, fiber, fat, fatty acids, cholesterol, protein, and amino acids. Consensus Report. Institute of Medicine of the National Academies. 5 Sept 2002. http://www.iom.edu/Reports/2002/Dietary-Reference-Intakes-for-Energy-Carbohydrate-Fiber-Fat-Fatty-Acids-Cholesterol-Protein-and-Amino-Acids.aspx. Last accessed 17 May 2013.
21. Fujioka K. Follow-up of nutritional and metabolic problems after bariatric surgery. Diabetes Care. 2005;28(2):481–4.
22. Signori C, Zalesin KC, Franklin B, Miller WL, McCullough PA. Effect of gastric bypass on vitamin D and secondary hyperparathyroidism. Obes Surg. 2010;20(7):949–52.
23. Davies DJ, Baxter JM, Baxter JN. Nutritional deficiencies after bariatric surgery. Obes Surg. 2007;17(9):1150–8. Review.
24. Buchwald H, Ikramuddin S, Dorman RB, Schone JL, Dixon JB. Management of the metabolic/bariatric surgery patient. Am J Med. 2011;124(12):1099–105.
25. Kellogg TA, Bantle JP, Leslie DB, Redmond JB, Slusarek B, Swan T, et al. Postgastric bypass hyperinsulinemic hypoglycemia syndrome: characterization and response to a modified diet. Surg Obes Relat Dis. 2008;4(4):492–9.
26. Jacques J. The latest on nutrition and hair loss in the bariatric patient. Bariatric Times. 19 Sept 2008. http://bariatrictimes.com/the-latest-on-nutrition-and-hair-loss-in-the-bariatric-patient/. Last accessed 17 May 2013.
27. Iglezias Brandao de Oliveira C, Adami Chaim E, da Silva BB. Impact of rapid weight reduction on risk of cholelithiasis after bariatric surgery. Obes Surg. 2003;13:625–8.
28. Méndez-Sánchez N, González V, Aguayo P, Sánchez JM, Tanimoto MA, Elizondo J, et al. Fish Oil (n-3) polyunsaturated fatty acids beneficially affect biliary cholesterol nucleation time in obese women losing weight. J Nutr. 2001;131(9):2300–3.
29. Maggard MA, Yermilov I, Li Z, Maglione M, Newberry S, Suttorp M, et al. Pregnancy and fertility following bariatric surgery: a systematic review. JAMA. 2008;300(19):2286–96.
30. de Zwaan M, Hilbert A, Swan-Kremeier L, Simonich H, Lancaster K, Howell LM, et al. Comprehensive interview assessment of eating behavior 18–35 months after gastric bypass surgery for morbid obesity. Surg Obes Relat Dis. 2010;6(1):79–85.
31. Gorin AA, Raftopoulos I. Effect of mood and eating disorders on the short-term outcome of laparoscopic Roux-en-Y gastric bypass. Obes Surg. 2009;19(12):1685–90.
32. Deitel M. Anorexia nervosa following bariatric surgery. Obes Surg. 2002;12(6):729–30.
33. Segal A, Kinoshita Kussunoki D, Larino MA. Post-surgical refusal to eat: anorexia nervosa, bulimia nervosa or a new eating disorder? A case series. Obes Surg. 2004;14(3):353–60.
34. Coates PS, Fernstrom JD, Fernstrom MH, Schauer PR, Greenspan SL. Gastric bypass surgery for morbid obesity leads to an increase in bone turnover and a decrease in bone mass. J Clin Endocrinol Metab. 2004;89(3):1061–5.
35. Bruno C, Fulford AD, Potts JR, McClintock R, Jones R, Cacucci BM, et al. Serum markers of bone turnover are increased at six and 18 months after Roux-en-Y bariatric surgery: correlation with the reduction in leptin. J Clin Endocrinol Metab. 2010;95(1):159–66.
36. Scopinaro N, Marinari GM, Pretolesi F, Papadia F, Murelli F, Marini P, et al. Energy and nitrogen absorption after biliopancreatic diversion. Obes Surg. 2000;10(5):436–41.
37. Holick MF. Vitamin D: importance in the prevention of cancers, type 1 diabetes, heart disease, and osteoporosis. Am J Clin Nutr. 2004;79:362–71. Erratum in: Am J Clin Nutr 2004;79:890.
38. Guyton KZ, Kensler TW, Posner GH. Vitamin D and vitamin D analogs as cancer chemopreventive agents. Nutr Rev. 2003;61:227–38.
39. Hayes CE, Nashold FE, Spach KM, Pedersen LB. The immunological functions of the vitamin D endocrine system. Cell Mol Biol (Noisy-le-Grand). 2003;49:277–300.
40. Mahlay NF, Verka LG, Thomsen K, Merugu S, Salomone M. Vitamin D status before Roux-en-Y and efficacy of prophylactic and therapeutic doses of vitamin D in patients after Roux-en-Y gastric bypass surgery. Obes Surg. 2009;19(5):590–4.
41. Ponsky TA, Brody F, Pucci E. Alterations in gastrointestinal physiology after Roux-en-Y gastric bypass. J Am Coll Surg. 2005;201(1):125–31. Review.
42. Shiffman ML, Kaplan GD, Brinkman-Kaplan V, Vickers FF. Prophylaxis against gallstone formation with ursodeoxycholic acid in patients participating in a very-low-calorie diet program. Ann Intern Med. 1995;122:899–905.
43. Sugerman HJ, Brewer WH, Shiffman ML, Brolin RE, Fobi MA, Linner JH, et al. A multicenter, placebo-controlled, randomized, double-blind, prospective trial of prophylactic ursodiol for the prevention of gallstone formation following gastric-bypass-induced rapid weight loss. Am J Surg. 1995;169:91–6; discussion 96–97.

Nutrition Care Across the Weight Loss Surgery Process

Julie M. Parrott and J. Scott Parrott

Chapter Objectives

1. To help the reader gain an understanding of the nutritional considerations of weight management during four critical phases of the weight loss surgery process, which we call preparing, healing, achieving, and maintaining
2. To identify the nutritional goals at each phase and address common patient concerns and challenges during each phase
3. To think about the weight loss process from a patient perspective rather than solely a surgical perspective

Introduction

The purpose of this chapter is to help the reader gain an understanding of the nutritional considerations of weight management during four critical phases of the weight loss surgery process, which we call preparing, healing, achieving, and maintaining. We recognize that this is a slight departure from the surgical approach more commonly encountered in the research literature: "preoperative," "early postoperative," and "later postoperative."

The reason for relabeling the phases of the weight loss surgery process is simple: we want to think about the weight loss process from a patient perspective rather than solely a surgical perspective. Focusing on the experience of the weight loss process from a patient's perspective may help us more clearly identify the changing role of diet and eating behaviors through the different phases of the process and provide the dietitian and other bariatric team members with tools for counseling, educating, and encouraging patients throughout this process.

In this chapter, we identify the nutritional goals at each phase and address common patient concerns and challenges during each phase. While we draw on the wealth of scientific research available on weight loss surgery, the goal of this chapter is practical (what can dietitians do to increase the likelihood that weight loss surgery patients will be successful?). So, we avoid the rigid style of a scientific research article. We do, however, point the reader toward research on the various topics we touch on. In areas where little research has been done, or research findings are inconsistent or ambiguous, we highlight that fact for the reader.

Before we go any further, we should address an important question that may be asked by dietitians not familiar with weight loss surgery. There is a huge (and growing) body of research on strategies for successful weight loss and weight maintenance: Does any of this apply to the weight loss surgery patient? Much of it does. However, because weight loss surgery patients have needs that set them off from the typical individual who is trying to lose weight, newcomers to the area of bariatric weight loss surgery dietetics should be aware of special considerations during the different phases of the weight loss process before and after surgery. Table 14.1 may help the reader get a sense of the degree to which the nutritional considerations of weight loss surgery patients may differ from those of the nonsurgical weight loss patient in the different phases of the process.

The question mark in the maintenance phase is meant to indicate that little research has been done on the nutritional considerations of patients several years out from weight loss surgery, as well as increasing differences among patients. For instance, we do not yet know whether (or to what degree) metabolic changes that occur immediately following surgery are maintained several years after surgery. To the extent that the physiological profile of bariatric surgery patients remains

---

J.M. Parrott, MS, RD, CPT (✉)
Central Jersey Bariatrics, 901 West Main Street, Suite 103 MAB, Freehold, NJ 07728, USA
e-mail: Julie.parrott@yahoo.com

J.S. Parrott, PhD
Department of Interdisciplinary Studies, SHRP, Newark, NJ, USA

Department of Quantitative Methods, School of Public Health, University of Medicine and Dentistry of NJ, Newark, NJ, USA
e-mail: scott.parrott@rutgers.edu

Table 14.1 Phases of the weight loss surgery process

Phase	How long is this phase?	How different are nutritional considerations from nonsurgical weight loss?
Preparation Goal: to prepare for surgery and lifestyle changes needed following surgery	Depends on many factors, such as insurance requirements, program characteristics, and patient readiness. Typically, within 3–6 months of surgery	Some special considerations
Healing Goal: to promote healing immediately following surgery	Surgical programs may vary somewhat but typically the first 6 weeks following surgery	Unique to weight loss surgery
Achieving Goal: to reach the target excess weight loss goal	Once the patient has fully healed and begun solid regular-type foods, this phase may last from 6 weeks after surgery to a full year or more	Special considerations
Maintaining Goal: to maintain target weight; manage weight regain	After the patient has reached their target weight or is outside the window (typically approximately 2 years) when the direct effects of the surgery are greatest, this phase becomes the patient's "new normal" for the rest of their life	Some special considerations?

distinct from patients who have not had weight loss surgery, dietitians working with these patients will want to account for that fact when working with patients. To the degree that, several years out, weight loss surgery patients are metabolically "the same" as patients who have not had weight loss surgery, then there is little rationale for treating them any different. However, at this point, we just do not know. More research is needed.

Preparation: Getting Ready for Surgery

There are two key goals in the preparation phase:
- Preparing the patient physiologically for surgery
- Educating the patient to begin their new life after weight loss surgery

Preparing the Patient Physiologically for Surgery

Weight Loss and Managing Comorbidities

While some programs emphasize presurgical weight loss, the research is not clear whether weight loss prior to surgery actually results in a greater amount of weight loss after surgery or just gives the patient a head start on the weight loss they can expect after surgery [1]. What is clear, however, is that weight loss prior to surgery can improve surgical outcomes for many patients. The American Association of Clinical Endocrinologists, the Obesity Society, and the American Society for Metabolic and Bariatric Surgery (AACE/TOS/ASMBS) Guidelines for the Perioperative Nutritional, Metabolic, and Nonsurgical Support of the Bariatric Surgery Patient, 2013 Update, recommend preoperative weight loss to reduce liver volume and to improve technical aspects of weight loss surgery [2]. Several researchers have published results indicating that (1) a preoperative prep with associated weight loss and subsequent (2) reduced fat in the liver creates a technically safer procedure by increasing the visual field and physical space for surgeons during a procedure [3–6]. If using a very-low-calorie diet (VLCD) approach prior to surgery, a minimum of 2 weeks "prep time" may be required to sufficiently reduce fat in the liver, with a maximum timeframe of 6 weeks to improve patient adherence [3, 7]. However, this is not recommended for all patients, but rather for higher risk patients (e.g., technically difficult cases, preoperative body mass index [BMI] >50 kg/m^2, etc.) at the discretion of the bariatric treatment team [8, 9].

Preparing the patient physiologically for surgery requires more than simply promoting weight loss. Directly addressing comorbidities is also a key component. Improving specific comorbidities, such as elevated blood glucose, poor oxygen perfusion, and poor healing prior to weight loss surgery, may improve early postoperative recovery (less recovery time with better managed comorbidities, e.g., diabetes and sleep apnea) and may be a necessity for weight loss surgery to proceed [2–7].

Nutrition Intervention Strategy

In light of the above, we provide two different nutrition intervention strategies. The first provides general strategies for the patient to begin a pattern of healthy diet, exercise, and behaviors that will be continued following surgery. The second, which we call a "liver prep diet," provides modifications to the general pre-weight loss surgery diet for use when a short-term intervention is needed to decrease liver fat and/or total weight prior to surgery. The diets are not mutually exclusive and may be used in tandem depending on the needs of the patient in preparing for both surgery and their life after surgery. Table 14.2 provides an overview of the basic pre-weight loss surgery diet and modifications that may be implemented for the liver prep diet. More details on selected aspects of this diet are provided below.

Importance of Medical Nutrition Therapy

Medical nutrition therapy—which includes a nutritional evaluation, labs, and education regarding lifestyle change—should be used to provide a patient with tools to appropriately control blood sugars and other targeted comorbidities as well as comply with program-specific weight loss. In some patients, preoperative weight loss may be an onerous task, due to mobility constraints, insulin resistance, and weight-promoting medications. Research indicates that preoperative weight loss with medical nutrition therapy can improve glycemic control and should therefore be utilized in obese patients with diabetes [10].

We should not assume that preoperative patients have good nutritional status or appropriate dietary intake. Many patients have numerous micronutrient deficiencies prior to surgery [11]. Additionally, the typical dietary intake of preoperative patients exceeds 50 % of energy intake from fat [12].

Additionally, research indicates that dietary counseling by a qualified dietetics professional [13] is associated with greater weight loss postoperatively, and adherence with follow-up appointments (missing less than 25 % of visits) is associated with greater percentage of excess weight loss (%EWL) and had more impact especially for AGB patients—ideally no fewer than 13 visits in 2 years for AGB [14].

Protein

An individual's protein requirement is significantly increased when energy (kcal) intake is not meeting individual needs. Nitrogen balance is severely compromised when dietary energy intake is less than 35 kcal/kg. Adding 100 g of carbohydrate per day decreases nitrogen loss by 40 % in modified protein fasts. When it occurs, protein malnutrition is generally observed at 3–6 months after surgery and is largely attributed to the development of food intolerance to protein-rich foods. All postoperative patients are at risk of developing protein-energy malnutrition related to decreased oral intake, but pre-surgery patients on a liver prep diet may be susceptible as well. Protein-deficient meals are common after RYGB and may also occur after AGB and LSG. Prevention of protein malnutrition requires regular assessment of protein intake and counseling regarding ingestion of protein from protein-rich foods and protein supplements. In general, dietary protein should be established first in any diet in proportion to body weight, and then carbohydrates and fats should be added as determined by energy needs [11, 15].

Energy/VLCD

Very-low-calorie diets (VLCDs) may be appropriate and effective for some patients preparing for surgery [16, 17]. However, even when a very-low-calorie diet is called for, it should not contain less than 45 g carbohydrates daily; otherwise adverse metabolic and emotional effects occur. Johnston et al. reported that patients undergoing a 6-week randomized controlled test were unable to exercise due to fatigue and increased symptoms of depression [18]. Additionally, decreasing caloric intake alone has not been correlated with decreased liver fat, but it may be that reduction in the patient's customary dietary intake of fat is enough to create significant changes in liver fat [3, 19]. Substituting one or more daily meals with meal replacements may be appropriate for patients needing to lose weight in preparation for surgery.

Preparing the Patient for Lifestyle Changes

Weight has been reported as an indicator of decreased liver mass, but may not be the best method (and is certainly not the only method) of evaluating how prepared for surgery or how successful a patient will be postoperatively with bariatric surgery. Since the cause of obesity is multifactorial, additional indicators should be considered when determining a bariatric surgery candidate's level of preparation, including other health indices (blood glucose control), behaviors (e.g., grazing), and self-efficacy (accomplishment of goals over time).

The main goal of the preoperative phase is to prepare the weight loss surgery patient for the lifestyle changes that are required after surgery. This will mean helping the patients to develop appropriate weight loss expectations, identifying areas in which additional support will be needed, and dispelling misconceptions (knowledge about nutritional lifestyle: what to eat? how much? when?). In other words, what can patients reasonably expect within the first postoperative year in terms of weight loss, behaviors, and challenges? Often, patients will come to the dietitian with questions that correspond to these key areas.

How Much Weight Can I Expect to Lose?

Research indicates that individuals who lose weight without surgery can expect to lose up to 5–10 % of their body weight [2]. A 10 % weight loss is associated with substantial improvement in risk profiles for diabetes and cardiovascular disease. However, weight loss surgery patients may expect to lose substantially more weight.

How much weight the bariatric surgery patient can expect to lose depends on the type of surgical procedure. A slightly dated meta-analysis [20] estimates the following average percent excess weight loss within the first year by type of surgery (95 % confidence intervals are in parentheses):

Table 14.2 Pre-weight loss surgery diets

	Pre-weight loss surgery diet	Liver prep diet
Goal	Begin pattern of healthy diet, exercise, and behavior patterns that will be continued following surgery	Decrease liver fat and/or total weight
Labs	Labs requested and evaluated vary by program but should follow the schedule recommended by the Endocrine Society and ASMBS Guidelines	
Diet	• Downplay the idea that the patient is following a diet. Rather, emphasize "intuitive" and "mindful" eating • Consider food intolerances, allergies, sensitivities, and patient finances	Emphasize that this diet is used only for a short time. Equate pre-WLS to bowel prep—just a little less pleasant and takes a little longer
Timing	Begins with the first visit with the dietitian	Begins at least 2 weeks prior to surgery, but no more than 6 weeks prior to surgery
Macronutrients		
Energy	Focus on making healthy changes to the patient's previous diet	Very-low-calorie diet
Protein	Increase lean protein ("loin" or "round" beef/pork)	Ensure sufficient protein in light of decreased energy intake
Carbohydrates	• Increase fiber • Carbs from fruits, vegetables, and grains	Not CHO/ketogenic (<45 g) Encourage additional fiber
Fats	Encourage healthy fats to increase satiety and HDL • Healthy fatty fish: salmon, herring, tuna • Plants: flax, almonds, walnuts • Monounsaturated—choose most often: olive and canola oil, nuts, and avocado • Polyunsaturated fats—choose more often: corn, soy, vegetable, and safflower oil • Trans fat—unhealthy—avoid some margarine and commercial foods • Saturated fat—limit fatty meats and whole milk dairy, processed foods	Check ingredients in order to avoid saturated and hydrogenated fats and choose more healthy fats from poly-unsaturated, mono-unsaturated or essential fats
Fluids	• Emphasize that calories should be eaten and not drunk except for liquid protein supplements • Increase water • Decrease milk, sodas, juices, fruit drinks, and alcoholic and caffeinated beverages	
Micronutrients	Begin or continue taking complete multivitamin	Discuss decreasing or condensing number of supplements if taking additional types
Meal patterns	While research indicates that more frequent meals may be associated with lower BMI in healthy individuals, it is unclear whether and under what conditions this applies to the weight loss surgery patient. For some patients, frequent eating can act as a trigger. Be judicious with recommendations regarding meal frequency	Eat/drink three times per day or enough to meet protein and kcals for VLCD
Portion size	• Educate patient regarding appropriate portion sizes • "My Plate" method may be useful	For meals (not substituted by meal replacements), use the plate method or bariatric food guide pyramid

Meal replacements	• Begin replacing one meal with a meal replacement from preapproved list of high-quality protein-rich "meals" • Provide various options (liquid and potential nonliquid) • See meal replacements section below	Options: • All liquid • 1 or more meals liquid meal replacement • Frozen prepackaged meals • Other RD approved patterns
Follow-up	Expectations vary by program, but research indicates that greater dietitian contact prior to surgery results in improved short-term weight outcomes	
Physical activity	• Exercise prior to either CHO or PRO meal • Walk further or gain access to a pool (depending on the size and physical condition of the patient, physical activities may be limited; tailor to patient ability and preferences) • Begin scheduled "activity," not exercise • If patient is able to walk, then begin with 10 min for 3–5 times/week working towards a daily goal of 30 min • If patient unable to be active, consider physical therapy for gait and balance evaluation and treatment • Increase activity slowly and with achievable goals (increase patient self-efficacy)	
Behavioral considerations	• Identify and avoid trigger environments (e.g., buffet restaurant) • Begin practicing mindful eating strategies • Provide some structure with diet, behaviors, and activity—planning skills • Is patient able to adhere—how to modify? • Is patient retaining information from visit to visit? If not, is teaching style or patient motivation barriers?	What changes will patient need to make after surgery—in light of obstacles experienced during "liver prep"?

- 47.5 % (40.7–54.2 %) for patients who underwent gastric banding
- 61.6 % (56.7–66.5 %) gastric bypass
- 68.2 % (61.5–74.8 %) gastroplasty
- 70.1 % (66.3–73.9 %) biliopancreatic diversion or duodenal switch

While these numbers may seem impressive, there are two key things to emphasize. First, these are sample averages—individual patient results will almost certainly be different. Assuming a normal distribution for weight loss following surgery, approximately half of the patients can realistically expect to lose less weight—perhaps substantially less. This leads to the second, and more important, point. If the numbers are correct, the unfortunate truth is that *most* patients will not reach their weight loss goal (assuming that is to lose *all* their excess weight). Notice that none of the averages (and, indeed, none of the 95 % confidence intervals) include 100 % of excess weight loss. So, a key (perhaps the most important) message regarding how much weight a patient can expect to lose is this: weight loss surgery, by itself, is no guarantee of losing all your excess weight. The patient should understand that weight loss surgery may help them reach their goals, but will not do it for them. The most honest answer to "How much can I expect to lose?" is probably that it depends on whether you make the lifestyle changes to take advantage of the benefits of the surgery to achieve your new "normal."

This dose of reality is not meant to discourage the patient (after all, approximately half of weight loss surgery patients can expect to lose *more* than the average). But, whether they fall in the upper or lower ends of this distribution depends on the patient putting in place a range of lifestyle changes. In the section on the achieving phase, we will review some strategies that the dietitian can use to help the patient identify and make these changes.

Will I Gain My Weight Back?

The short answer, based on the research, is that you stand a good chance of regaining at least some weight [12, 21]. Research on longer-term outcome (e.g., 5–10 years after surgery) consistently shows that many patients regain at least a portion of the weight they lost; in fact, by 10 years many patients have regained 25 % of their lost weight [15]. Whether and how much weight a patient may regain differs by surgical procedure as well as by a number of lifestyle factors.

Recent research suggests that as obesity develops, a number of metabolic changes occur, which may not completely reverse when weight is lost. This means, in practical terms, that once a patient has gained a significant amount of weight, their body will always be primed to gain it back. In short, it is easier to regain weight once you have been obese.

This highlights an important point for helping the patient to develop realistic and strategic expectations. If the patient understands that his or her body will always be "eager" to regain the lost weight, then they can grasp the fact that achieving and maintaining a healthy weight is something they must work at for the rest of their lives. Some patients may find this discouraging—after all, haven't they tried losing weight and been unsuccessful up until now? The point to emphasize is that weight loss surgery and the concomitant skills they learn provide a powerful new set of tools to increase their odds of success. We will review the healthy lifestyle skills that increase the likelihood of success in the section on achieving phase.

Will I Need to Exercise?

The benefits of exercise are well established. However, merely educating the patient on the benefits of exercise is not enough. Most, if not all, patients will have at least a vague awareness of why they should exercise. The hurdle is less likely to be their understanding than it is their ability, motivation, or opportunity. For many very heavy patients, it is not simply that they do not want to be physically active—they simply may not be physically able to participate in activities they think of as "exercise." In this case, modified activity plans may be ideal (e.g., low impact that emphasizes stretching, flexibility, and balance).

Another problem is a patient's preconception of "exercise." While sedentary individuals may have negative associations with the term "exercise" (perhaps tied to painful memories of sports or "the gym"), they may be more positively disposed to "physical activity." Framing is key. Find out what associations individuals have with physical activity and exercise. The reality is that weight loss surgery will enable patients to participate in activities they may have found difficult or impossible previously. Presenting the range of opportunities to participate in activities they may enjoy (with people they want to be with) may help shift the attitude from "I *have* to exercise" to "I get to do fun things I couldn't do before!"

What Behavioral Changes Will I Need to Make?

Patients may be aware that they need to make *some kind* of behavioral changes but have little understanding of what these changes are, why they need to make them, or strategies for making them. Indeed, many patients are deeply unaware of the underlying problem. The problem may be cast, simplistically, as a problem with food: "I eat because I'm always hungry." So, they think, "If I'm not hungry I won't eat." Indeed, they may perceive themselves to be hungry, but this may actually mask what are deeper and more pathological aspects of their relationship to food. Research indicates that personality disorders [1], disinhibition [22], and a range of maladaptive behaviors [23] of which the patient may be vaguely aware (if at all) are all associated with lack of success with losing weight.

While dietetics professionals can focus on behaviors associated with eating, addressing the deeper psychological and social motivations for eating may fall well outside their scope of knowledge and practice. Including a psychologist or psychotherapist trained in dysfunctional eating into the treatment team may greatly improve a patient's chances of success [24].

Healing: Nutrition to Recover from Surgery

Even before the patient has completely recovered from their surgery, dietitians can begin to work with the patient to begin to put into practice topics covered in nutrition counseling prior to surgery and strengthen those concepts and strategies through further education. Indeed, depending on program or insurance requirements, the period shortly after surgery may provide the dietitian with the most intensive patient contact. So, even though the nutritional focus may be somewhat different in this phase compared to the other phases, time spent in nutrition counseling sessions should also focus on strategies the patient will put into practice more intensively in the achieving phase (discussed later in this chapter).

During the brief period shortly following surgery, dietary needs and limitations are unique for weight loss surgery patients. Resources for helping to design patient diet and diet progression during this period are available [25]. Most bariatric surgery programs have their own methods, nuances, or strategies. It is critical for the treating clinicians and team to be on the same page. We highlight some common features that have a modicum of research support.

Additionally, this is the first phase in which the patient will begin to get used to their "new stomach"—discovering what they can and cannot comfortably tolerate. So, although food tolerance is an important issue the patient will face through the first year or so after surgery, we introduce the topic of food tolerance in this phase.

Main Nutritional Goals

The main nutritional goals immediately following surgery focus on hydration, obtaining adequate protein and adequate micronutrients. In order to prevent unwanted gastrointestinal symptoms (nausea, vomiting, and dumping) and subsequent complications (such as nutritional deficiencies and weight regain), patients who have undergone a bariatric procedure are required to make substantial changes to diet and eating behavior including consuming small portions, avoiding high-fat or sugar-full foods, eating slowly, and chewing food well. See Frank [25] and Aills [11] for diet progression recommendations.

Hydration: The patient should take small sips, typically within the first 3 days after surgery: 30 ml every 15–30 min as tolerated. Adequate hydration can also be assessed via fluid intake and output with patient observation of fluids consumed and urine concentration and frequency.

Protein: Obtaining adequate protein is a major concern during the clear liquid phase and clinician should be alert to any protein intolerances or aversions are present before surgery or develop afterward. Patients will need to use supplements of high-quality powdered or liquid protein sipped slowly. All solid foods should be eaten in small bites of food chewed thoroughly.

Vitamins: Micronutrient supplements are needed to avoid micronutrient deficiencies. Typically, chewable or liquid micronutrient supplements are tolerated well in the first 4 weeks after surgery. Avoid "incomplete" gummy-type vitamins lacking specific nutrients, e.g., thiamin or vitamin B1. See Aills [11] or Mechanick [2] for recommendations.

Dietary Strategies: Food Tolerance

Research comparing adjustable gastric banding (AGB), Roux-en-Y gastric bypass (RYGB), and sleeve gastrectomy (SG) indicates that the degree of food tolerance varies by surgical procedure [26]. Patients who have had the SG are likely to have superior food tolerance relative to other procedures with patients who have underdone the RYGB having marginally lower tolerance. Patients who underwent the AGB had the lowest measures of food tolerance. The researchers also concluded that "a clear relationship exists between improved food tolerance and gastrointestinal quality of life" [26].

Physical Activity

During this period of rapid weight loss, the general exercise goals are to avoid cardiopulmonary complications and preserve lean muscle mass. The Physical Activity Toolkit for Registered Dietitians[1] recommends two key resources to help the dietetics professional integrate physical activity into the patient's new healthy lifestyle:

- *The 2008 Physical Activity Guidelines for Americans*, US Department of Health and Human Services.[2] This evidence-based document provides general information and guidance for achieving the health benefits of regular physical activity. It may serve as a useful point of departure for developing individualized physical activity plans for weight loss surgery patients.
- *Exercise is Medicine*® (EIM). This is a multi-organizational initiative resource that provides a guide for health

---

[1] Available at http://www.eatright.org/WorkArea/linkit.aspx?LinkIdentifier=id&ItemID=6442474633&libID=6442474610

[2] http://www.health.gov/paguidelines

and fitness professionals (sponsored by the American College of Sports Medicine, the American Medical Association, and the American College of Sports Medicine).[3]

While these resources may be helpful, an important reality to take into account is that while weight loss surgery patients often intend to engage in regular physical activity, these intentions are, more often than not, unrealized. In one study, "lack of time" was the most commonly selected barrier to physical activity, followed by "too tired" and "pain and discomfort" [27]. So, when designing a physical activity plan for weight loss surgery patients, these common barriers need to be taken into account. Shifting the focus from "something you have to do" to "something your new body allows you to do" may be a key motivational strategy for dietetics professionals.

Achieving: Creating the New Normal

After the patient has fully recovered from surgery, they now begin to put into practice the principles and behaviors to create their new lifestyle. Unfortunately, many weight loss surgery outcome studies do not report the inclusion of dietary interventions or other strategies used to help optimize weight loss outcomes. Yet, research outside of bariatric surgery makes clear that patients can affect these weight loss outcomes by devoting their time and energy toward making lifestyle changes in nutritional, physical, and behavioral health areas. Some weight regain is "normal" after 2–3 years post-op, and waiting for weight regain is not the time to begin making lifestyle changes. Change should begin in the first year postoperatively with some "practice" lifestyle changes preoperatively in three key areas: nutrition and diet, behaviors, and physical activity.

A New Dietary Lifestyle

After the weight loss patient's diet has progressed to the new normal, they need to understand that they are no longer "dieting" in the sense of eating to quickly lose weight. Rather, the goal is to develop healthy diet, exercise, and behavior patterns that will last them the rest of their lives. There are a few modifications to a healthy diet for the general population that can be made to adjust these diets to some special considerations for weight loss surgery patients.

We will present some general resources for healthy eating patterns and then provide some guidance on how these healthy diets may be modified to maximize success in the bariatric patient. We pay special attention to dietary modifications to increase satiety.

Evaluate and Change Diet Composition to "More Healthy" Focus

There are a number of existing resources that, with appropriate changes, can be applied to weight loss surgery patients. The following are some resource that the dietetics professional may find helpful:

AHA Recommendations for a Weight Loss Surgery Patient

As part of a healthy diet, an adult consuming 2,000 cal daily should aim for:

- *Fruits and vegetables*: At least 4.5 cups a day
- *Fish* (*preferably oily fish*): At least two 3.5 oz servings a week
- *Fiber-rich whole grains*: At least three 1 oz-equivalent servings a day
- *Sodium*: Less than 1,500 mg a day
- *Sugar-sweetened beverages*: No more than 450 cal (36 oz) a week
- *Other dietary measures*:
  - *Nuts, legumes, and seeds*: At least four servings a week
  - *Processed meats*: No more than two servings a week
  - *Saturated fat*: Less than 7 % of total energy intake

American Society of Metabolic and Bariatric Surgery

A range of resources are available at http://asmbs.org/resources.

Academy of Nutrition and Dietetics

The Academy has several resources including:

- The Bariatric Surgery Nutrition Care Evidence Analysis Library: http://andevidencelibrary.com/topic.cfm?cat=1406.
- The ADA Pocket Guide to Bariatric Surgery: https://www.eatright.org/shop/product.aspx?id=5007.
- The Weight Management Dietetic Practice Group has a Bariatric Surgery Subunit and provides a number of different resources: http://wmdpg.org.

"My Plate" Tools

- Another option to provide basic healthy nutrition, physical activity, and behaviors for an overall healthy lifestyle with a tracking option (http://www.choosemyplate.gov).
- There is a "SuperTracker" option, which allows individuals to tailor the program for their own goals and monitor progress.

These general dietary targets should be modified based on special food source considerations for weight loss surgery patients. Table 14.3 provides a list of some diet modifications found to be helpful for weight loss surgery patients.

---
[3] Available at http://www.exerciseismedicine.org

Table 14.3 Special modifications of healthy diet for post-weight loss surgery patients

Post-weight loss surgery diet modifications		
Timing		Education on the characteristics of the postsurgical diet should begin prior to surgery; patients should begin to implement the following general principles
Macronutrients		
	Energy	Kcal <1,300 + kcal after the first post-op year

	Protein	• PRO >60 g per day: protein ≥1.3–1.5 g/kg IBW
		• PDCAAS: consider the quality and amount of protein per serving
		• Include BCAA, e.g., leucine from foods and supplements
		  – The stimulatory effect of AAs on muscle protein synthesis is primarily due to indispensable/essential AAs, with leucine being the MOST effective
		  – Increased concentrations of leucine have the potential to stimulate MPS during catabolic conditions associated with food restriction or after exhaustive exercise

	Carbohydrates	• Keep CHO <130 g • Low glycemic load CHO • Decrease intake of simple CHO foods (decrease trigger foods and cycle of food cravings) [43] • Carbohydrates: protein ratio ~1.5: 1.0
	Fats	Decrease saturated fat and replace with poly- or monounsaturated fats
	Fluids	• Fluids: vary with duration, environment, training • Pre- and postexercise: fluids, carbs, leucine (BCAA) • During exercise: fluids and carbs
Micronutrients		• Multivitamins with thiamin, selenium, zinc, copper (15 mg zinc: 1 mg copper) • Calcium citrate without meals, calcium carbonate with meals • Vitamin D • Vitamin B 12 • Iron • Other fat soluble nutrients • Other minerals • Probiotics • Omega-3 fatty acids • Fiber
Stimulate satiety		• Do not eat and drink at the same time (due to increased gastric emptying of solids with liquids) • Increase protein: carbohydrate ratio • Improve quality of protein • Decrease intake of sugars to avoid dumping syndrome in patients with gastric bypass • Decrease intake of excess kcal via nonnutritious snacks and beverages (juices, soda, alcohol, whole milk vs. 1 % or fat-free) • Healthy fats (poly- and monounsaturated) help increase satiety and HDL
Meal patterns		• Decrease kcal intake in later part of the day • Incorporate consistent protein-rich breakfast • Increase non-kcal fluids after specified time of the day (dinner)
Functional foods		• Choose carbohydrates from fruits, vegetables, and grains • Increase fiber to increase short-chain fatty acids (SCFA) production [44] • Incorporate the following plant foods: flax, almonds, walnuts

BCAA = branch chain amino acid
AA=amino acids
MPS= muscle protein synthesis
PDCAAS = protein digestibiity corrected amino acid score

Meal Replacements and Eating Frequency

In addition to recommended foods (and portion sizes), use of meal replacements and recommendations regarding eating frequency may aid some patients during this period of rapid weight loss. While research shows that both use of meal replacements and more frequent meals (approximately five times per day) may be associated with weight loss or maintenance of a healthy weight among individuals who have not had weight loss surgery [28], this has not been well researched among patients who struggle with obesity and/or candidates for weight loss surgery.

While more frequent smaller meals and/or snacks may help some patients (by increasing satiety), this may not be appropriate for all patients. For patients who tend to be "grazers" or for whom certain foods may act as triggers and thus predispose the patient to binging episodes [29], the dietetic professional is cautioned to take a highly judicious and individualized approach. As disordered eating patterns appear to be frequent among weight loss surgery patients, we want to avoid recommending eating patterns that could feed into those disordered patterns [30].

Increase Satiety
When is enough, enough? Unfortunately, the body's ability to exquisitely balance energy needs and intake (and so maintain a remarkably stable weight in the face of substantial fluctuations in intake) is thrown off in many individuals who struggle with obesity [31]. So, a key component of the new dietary lifestyle is recalibrating what the patient perceives as "being full." In other words, the goal is to increase satiety with lower intake. The challenge is that satiety is a complex process comprising purely physiological pathways (neural and humoral signals that originate from multiple sites; e.g., stomach, proximal and distal small intestine, colon, and pancreas) in response to both mechanical and chemical properties of food, as well as higher cognitive centers that regulate feeding (such as the perception of fullness). In many individuals with obesity, there appears to be a breakdown in this "gut-brain" circuit. In order to help the patient, it is important to have a basic understanding of the key regulators of feeding via gastric, intestinal, and pancreatic signals.

Emerging Research on the Role of Gut Hormones
The interaction between dietary pattern and the role of gut hormones in obesity and the regulation of satiety is an emerging area of research. Food composition, macronutrients, and other non-nutrient components as well as the physical properties of food not only affect the secretion of gut peptides but also their transcription and the differentiation of enteroendocrine cells, which ultimately modifies gut hormone responses. Gut hormones, such as GIP, CCK, GLP-1, and PYY, play a key role in glucose homeostasis, lipid metabolism, energy expenditure, and food intake [32]. In bariatric surgeries, such as Roux-en-Y gastric bypass or sleeve gastrectomy, the observed improvement in patients is accompanied by modifications in the gut hormone profile, suggesting a link between the observed weight reduction and the metabolic improvement of gut hormones. However, these relationships are complex, and it is still too early to make concrete dietary composition recommendations to influence these hormones. We encourage dietetic professionals to keep an eye on this area of research.

A New Physical Activity Lifestyle

As weight loss surgery patients begin to lose their weight, they should have increasing ability to participate in a variety of physical activities. While physical activity recommendations for healthy adults is the target, remaining weight, patient preference, and lack of conditioning from (possibly) long periods of inactivity and other health concerns may mean that exercise goals should be both personalized and integrated gradually. Again, it is important to emphasize that some patients may have negative associations with "exercise." Patients may be more amenable to approaches that emphasize participation in active pursuits the patient finds enjoyable.

As patients begin to become more active, the types and intensities of physical activity plans may begin to vary widely among patients. For instance, some patients may begin to actively train for marathons or bodybuilding, while others may prefer less intense forms of physical activity like yoga or walking. Tailoring nutritional intake to patient exercise goals becomes increasingly important, and individualized recommendations are likely to become more diverse as patients approach their target healthy weight.

New Behaviors and Ways of Thinking

A patient's relationship to food prior to weight loss surgery is intimately enmeshed in the patient's psychological and social fabric. So, building a "new normal" may require more than simply changing the way the patient eats and exercises. Patients may need support to make the psychological and social adjustments necessary to support their new life. A recent systematic review reports that participation in psychotherapeutic interventions and support groups is associated with increased weight loss [33]. Without appropriate psychological and social support, the patient may not be equipped to overcome some of the more common maladaptive behaviors (discussed later).

Additionally, patients have spent years ignoring hunger pains through various diet attempts and overriding the sensation of fullness through binge eating or other disordered eating. The feeling of "fullness" changes after weight loss surgery. Instead of the distension felt from a full stomach and further fullness creating pressure on the diaphragm with resulting heartburn and a bloated sensation, "full" after bariatric surgery occurs higher in the chest, above the sternum. So, beyond new behaviors and new ways of thinking, the patient will benefit from the help and support of other patients and bariatric team members to understand a new set of physical sensations—the "new normal." In short, the patient will need to learn what "feeling full" feels like with their new stomach.

Maintaining: Managing Postsurgery Weight Regain

As we noted previously, longer-term weight regain is common among weight loss patients. On average, patients may be expected to regain 20–25 % of the weight lost in the first 2 years after surgery over a 10-year period [12]. Therefore, it is important to identify factors that are associated with and could enhance the self-regulation of food intake and other behaviors related to weight management.

Identify Maladaptive Behaviors

Maladaptive behaviors are major contributors to weight regain. We do not yet know whether patients revert to maladaptive behaviors after making healthy behavioral changes shortly after surgery, or if these behaviors have always been present to some degree, but their effects are blunted due to the physiological changes after surgery. We suspect that different patients have different profiles in this respect.

While we do not expect that the dietetics professional will be an expert in the psychological dynamics underlying these behaviors, the dietitian can and should be aware of these behaviors. For some of the following topics, the research is extensive and so beyond the scope of this chapter to thoroughly review. We cannot here address the range of reasons that individuals may exhibit these behaviors. In order to address the psychological and motivational influences on these behaviors, we recommend that the patient be referred for psychotherapeutic interventions.

Research indicates that the following maladaptive behaviors are associated with weight regain:

- *Excessive intake of calories* via snacks and fast foods including:
  - Increased dietary intake of sweets
  - Increased dietary intake of fatty foods and less healthy foods such as simple carbohydrates
- *Eating patterns*:
  - *Breakfast skipping* (sometimes also accompanied by night eating syndrome): This is associated with poorer weight status [34], though it is not clear that, metabolically, skipping breakfast causes weight increase. At the very least, indication of breakfast skipping in the patient may serve as a signal for other maladaptive behaviors.
  - *Night eating syndrome*: A persistent pattern of late-night eating is present in an estimated 17 % of postsurgical patients. One study estimated that night eating episodes were associated with an average 1,134 kcal intake per episode [35].
  - *Late eating*: >50 % kcal after dinner meal with or without night eating.
  - *Grazing*: More or less continuous eating or snacking throughout the day is a fairly common postsurgical behavior (one study estimates that 38 % of postsurgical weight loss patients engage in this pattern of eating [36]). This eating pattern is associated with both poorer weight outcomes as well as increased psychological stress.
  - *Binge eating*: Unlike grazing, binge eating is not identified primarily on the basis of eating frequency, but involves recurring episodes of excessive eating marked by feeling a lack of control, and is classified as an eating psychopathology [37].
  - *Decreased mindful eating*: Increased disinhibition—a lack of restraint or increased impulsivity. This is also described as a *lack of control* (LOC) with food urges [36] and is common among preoperative patients (with one estimate at 40 % of patients experiencing at least one episode of LOC [38]). Research indicates that there may be a cyclical relation between negative emotional states and various forms of disinhibited eating (like binge eating or grazing). A patient may eat mindlessly as a way to assuage negative feelings but then feel guilty or depressed because of the disordered eating predisposing them toward yet another mindless eating episode.
- *Decreased well-being*: If, as is common among weight loss patients, eating is a coping or self-comforting behavior associated with stress or negative emotional states, then patients may revert to maladaptive behaviors as a way to manage negative emotions [39].
- *Addictive behaviors* (alcohol or drug use, etc.): Patients who show signs of addictive behaviors should be referred immediately to an appropriate health professional [40].
- *Sedentary lifestyle*: Beyond simply depriving the patient of the metabolic benefits of physical activity, indication that a patient is not (or no longer) engaging in physical activity can serve as a flag for a possible negative emotional state (which can be a flag for the maladaptive behaviors described previously).

Dietary Strategies for Managing Weight Regain

Food frequency questionnaire results [41] of patients following the RYGB showed an insufficient intake of good quality foods such as fruits, vegetables, meats and eggs, dairy products, beans, and carbohydrate in all groups, although the intake of snack and sweets was higher than the recommendation. As expected by the surgery-imposed restrictions and dumping syndrome, frequency of snacks and sweets and oils and fatty foods was lower in patients with less than 5 % excess weight regain within the two first years after surgery compared to patients who regained more than 5 % excess weight.

The dietetics professional should continue to work with the patient to increase the quality of their diet, and if the patient begins to exhibit any of the maladaptive behaviors listed previously, additional nutritional and/or psychological counseling may be needed to get the patient "back on track."

Dietary strategies in the maintaining phase are the same as those listed in the achieving phase but with continued monitoring and support to intervene when a patient appears to exhibit behaviors or eating patterns that could derail their new healthy lifestyle.

Physical Activity Strategies for Managing Weight Regain

The general goal with respect to long-term physical activity in the bariatric patient is to *increase energy expenditure*. Exercise is a key component of the post-weight loss surgery lifestyle and may be associated with lower weight regain [22]. Unfortunately, regular physical activity is not likely to have been a part of the patient's presurgery lifestyle, so developing and maintaining these habits may require substantial changes in the patient's schedule. In general, the patient should be encouraged to:

- *Increase energy expenditure*—Research is showing promising "reversal" of impaired fatty acid oxidation in skeletal muscle and insulin resistance. Research indicates that patients with obesity exhibit a defect in lipid oxidation within skeletal muscle, but this defect can be corrected with exercise training after 10 days but not with weight loss alone [42].
- *Move more* (minimum 150 min per week) and sit less—The patient may need help developing strategies for achieving that fit into their work and home schedules. An increasing number of companies are instituting workplace wellness programs that integrate healthy lifestyle practices into the daily work routine. Patients may have the opportunity to take advantage of resources such as these.
- *Improve body composition* (for instance, by strength training two to three times per week)—Increases in lean mass to increases resting energy expenditure.

Again, it is important to individualize patient exercise goals and allocate nutrition according to length and intensity of each patient's physical activity.

What Is the Big Picture?

What is happening with patients who are failing bariatric surgery? Studies have shown that individuals with poor weight loss after gastric bypass operations may have an attenuated release and response to GLP-1 and PYY. Table 14.4 provides a general overview of factors associated (both positively and negatively) with weight regain in weight loss surgery patients.

Conclusion

Weight Regain

After having achieved some degree of success following surgery, it can be particularly discouraging to weight loss surgery patients to begin to regain some of the weight they worked so hard to lose [41]. However, even though some weight regain is "normal" (in the sense that it is very common), it does not have to be viewed as a sign of failure (either of the procedure or of the patient). In fact, it may be an important part of weight maintenance education to help the patient understand that since their bodies are metabolically primed to regain weight, they can expect to see some short-term fluctuations in weight. Moreover, if patients have a sense that they are not condemned to fail (as they may have many times before weight loss surgery) and that the lifestyle tools and concerned healthcare professionals are available, then they may be able to avoid a vicious cycle of increasing discouragement and increasing weight.

As we noted, many of the factors that predispose patients to regain weight are behavioral. Some of the gains made by patients may disappear or attenuate over time. So, periodic assessment to prevent or treat eating or other psychiatric disorders is recommended [2]. In some severe cases, revisional surgery may be needed, but this should never be a first line of defense against weight regain.

Question and Answer Section

Questions

1. A key goal of presurgery nutrition counseling is:
   A. Patients should plan to lose 10 % of their excess body weight prior to surgery.
   B. To educate the patient that weight loss surgery, by itself, is no guarantee of losing all a patient's excess weight and lifestyle changes are crucial for success.
   C. Patients should substitute one to two meals per day with a liquid meal replacement.
   D. A and B.
   E. All of the above.
2. During the "achieving" phase of the weight loss process, patients should:
   A. Be encouraged to eat five small meals a day.
   B. Achieve the goal 75 min per week of vigorous physical activity.

Table 14.4 Summary chart of factors contributing to or preventing weight regain

Impact	Food/nutrient	Effects
Positive (+)	Dairy/calcium	2–3 servings per day found in dairy and meat
		Conjugated linoleic acid (CLA): number of potential health effects in animal studies, including ability to reduce body fat
+	Fiber	Insulin
		Improves satiety
+	Omega-3 fatty acids	EPA/DHA decrease inflammatory process of adipocyte
+	Protein	Complete proteins made of the indispensable and conditionally indispensable amino acids increase satiety and may increase energy expenditure
+	BCAA, leucine	Preserve lean mass, stimulate muscle growth
+	Pro-/prebiotics	Favorable impact on gut biome: composition of gut microbiota may affect amount of energy extracted from the diet [45]
+	Meal replacements	Substituting one or two daily meals with meal replacements is a successful weight loss and weight maintenance strategy
+	Mandatory preoperative weight loss	Increases total excess weight loss post-op
+	Carbs	Low glycemic load (GL) may reduce late dumping
+	Nutrition recommendations	CHO spares lean mass (45 % CHO, 35 % pro, 20 % fat ~16 kcal/kg) [2]
+	Moderate physical activity	Improves fat handling defects by:
		Increasing fat oxidation
		Decreasing fat storage
		Decreasing fat-promoting hormones such as cortisol
		Increasing energy expenditure—partly via preserving lean muscle mass
		Decreasing energy intake
		Improving mood
Negative (−)	Saturated/trans fats	Increase LDL, decrease HDL
−	Processed foods	BPA, GMO, chemicals, dyes, preservatives
−	Addiction	Increased hunger
	Sugars	Lowered satiety
	Fructose	
	Liquid calories	
−	Carbohydrates	Emphasizing carbs during early postoperative phase will increase CHO intake and decrease protein intake
		Increasing simple CHO postoperatively associated with weight regain
−	Skipping breakfast	Stimulates more impulsive snacking and eating at later meals; a meal replacement works well for patients who do not tolerate solid foods in morning
−	Eating and drinking fluid in same meal	Drinking during meals will result in more rapid transition of solid food from the gastric pouch, eliminating the sensation of fullness and resulting in ingestion of larger portions and/or more frequent meals
−	Specific psych medications	Promotes weight gain and/or regain
−	Psychiatric conditions (presence of 2 or more)	Inadequate weight loss or weight regain

C. Focus on eating strategies that will increase satiety, i.e., satisfied, but not full beyond capacity and minimize frequent hunger.
   D. Seek psychological counseling.
   E. All of the above.
3. In the "maintaining" phase of the weight loss process:
   A. The patient's body will adapt to the new gut, and so the immediate physiological effects of the surgery will decrease in importance.
   B. Maladaptive eating patterns present a significant threat for weight regain.
   C. The role of exercise in weight loss becomes less important.
   D. A and B.
   E. All of the above.

Answers

1. Correct answer: **B**. Research indicates that most patients will not lose all their excess body weight after surgery and that substantial lifestyle changes are a necessary component of the weight loss process to manage weight long term.

   Incorrect answers:
   Response for A: The main goal of pre-weight loss counseling is to prepare the patient for surgery and for the lifestyle changes they will need to make in order to achieve successful weight loss. Weight loss prior to surgery may be appropriate for some, but not all, patients to prepare them for surgery.
   Response for C: Patient needs for surgery preparation differ. While meal substitution may help some patients achieve weight loss in preparation for surgery, it may not be needed for all patients. Program requirements will differ, and while a universal program requirement of meal substitution may homogenize dietary counseling strategies, it is no substitute for qualified, individualized dietary intervention.

2. Correct answer **C**. Research shows that particular types of foods and eating strategies can increase a feeling of fullness and thus prevent eating purely from feelings of hunger. As part of this strategy, patients may need to "relearn" what satiety (including fullness, hunger, and satisfied) feels like.

   Incorrect answers:
   Response to A: Research is controversial regarding the number of meals appropriate for optimal weight loss. While more frequent, smaller meals may be associated with decreased weight in the nonsurgical population, it has not been clearly demonstrated in the weight loss surgery population. In fact, research on bariatric surgery patients indicate that a number of maladaptive eating behaviors include frequent eating and thus counseling the patient to eat more frequently may feed into these maladaptive behaviors.
   Response to B: Regular physical activity plays a vital role in the weight loss and weight maintenance process. However, while the level of physical activity specified for the general public in national guidelines may be an ultimate goal, many weight loss patients may not be able to achieve these goals for a number of reasons (including a fear or distaste for "exercise," inability to meet the goals due to physical limitations, restrictions on the patient's weekly schedules, etc.). The black-and-white standard of meeting the national exercise goals or not may lead patients who cannot realistically meet these goals to perceive themselves as "failures" and so give up on physical activity altogether.
   Response to C: Psychological counseling may play a vital role in the weight loss success of many patients—especially patients whose maladaptive eating behaviors stem from underlying and unrecognized emotional issues. However, there is no research to indicate that a recommendation for universal psychological counseling is warranted.

3. Correct answer: **D**. The gut does adapt and while the effects of surgery may not disappear entirely (research indicates that long-term metabolic changes may result), the rapid weight loss that is a hallmark of the immediate effects of surgery will end within 1–2 years. As the immediate effects of surgery subside, the relative importance of behavioral changes will increase. The effects of maladaptive eating behaviors, which either develop during this period or were never adequately addressed in the previous weight loss phases, are strongly associated with weight regain during this period.

   Incorrect answer:
   Response to C: Because of the waning immediate effects of surgery, the role of regular physical activity (as a component of a comprehensive lifestyle change) actually increases during the weight maintenance phase. Change in metabolism resulting from regular physical activity can help maintain initial weight loss.

References

1. Livhits M, Mercado C, Yermilov I, Parikh JA, Dutson E, Mehran A, et al. Preoperative predictors of weight loss following bariatric surgery: systematic review. Obes Surg. 2012;22(1):70–89.
2. Mechanick JI, Youdim A, Jones DB, Garvey WT, Hurley DL, McMahon MM, et al. Clinical practice guidelines for the periopera-

tive nutritional, metabolic, and nonsurgical support of the bariatric surgery patient-2013 update: cosponsored by american association of clinical endocrinologists, the obesity society, and american society for metabolic & bariatric surgery. Endocr Pract. 2013;19(2):337–72.
3. Colles SL, Dixon JB, Marks P, Strauss BJ, O'Brien PE. Preoperative weight loss with a very-low-energy diet: quantitation of changes in liver and abdominal fat by serial imaging. Am J Clin Nutr. 2006;84(2):304–11.
4. Benotti PN, Still CD, Wood GC, Akmal Y, King H, El Arousy H, et al. Preoperative weight loss before bariatric surgery. Arch Surg. 2009;144(12):1150–5.
5. Browning JD, Baker JA, Rogers T, Davis J, Satapati S, Burgess SC. Short-term weight loss and hepatic triglyceride reduction: evidence of a metabolic advantage with dietary carbohydrate restriction. Am J Clin Nutr. 2011;93(5):1048–52.
6. Alvarado R, Alami RS, Hsu G, Safadi BY, Sanchez BR, Morton JM, et al. The impact of preoperative weight loss in patients undergoing laparoscopic roux-en-y gastric bypass. Obes Surg. 2005;15(9):1282–6.
7. Busetto L, Tregnaghi A, De Marchi F, Segato G, Foletto M, Sergi G, et al. Liver volume and visceral obesity in women with hepatic steatosis undergoing gastric banding. Obes Res. 2002;10(5):408–11.
8. Mechanick JI, Youdim A, Jones DB, Garvey WT, Hurley DL, McMahon MM, et al. Clinical practice guidelines for the perioperative nutritional, metabolic, and nonsurgical support of the bariatric surgery patient-2013 update: cosponsored by American Association of Clinical Endocrinologists, the Obesity Society, and American Society for Metabolic & Bariatric Surgery*. Obesity. 2013;21 Suppl 1:S1–27.
9. Apovian CM, Cummings S, Anderson W, Borud L, Boyer K, Day K, et al. Best practice updates for multidisciplinary care in weight loss surgery. Obesity. 2009;17(5):871–9.
10. Liu RC, Sabnis AA, Forsyth C, Chand B. The effects of acute preoperative weight loss on laparoscopic roux-en-y gastric bypass. Obes Surg. 2005;15(10):1396–402.
11. Allied Health Sciences Section Ad Hoc Nutrition C, Aills L, Blankenship J, Buffington C, Furtado M, Parrott J. Asmbs allied health nutritional guidelines for the surgical weight loss patient. Surg Obes Relat Dis. 2008;4(5 Suppl):S73–108.
12. Sjostrom L, Lindroos AK, Peltonen M, Torgerson J, Bouchard C, Carlsson B, et al. Lifestyle, diabetes, and cardiovascular risk factors 10 years after bariatric surgery. N Engl J Med. 2004;351(26):2683–93.
13. Parrott JM, Parrott JS, Sowemimo S, Adeyeri A, editors. Specialized bariatric rd counseling improves pre-surgery weight loss and post-surgical excess weight loss Food and Nutrition Conference and Expo. Philadelphia: Academy of Nutrition and Dietetics; 2012.
14. Sarwer DB, Moore RH, Spitzer JC, Wadden TA, Raper SE, Williams NN. A pilot study investigating the efficacy of postoperative dietary counseling to improve outcomes after bariatric surgery. Surg Obes Relat Dis. 2012;8(5):561–8.
15. Heber D, Greenway FL, Kaplan LM, Livingston E, Salvador J, Still C, et al. Endocrine and nutritional management of the post-bariatric surgery patient: an endocrine society clinical practice guideline. J Clin Endocrinol Metab. 2010;95(11):4823–43.
16. Lewis MC, Phillips ML, Slavotinek JP, Kow L, Thompson CH, Toouli J. Change in liver size and fat content after treatment with optifast very low calorie diet. Obes Surg. 2006;16(6):697–701.
17. Westerbacka J, Lammi K, Hakkinen AM, Rissanen A, Salminen I, Aro A, et al. Dietary fat content modifies liver fat in overweight nondiabetic subjects. J Clin Endocrinol Metab. 2005;90(5):2804–9.
18. Johnston CS, Tjonn SL, Swan PD, White A, Hutchins H, Sears B. Ketogenic low-carbohydrate diets have no metabolic advantage over nonketogenic low-carbohydrate diets. Am J Clin Nutr. 2006;83(5):1055–61.
19. Tiikkainen M, Bergholm R, Vehkavaara S, Rissanen A, Hakkinen AM, Tamminen M, et al. Effects of identical weight loss on body composition and features of insulin resistance in obese women with high and low liver fat content. Diabetes. 2003;52(3):701–7.
20. Buchwald H, Avidor Y, Braunwald E, Jensen MD, Pories W, Fahrbach K, et al. Bariatric surgery: a systematic review and meta-analysis. JAMA. 2004;292(14):1724–37.
21. Adams TD, Davidson LE, Litwin SE, Kolotkin RL, LaMonte MJ, Pendleton RC, et al. Health benefits of gastric bypass surgery after 6 years. JAMA. 2012;308(11):1122–31.
22. Bond DS, Phelan S, Leahey TM, Hill JO, Wing RR. Weight-loss maintenance in successful weight losers: surgical vs non-surgical methods. Int J Obes. 2009;33(1):173–80.
23. Rudolph A, Hilbert A. Post-operative behavioural management in bariatric surgery: a systematic review and meta-analysis of randomized controlled trials. Obes Rev. 2013;14:292–302.
24. Shaw K, O'Rourke P, Del Mar C, Kenardy J. Psychological interventions for overweight or obesity. Cochrane Database Syst Rev. 2005(2):CD003818.
25. Frank LL. Nutritional management of bariatric surgery patients. Clarksville: Wolf Rinke Associates; 2012.
26. Overs SE, Freeman RA, Zarshenas N, Walton KL, Jorgensen JO. Food tolerance and gastrointestinal quality of life following three bariatric procedures: adjustable gastric banding, roux-en-y gastric bypass, and sleeve gastrectomy. Obes Surg. 2012;22(4):536–43.
27. Bond DS, Thomas JG, Ryder BA, Vithiananthan S, Pohl D, Wing RR. Ecological momentary assessment of the relationship between intention and physical activity behavior in bariatric surgery patients. Int J Behav Med. 2013;20(1):82–7.
28. Bachman JL, Phelan S, Wing RR, Raynor HA. Eating frequency is higher in weight loss maintainers and normal-weight individuals than in overweight individuals. J Am Diet Assoc. 2011;111(11):1730–4.
29. Colles SL, Dixon JB. Night eating syndrome: impact on bariatric surgery. Obes Surg. 2006;16(7):811–20.
30. Kruseman M, Leimgruber A, Zumbach F, Golay A. Dietary, weight, and psychological changes among patients with obesity, 8 years after gastric bypass. J Am Diet Assoc. 2010;110(4):527–34.
31. Cummings DE, Overduin J. Gastrointestinal regulation of food intake. J Clin Invest. 2007;117(1):13–23.
32. Moran-Ramos S, Tovar AR, Torres N. Diet: friend or foe of enteroendocrine cells—how it interacts with enteroendocrine cells. Adv Nutr. 2012;3(1):8–20.
33. Beck NN, Johannsen M, Stoving RK, Mehlsen M, Zachariae R. Do postoperative psychotherapeutic interventions and support groups influence weight loss following bariatric surgery? A systematic review and meta-analysis of randomized and nonrandomized trials. Obes Surg. 2012;22(11):1790–7.
34. Cho S, Dietrich M, Brown CJ, Clark CA, Block G. The effect of breakfast type on total daily energy intake and body mass index: results from the Third National Health and Nutrition Examination Survey (nhanes iii). J Am Coll Nutr. 2003;22(4):296–302.
35. Birketvedt GS, Florholmen J, Sundsfjord J, Osterud B, Dinges D, Bilker W, et al. Behavioral and neuroendocrine characteristics of the night-eating syndrome. JAMA. 1999;282(7):657–63.
36. Colles SL, Dixon JB, O'Brien PE. Grazing and loss of control related to eating: two high-risk factors following bariatric surgery. Obesity. 2008;16(3):615–22.
37. Wilfley DE, Bishop ME, Wilson GT, Agras WS. Classification of eating disorders: toward dsm-v. Int J Eat Disord. 2007;40(Suppl):S123–9.

38. White MA, Kalarchian MA, Masheb RM, Marcus MD, Grilo CM. Loss of control over eating predicts outcomes in bariatric surgery patients: a prospective, 24-month follow-up study. J Clin Psychiatry. 2010;71(2):175–84.
39. Mitchell JE, Steffen K. The interface between eating disorders and bariatric surgery. Eat Disord Rev. 2009;20(1):1.
40. Odom J, Zalesin KC, Washington TL, Miller WW, Hakmeh B, Zaremba DL, et al. Behavioral predictors of weight regain after bariatric surgery. Obes Surg. 2010;20(3):349–56.
41. Freire RH, Borges MC, Alvarez-Leite JI, Toulson Davisson Correia MI. Food quality, physical activity, and nutritional follow-up as determinant of weight regain after roux-en-y gastric bypass. Nutrition. 2012;28(1):53–8.
42. Berggren JR, Boyle KE, Chapman WH, Houmard JA. Skeletal muscle lipid oxidation and obesity: influence of weight loss and exercise. Am J Physiol Endocrinol Metab. 2008;294(4): E726–32.
43. Page KA, Chan O, Arora J, Belfort-Deaguiar R, Dzuira J, Roehmholdt B, et al. Effects of fructose vs glucose on regional cerebral blood flow in brain regions involved with appetite and reward pathways. JAMA. 2013;309(1):63–70.
44. Schwiertz A, Taras D, Schafer K, Beijer S, Bos NA, Donus C, et al. Microbiota and SCFA in lean and overweight healthy subjects. Obesity. 2010;18(1):190–5.
45. Backhed F, Ding H, Wang T, Hooper LV, Koh GY, Nagy A, et al. The gut microbiota as an environmental factor that regulates fat storage. Proc Natl Acad Sci U S A. 2004;101(44):15718–23.

Part III

Obesity Medicine

Lifestyle Modification for the Treatment of Obesity

David B. Sarwer, Meghan L. Butryn, Evan Forman, and Lauren E. Bradley

Chapter Objectives

At the end of this chapter the reader will be able to list the components of an effective lifestyle modification program for weight loss. The reader will also be able to identify examples of the efficacy of lifestyle modification programs. This chapter will provide the reader with the knowledge to explain how lifestyle modification relates to weight loss, bariatric surgery, as well as weight maintenance.

Lifestyle Modification for Weight Loss

Lifestyle modification is considered the first line of treatment for individuals with a body mass index (BMI) of 25 kg/m^2 or greater, which classifies them as overweight. Lifestyle modification also is recommended for use with individuals who may use pharmacotherapy to control their weight. The terms *lifestyle modification*, *behavioral treatment*, and *behavioral weight control* are often used interchangeably. They all include three principal components: (1) diet, (2) physical activity (PA), and (3) behavioral modification. Lifestyle modification, as applied to weight control, refers to a set of principles and techniques to help patients adopt new eating and activity habits, replacing maladaptive habits that likely contributed to the development of obesity.

D.B. Sarwer, PhD (✉)
Department of Psychiatry, Director of Clinical Services Center for Weight and Eating Disorders, Perelman School of Medicine at the University of Pennsylvania, Philadelphia, PA, USA
e-mail: dsarwer@mail.med.upenn.edu

M.L. Butryn, PhD • E. Forman, PhD • L.E. Bradley, MS
Department of Psychology, Drexel University,
3201 Chestnut Street, Philadelphia, PA 19104, USA
e-mail: mlb34@drexel.edu; evan.forman@drexel.edu;
leb57@drexel.edu; laur.bradley@gmail.com

These lifestyle modification strategies are used in some, if not all, forms of weight control. For example, self-directed diets obtained from books, magazines, and Web sites typically include recommendations to avoid certain foods and consume others. Commercial weight-loss programs include behavioral modification strategies in both their in-person groups and their online programs. Pharmacological treatments for obesity, even with their checkered past and uncertain future, often include behaviorally based programs designed to maximize weight losses. These strategies also are believed to play an important role in long-term success after bariatric surgery, as discussed in detail below.

The elements of lifestyle modification for weight loss and maintenance are based on social cognitive theory [1–4]. Social cognitive theory emphasizes that self-efficacy—the perceived ability to execute actions in support of a behavior—is a crucial determinant of the initiation and maintenance of an adaptive behavior. Central to the formulation of self-efficacy is the successful implementation of self-regulation strategies important for the management of chronic illness [2–4]. As applied to weight control, these strategies include altering eating and exercise behaviors, as well as restructuring environmental cues to enhance the likelihood of adherence. Lifestyle modification also includes education about nutrition and physical activity.

Ideally, patients receive medical clearance from their primary care physician or other medical provider to confirm that the patient is appropriately healthy for weight reduction. It also is recommended that patients undergo a comprehensive behavioral evaluation prior to the onset of treatment [5]. This evaluation reviews patient's weight history, current diet composition, eating behaviors, and activity patterns.

Most lifestyle modification programs utilize a structured treatment protocol. These protocols are often delivered to patients by nutritionists, registered dietitians, and other behavioral health providers, but they also can be found in self-help books and as part of Internet-based programs. Treatment is often conducted individually but also can be provided in small groups that meet weekly in order to facilitate adherence and weight loss.

Lifestyle modification programs typically consist of several main components. These include self-monitoring of behavior, caloric restriction, increased physical activity, and cognitive-behavioral strategies to identify maladaptive eating and activity behaviors and promote the development of healthy behaviors.

Self-Monitoring

Self-monitoring of food intake and physical activity is likely the most important skill to help patients successfully engage in self-regulation. Patients are typically asked to monitor their weight on a regular basis (at least weekly but in some programs daily) but also keep records of their daily food intake, total calories, and physical activity. Self-monitoring provides patients with feedback on their targeted behavior as well as opportunity to modify these behaviors as appropriate. Regular self-monitoring of food intake and weekly weighing is perhaps the strongest predictor of initial weight loss as well as larger weight losses at the end of treatment.

Sessions with the treatment provider typically begin with a review of participants' food and activity records. The provider helps participants identify strategies to cope with problems identified and, thus, increase their adherence to the prescribed eating and activity plans. Although the provider focuses on a new topic each week, sessions focus more on participants' reviewing their progress than on the practitioner's lecturing.

Caloric Restriction

Lifestyle modification programs typically prescribe a balanced deficit diet that ranges from 1,200 to 1,800 cal per day. Patients who begin treatment with a relatively lower body weight are given a calorie goal at the lower end of this range than individuals with a higher BMI. Calorie goals are based on the assumption that reducing daily intake to 500 cal below baseline levels will produce approximately 0.5 kg per week of weight loss. Through trial and error, the patient and treatment provider can determine a more specific calorie goal to promote this rate of weight loss, which is thought to minimize the potential risk of any negative health consequences related to a more rapid weight loss. Formulas also can be used to more precisely estimate energy needs based on sex, age, weight, and activity level. Adherence to the prescribed calorie goal is the key to achieving weight loss. Focusing on calorie intake goals, rather than following a plan outlining more specific changes to the composition of the diet, allows patients to be flexible and make self-selected food choices that are sustainable over the long-term. Balanced deficit diets like this typically do not require ongoing medical supervision.

Overweight and obese individuals in lifestyle modification programs are usually encouraged to consume a high-carbohydrate, low-fat diet (i.e., fewer than 30 % of calories from fat) that emphasizes consumption of fruits, vegetables, and whole grains [6]. This diet is consistent with recommendations of the US Department of Agriculture [7]. Lifestyle modification, however, can be combined with a variety of other dietary approaches, including those that encourage a reduction in the consumption of carbohydrates and sugars.

Many lifestyle modification programs also include or encourage the use of meal replacement products as a means to promote adherence to the recommended caloric targets. Many of these products are readily available in grocery stores; others are available directly from the company and can be ordered over the Internet. These approaches appear to produce superior weight losses compared to those seen with isocaloric diets composed of conventional foods [8].

Physical Activity

Physical activity is another tenant of lifestyle modification programs for weight loss. Patients can increase their energy expenditure in two ways: with programmed or lifestyle activity. Programmed activity is synonymous with "exercise" and is typically planned and completed in a discrete period of time (i.e., 30–60 min) at a relatively high-intensity level (i.e., 60–80 % of maximum heart rate). Examples of programmed activity include jogging, biking, or swimming. Lifestyle activity, by contrast, involves increasing energy expenditure throughout the course of the day, without concern for the intensity or duration of the activity [9]. Patients can increase their lifestyle activity by parking further away from store entrances or taking stairs rather than escalators.

Physical activity alone (in the absence in the reduction of caloric intake) is of limited benefit in inducing weight loss [10]. This is surprising and disappointing to patients and providers, who often assume that high levels of physical activity, regardless of changes in diet and eating behavior, can produce a substantial weight loss. In reality, most individuals simply cannot find the time or motivation to engage in the high volume of activity (e.g., 35 miles of walking a week) required to lose a mere 0.5 kg a week. This rate of weight loss is more easily achieved by participants' simply restricting their food intake by 500 kcal/d.

The greatest contribution of physical activity to successful weight control may be related to long-term weight maintenance. The long-term benefits of physical activity for weight management have been demonstrated by numerous studies [11–14]. To achieve optimal long-term weight control, patients are encouraged to expend 2,500–3,000 kcal/week, the equivalent of walking 25–30 miles a week.

Cognitive-Behavioral Strategies

Lifestyle modification programs also teach patients cognitive-behavioral skills. Patients practice setting short-term, reasonable, specific, and measurable goals for the development of more adaptive and healthy behaviors. Assessing progress toward these goals on a weekly basis is a cornerstone of treatment. Functional analysis teaches patients to identify the events or cues that occur before and after a targeted behavior to determine what is causing and maintaining the maladaptive behavior and make changes in these events or cues accordingly and to promote the engagement in healthier behaviors. Stimulus control principles also are used to change the internal and external cues associated with targeted eating and activity behaviors. Patients are taught to change their immediate environments (e.g., the home and workplace) so that they facilitate, rather than hinder, positive behavior change. For example, stimulus control can focus on reducing exposure to particularly tempting high-calorie foods, increasing the availability and visibility of healthy food, and creating cues for physical activity.

Problem solving is another core behavioral skill. Patients identify a problem in detail, brainstorm potential solutions to the problem, consider the pros and cons of each option, choose a solution, develop a plan to implement it, and evaluate the effectiveness of the chosen solution once the behavior has been implemented. Relapse prevention skills help patients to anticipate and develop strategies for dealing with high-risk situations, such as a stressful project at work or a vacation, and plan how they will respond to lapses in adherence. Most lifestyle modification programs also teach cognitive restructuring, in which patients identify and modify automatic thoughts and develop rational responses to these thoughts as a way of changing behavior.

Efficacy of Lifestyle Modification

Individuals treated by a comprehensive lifestyle modification using the tenants detailed above lose approximately 7–10 % of their initial weight within 4–6 months of active treatment. Approximately 80 % of patients who begin treatment complete it, suggesting the acceptability of treatment to the vast majority of patients. Thus, lifestyle modification yields favorable results as judged by the criteria for success (i.e., a 5–10 % reduction in initial weight) proposed by the World Health Organization, the National Institutes of Health, and the Dietary Guidelines for Americans [7, 15, 16]. These findings are associated with significant improvements in weight-related comorbidities, such as type 2 diabetes and hypertension.

Three large studies have provided perhaps the most important evidence for the efficacy and effectiveness for lifestyle modification in the treatment of obesity. These studies include the Diabetes Prevention Program, Look AHEAD, and the recently completed Power Trials.

Diabetes Prevention Program

The Diabetes Prevention Program was a large, nationwide randomized controlled trial of more than 3,200 overweight or obese men and women with impaired glucose tolerance. Participants were randomly assigned to one of three treatment conditions: (1) placebo, (2) metformin, or (3) a lifestyle modification intervention designed to achieve a weight loss of 7 % of initial body weight [17]. After almost 3 years of active treatment, persons who received lifestyle modification lost 5.6 kg, which was significantly greater than the 2.1 kg weight loss in the metformin group and the negligible weight change experienced by the placebo group. More impressively, the lifestyle modification group experienced a 58 % decreased risk of developing type 2 diabetes as compared to placebo, which was almost double the 31 % decreased risk experienced by those who were treated with metformin and as compared to placebo.

A number of reports have highlighted the impressive long-term results from the trial. Following active treatment, participants in all three treatment groups were offered quarterly support groups designed to maintain the benefits of treatment. The benefits of lifestyle modification were well maintained over a 10-year period; diabetes incidence was reduced by 34 % in the lifestyle group and by 18 % in the metformin group, as compared to placebo [18].

Look AHEAD

The Look AHEAD (Action for Health in Diabetes) study provides additional evidence that lifestyle modification can produce clinically significant weight loss and long-term improvements in cardiovascular risk factors and fitness [19]. Look AHEAD enrolled 5,145 overweight and obese individuals (age 55–74 years) with type 2 diabetes. They were randomly assigned to an intensive lifestyle intervention (ILI) or a usual care group, referred to as Diabetes Support and Education (DSE). Participants in ILI attended group and individual sessions on an approximately weekly basis in year 1. Sessions continued with less frequency in years 2–4. ILI participants were encouraged to exercise at least 175 min per week, limit calorie and fat intake, and use portion-controlled meals and meal replacements. DSE participants attended three educational sessions per year. At the end of year 1, ILI participants lost 8.6 % of initial weight, compared to 0.7 % for DSE. At the end of year 4, ILI participants maintained a weight loss of 4.7 % of initial weight, compared with 1.1 % for DSE. At year 4, ILI participants also maintained significantly greater improvements than DSE participants in cardiovascular fitness, hemoglobin A(1c) levels, blood pressure, and HDL cholesterol.

Power-Up Trials

Recently, three studies investigated the efficacy of lifestyle modification, along with other weight-loss interventions, delivered in primary care practices.

At the University of Pennsylvania, 390 obese adults were assigned to one of three types of interventions: usual care, brief lifestyle counseling (which included in-person monthly coaching sessions with a medical professional in the physician's office), and enhanced brief lifestyle counseling (which also included the use of meal replacements or weight-loss medications) [20]. At the end of the 2-year trial, mean weight losses were 1.7±0.7, 2.9±0.7, and 4.6±0.7 kg, respectively. The weight loss seen with enhanced brief lifestyle counseling was significantly greater than the loss seen with usual care. More frequent attendance at counseling sessions was associated with greater weight loss, providing additional evidence of the importance of continued patient-provider for facilitating long-term weight maintenance.

In a study done by Appel and colleagues at Johns Hopkins University, 415 obese patients with at least one cardiovascular risk factor were recruited from six primary care offices [21]. The participants were divided into one of three interventions. One intervention provided patients with weight-loss support remotely (telephone, study-specific Web site, and email). The other intervention provided in-person support during group and individual sessions along with the three remote means of support. There was also a control group in which weight loss was self-directed. At the end of the 24-month intervention, the mean weight losses were 0.8 kg in the control group, 4.6 kg in the group receiving remote support only, and 5.1 kg in the group receiving in-person support. The weight losses in both intervention groups were significantly greater than the weight losses in the control group. This study showed that a lifestyle intervention delivered remotely was as effective as the more traditional approach to treatment, which incorporated more face-to-face contact between participants and weight-loss coaches.

The third study from this program of research was conducted at Harvard University [22] Investigators randomized 222 adults with long-duration, poorly controlled diabetes, into three groups. One group (structured behavioral arm) received a 5-session, manual-based, educator-led, structured group intervention with cognitive-behavioral strategies. Another group (group attention control) received an educator-led education program. The third group (individual control) received unlimited individual nurse and dietitian education sessions for 6 months. The structured behavioral arm was more effective than the two control interventions in improving glycemia in the participants by showing greater improvements in HbA (1c) than the group and individual control arms (3-month HbA (1c) concentration changes: 0.8 % versus −0.4 % and −0.4 %, respectively). This study showed that structured, cognitive-behavioral programs using psychological and behavioral strategies can be used to improve glycemia in patients with long-duration diabetes.

Long-Term Weight Maintenance

Despite the impressive results from the clinical trials described, weight regain is a significant threat to the long-term success of lifestyle modification. Patients treated by lifestyle modification for 20–30 weeks typically regain about one-third of their lost weight in the year following treatment. Weight regain slows after the first year, but by 5 years the vast majority of patients are likely to have returned to their baseline weight [23].

There are likely a number of factors that contribute to weight regain. Compensatory metabolic responses to weight loss, including reductions in resting energy expenditure and changes in appetite hormones such as leptin and increases in ghrelin, protect against the adverse effects of starvation, which the body cannot distinguish from intentional dieting [24]. A number of environmental and behavioral factors also play a role in weight regain. For example, once patients stop active participation in lifestyle modification, they encounter an environment filled with countless, convenient eating opportunities (particularly for high-calorie foods) and which also discourages engagement in physical activity.

Despite these disheartening observations, data from the National Weight Control Registry [25] suggests that some individuals are successful maintaining weight losses over extended periods of time. The Registry, which includes individuals who have maintained at least a 30 lb weight loss for at least 1 year, suggests that continued application of the tenants of lifestyle modification strategies described above is associated with weight maintenance. Individuals in the Registry report eating a reduced calorie diet (approximately 1,400 kcal/d) which is low in fat and high in carbohydrates. At the same time, they engage in high levels of lifestyle and programmed activity (approximately 2,800 kcal/wk). A large percentage of Registry patients also continue to self-monitor their food intake and daily calories. Many registry members report that they regularly weigh themselves; 44 % weigh themselves at least once a day and 31 % weigh themselves weekly [26].

Continued, regular contact between the patient and a treatment provider also appears to be associated with weight maintenance. This contact provides participants the support and motivation needed to continue to practice weight control behaviors. Within the past decade, there has been increased attention to the use of electronically provided treatment, both for initial weight loss as well as weight maintenance [21, 27–30]. The use of telephone, mail, or email contact could decrease the burden of participants' attending on-site maintenance sessions.

The Application of Lifestyle Modification to Bariatric Surgery

There is little debating the superiority of bariatric surgery to lifestyle modification interventions when they are compared on the size of weight loss as well as improvements in morbidity and mortality. However, the impressive outcomes seen with surgery must be balanced by reports suggesting that 20–30 % of patients fail to reach the typical postoperative weight loss or begin to regain large amounts of weight within the first 2 years of surgery [31, 32]. These suboptimal results are usually attributed to behavioral factors, including dietary intake, disordered eating, and low levels of physical activity [33]. As a result of these treatment "failures," a number of patients are returning for further surgical procedures, when application of lifestyle modification may be a more appropriate first-line intervention.

The current standard of care in bariatric surgery does not provide the long-term behavioral support necessary to follow the rigorous postoperative dietary regimen or adaptive eating behaviors necessary for lifelong success. At the same time, while bariatric surgery programs typically encourage their patients to increase their physical activity after surgery, few provide specific recommendations, training, or monitoring of patients' progress. Recent studies using objective measures show most patients are inactive or insufficiently active preoperatively and do not make substantial changes in their PA postoperatively [34–37]. Physical activity after bariatric surgery is discussed in more detail in Chap. 22.

These findings highlight the struggles that bariatric surgery patients experience in adopting a habitual postoperative PA program. Without additional support, patients with low levels of PA preoperatively are unlikely to make significant changes in their PA postoperatively, thus placing them at higher risk for experiencing poorer initial weight losses and weight regain [38]. Encouragingly, a recent study of 33 bariatric surgery patients, randomized to either standard postoperative care or a 12-week program in which patients were instructed to expend >2,000 kcal/week in PA found that 53 % of patients could meet that activity goal and 82 % expended >1,500 kcal/week [39]. While those in the intervention condition engaged in higher levels of PA, the two groups did not differ in weight change over the 12 weeks. This may be the result of the brief nature of the intervention and lack of specific dietary counseling in the intervention group.

Furthermore, bariatric patients struggle to routinely follow-up with their programs, either through annual visits or attendance at support groups.

A number of studies have found that more frequent postoperative follow-up and/or attendance at support groups is associated with greater weight loss [40–43]. These observations, coupled with the maladaptive changes in dietary adherence and low levels of PA seen in the studies detailed above, underscore the need for the development and investigation of lifestyle interventions to promote long-term success after surgery.

Recently, investigators have begun to apply lifestyle modification interventions to the postoperative care of bariatric patients and to improve postoperative outcomes. Papalazarou and colleagues completed a pilot study of 30 women who underwent laparoscopic adjustable gastric banding and were randomly assigned to usual postoperative care or a lifestyle intervention of standard behavior modification strategies delivered by a dietitian in monthly visits during the first postoperative year [44]. The intervention led to significantly greater weight loss and weight maintenance 12, 24, and 36 months after surgery (45.3 kg versus 30.8 kg at postoperative year 3).

At least two studies have described "rescue" interventions designed to promote weight loss in individuals who either failed to lose an anticipated amount of weight after surgery or who regained weight. In a pilot study of 33 individuals, Faria and colleagues used a low glycemic load diet to promote a 4.3 ± 1.3 kg weight loss in 3 months [45]. Kalarchian and colleagues reported on 36 patients who had lost <50 % of their excess weight at least 3 years postoperatively [46]. They were randomly assigned to a behavioral weight control program or wait list control group for approximately 6 months. Individuals who received the intervention lost more weight than those in the control group (5.8 ± 3.5 % v. 0.9 ± 3.2 %), but the difference between the groups was not significant.

Sarwer and colleagues recently completed a pilot study designed to investigate the hypothesis that the provision of postoperative dietary counseling, delivered by a registered dietitian, would lead to greater weight loss, as well as more positive improvements in dietary intake and eating behavior, as compared to standard postoperative care [47]. Eighty-four patients were randomized to one of two postoperative treatment conditions. Forty-one patients were assigned to brief (15 min), every-other-week, in-person postoperative dietary counseling sessions with a dietitian for the first 4 months after surgery. The other individuals ($n=43$) received standard postoperative care, in which they were encouraged but not required to attend the program's monthly support group (standard care).

Participants who received dietary counseling lost 20.7 ± 1.1 % of their initial weight at the end of the intervention (month 4), which was greater than the 18.5 ± 1.1 % loss in the standard care group. Participants who received dietary counseling maintained a greater weight loss at month 24, but the difference between the groups did not reach statistical significance. At each postoperative assessment, individuals who received dietary counseling had lower mean consumption of calories, sweets, and fat and higher mean protein consumption as compared to individuals in standard care. However, these differences did not reach statistical significance [47].

Results of this pilot study provide support for the potential utility of postoperative dietary counseling to improve outcomes following bariatric surgery. However, the study also suffered from a number of limitations. First, the relatively small sample sizes of the two groups may have prevented the detection of statistically significant differences between them. Second, the delivery of the intervention may have been premature. That is, the dietary counseling took place during the period of greatest weight loss and when the physiological effects of bariatric surgery may be most potent. The intervention may be of greater benefit to patients if it is extended throughout the postoperative period. Third, patients had trouble completing their in-person visits. While participants reported that they found the sessions helpful, several indicted that they could not complete these session as they had used most of their sick, personal, and vacation time completing their preoperative clinical assessments. Encouragingly, a post hoc analysis revealed that those who received four or more counseling sessions lost more weight than those who participated in fewer sessions, including a 7.2 % difference in weight loss 24 months after surgery [47].

The findings from these pilot studies provide some evidence for the potential efficacy of postoperative lifestyle modification interventions after surgery. Larger studies of this issue are clearly needed and may need to consider to include the use of electronically delivered (i.e., telephone, electronic mail and text messaging, as well as Internet sites) to reduce the burden of in-person treatment visits.

New Developments in Lifestyle Modification

Given the insufficiencies of lifestyle modification treatments to provide long-lasting weight losses, some investigators are incorporating innovative psychological components to increase adherence to eating and physical activity recommendations. These include the use of Internet interventions [48], financial incentives [49], and motivational interviewing [50]. One approach that appears especially promising incorporates aspects from third-wave cognitive-behavioral treatments that emphasize mindful acceptance of one's internal experiences (e.g., hunger, food cravings), rather than changing or eliminating these experiences, in the service of desired goals and values [51]. Some programs also focus on raising awareness of decision-making processes to increase deliberate health-related decisions despite of an implicit drive for reward (e.g., consumption of palatable foods) [52].

Early research supports the efficacy of acceptance-based behavioral interventions. Results from several analog studies suggest the superiority of acceptance-based versus standard cognitive-behavioral strategies for managing food cravings, particularly in those with higher levels of disinhibited eating and greater responsivity to the food environment [53, 54]. Other studies have demonstrated the efficacy of acceptance-based interventions for weight loss. For example, studies have found promising effects of Acceptance and Commitment Therapy (ACT) workshops on weight loss and weight-loss maintenance as compared to control conditions [55].

Recent research has expanded upon these initial findings by evaluating longer-term interventions with an emphasis on acceptance-based strategies. For example, Niemeier and colleagues found that a 24-week acceptance-based intervention resulted in particularly large weight losses (10.2 kg) at 9-month follow-up [56]. Forman and colleagues reported substantial weight loss at both posttreatment and 6-month follow-up (8.1 % and 10.3 %, respectively) in 19 overweight women who participated in a 12-session acceptance-based intervention [57]. In an extension of this study, 128 participants were randomly assigned to receive a 40-week standard behavioral intervention or an acceptance-based behavioral intervention. Although both groups displayed comparable and significant weight losses, when interventions were administered by expert clinicians, those in acceptance-based behavioral therapy (ABT) lost significantly more weight compared to those in standard behavioral treatment (SBT) at posttreatment (13.2 % versus 7.5 %) and 6-month follow-up (11.0 % versus 4.8 %). ABT was found to be substantially more effective at follow-up in those with higher levels of depression at baseline, greater responsiveness to food cues, higher levels of disinhibition, and greater emotional eating. Combined, the current research suggests that the addition of acceptance-based components to lifestyle modification programs may be beneficial, especially for those with greater responsivity to the food environment and with higher levels of disinhibited eating.

There are theoretical reasons for hypothesizing that acceptance-based interventions may be particularly beneficial for individuals post-bariatric surgery. For instance, hunger and food cravings are implicated in weight regain among bariatric surgery patients [58], and better tolerating these types of aversive internal experiences is a focus of acceptance-based approaches. Recent research provides initial support for this theoretical model. For example, one case study has reported on the success of a mindfulness-based intervention postsurgery in continued weight loss and decreased emotional eating and grazing [59]. Also, a standard cognitive-behavioral intervention that incorporated mindfulness strategies targeting binge eating resulted in sustained weight loss after bariatric surgery [60]. Research also shows additional benefits of acceptance-based interventions in this population apart from weight outcomes. Weineland and colleagues found decreases in eating disordered behavior and body dissatisfaction and improved quality of life in those randomly assigned to an ACT intervention compared to those assigned to treatment as usual [61]. Taken together, these results show promise of incorporating acceptance-based strategies when treating the post-bariatric surgery population; however, more research is necessary.

Conclusion

This chapter has provided an overview on the use of lifestyle modification for weight loss. Lifestyle modification involves a number of behavioral strategies designed to improve diet quality, change maladaptive eating behaviors, and promote increased levels of physical activity. These interventions typically produce a weight loss of 7–10 % of initial body weight and which is associated with improvements in weight-related health problems. Recent studies have suggested that these interventions also have the ability to be translated to both primary care practice as well as different modalities such as telephone counseling and the Internet. Patients who continue to engage in the lifestyle modifications strategies that promoted the initial weight loss appear to have some success in maintaining these losses over extended periods of time. Unfortunately, physiological changes, environmental factors, and the difficulty in making these changes a regular part of daily living make long-term maintenance difficult for most.

The relatively modest size of the weight losses seen with lifestyle modification, coupled with the challenges of long-term weight maintenance, lead many professionals who typically work with bariatric patients to quickly discount the value of lifestyle modification for weight loss. This is unfortunate. In the past few years, a number of small studies have begun to look at the potential utility of lifestyle interventions to promote lifelong success after bariatric surgery, particularly for those individuals who experience smaller-than-expected early weight losses or sizable weight regain. Furthermore, newer models of behavioral change, such as Acceptance and Commitment Therapy, show promise when their potential application to bariatric surgery is considered. For these reasons, lifestyle modification is likely to play an important role in the further development and refinement of bariatric surgery in the years to come.

Question and Answer Section

Questions

1. Lifestyle modification for weight loss includes all of the following except:
   A. Physical activity
   B. Weight-loss surgery
   C. Diet
   D. Behavioral modification
2. Data from the National Weight Control Registry suggests that individuals who are successful at maintaining weight losses over extended periods of time apply which of the following behaviors:
   A. Consume a low-carbohydrate diet
   B. Play a sport
   C. Keep a daily dairy of food intake
   D. Weigh themselves only at annual checkups with their physician

Answers

1. Answer: **B**. Lifestyle modification does not include surgical treatment for overweight/obesity, although lifestyle modification is recommended both before and after a patient has weight-loss surgery.
2. Answer: **C**. A large percentage of Registry patients self-monitor their food intake and daily calories.

Acknowledgments Completion of this chapter was supported, in part, by grants:
NIH Grant HL109235
NIDDK Grant 1RC1DK086132
University of Pennsylvania Diabetes Research Center Grant 2P30DK019525-36
NIH Grant R01-DK072452
NIH Grant NCT00721838

Disclosures Dr. Sarwer has received consulting compensation from Allergan, BAROnova, EnteroMedics, and Ethicon Endo-Surgery, which are manufacturers of products for obesity. None of these entities provided financial support for his work on this manuscript.

References

1. Bandura A. Self-efficacy: toward a unifying theory of behavioral change. Psychol Rev. 1977;84(2):191–215.
2. Glanz K, Rimer BK, Viswanath K. Health behavior and health education: theory, research, and practice. 4th ed. San Francisco: Jossey-Bass, Inc.; 2008.
3. Painter JE, Borba CP, Hynes M, Mays D, Glanz K. The use of theory in health behavior research from 2000 to 2005: a systematic review. Ann Behav Med. 2008;35(3):358–62. Epub 2008 Jul 17.

4. Rothman AJ. Toward a theory-based analysis of behavioral maintenance. Health Psychol. 2000;19:64–9.
5. Kushner RF, Sarwer DB. Medical and behavioral evaluation of patients with obesity. Psychiatr Clin North Am. 2011;34(4):797–812.
6. Diabetes Prevention Program Research Group. The Diabetes Prevention Program: description of lifestyle intervention. Diabetes Care. 2002;25(12):2165–71.
7. U.S. Department of Agriculture, U.S. Department of Health and Human Services. Dietary Guidelines for Americans. Washington, DC (2010). Available from: http://www.health.gov/dietaryguidelines/2010.asp.
8. Heymsfield SB, van Mierlo CA, van der Knaap HC, Heo M, Frier HI. Weight management using a meal replacement strategy: meta and pooling analysis from six studies. Int J Obes. 2003;27(5):537–49.
9. Blair SN, Leermakers EA. Exercise and weight management. In: Wadden TA, Stunkard AJ, editors. Handbook of obesity treatment. New York: Guilford Press; 2002. p. 283–300.
10. Wadden TA, Butryn ML, Byrne KJ. Efficacy of lifestyle modification for long-term weight control. Obes Res. 2004;12(Suppl):151S–62.
11. Jakicic JM, Winters C, Lang W, Wing RR. Effects of intermittent exercise and use of home exercise equipment on adherence, weight loss, and fitness in overweight women: a randomized trial. J Am Med Assoc. 1999;282(16):1554–60.
12. Jeffery RW, Wing RR, Sherwood NE, Tate DF. Physical activity and weight loss: does prescribing higher physical activity goals improve outcome? Am J Clin Nutr. 2003;78(4):684–9.
13. Wing RR, Hill JO. Successful weight loss maintenance. Annu Rev Nutr. 2001;21:323–41.
14. Wing RR. Physical activity in the treatment of the adulthood overweight and obesity: current evidence and research issues. Med Sci Sports Exerc. 1999;31(11 Suppl):S547–52.
15. World Health Organization. Obesity: preventing and managing the global epidemic. Geneva: World Health Organization; 1998.
16. National Institutes of Health/National Heart, Lung, and Blood Institute. Clinical guidelines on the identification, evaluation, and treatment of overweight and obesity in adults. Obes Res. 1998;6:51S–210.
17. Diabetes Prevention Program Research Group. Reduction in the incidence of type 2 diabetes with lifestyle intervention or metformin. N Engl J Med. 2002;346(6):393–403.
18. Diabetes Prevention Program Research Group. Effects of withdrawal from metformin on the development of diabetes in the diabetes prevention program. Diabetes Care. 2003;26(4):977–80.
19. Look AHEAD Research Group. Long term effects of a lifestyle intervention on weight and cardiovascular risk factors in individuals with type 2 diabetes: four year results of the Look AHEAD trial. Arch Intern Med. 2010;170(17):1566–75.
20. Wadden TA, Volger S, Sarwer DB, Vetter ML, Tsai AG, Berkowitz RI, et al. A two-year randomized trial of obesity treatment in primary care practice. N Engl J Med. 2011;365(21):1969–79.
21. Appel L, Clark J, Yeh H, Wang NY, Coughlin JW, Daumit G, et al. Comparative effectiveness of weight-loss interventions in clinical practice. N Engl J Med. 2011;365(21):1959–68.
22. Weinger K, Beverly EA, Lee Y, Sitnokov L, Ganda OP, Caballero AE. The effect of a structured behavioral intervention on poorly controlled diabetes: a randomized controlled trial. Arch Intern Med. 2011;171(22):1990–9.
23. Perri MG, Corsica JA. Improving the maintenance of weight lost in behavioral treatment of obesity. In: Wadden TA, Stunkard AJ, editors. Handbook of obesity treatment. New York: Guilford Press; 2002. p. 357–79.
24. Vetter ML, Ritter S, Wadden TA, Sarwer DB. Comparison of bariatric surgical procedures on diabetes remission: efficacy and mechanisms. Diabetes Spectr. 2012;25:200–10.
25. National Weight Control Registry. http://www.nwcr.ws/. Accessed 28 Feb 2013.
26. Wing RR, Tate DF, Gorin AA, Raynor HA, Fava JL. A self-regulation program for maintenance of weight loss. N England J Med. 2006;355(15):1563–71.
27. Donnelly JF, Smith BK, Dunn L, Mayo MM, Jacobsen DJ, Stewart EE, et al. Comparison of a phone vs. clinic approach to achieve 10% weight loss. Int J Obes. 2007;31:1270–6.
28. Eakin E, Reeves M, Lawler S, Graves N, Oldenburg B, Del Mar C, et al. Telephone counseling for physical activity and diet in primary care patients. Am J Prev Med. 2009;36(2):142–9.
29. Perri M, Limacher M, Durning P, Janicke JM, Lutes LD, Bobroff LB, et al. Extended-Care programs for weight management in rural communities. Arch Intern Med. 2008;168(21):2347–54.
30. Sherwood N, Crain A, Martinson B, Hayes MG, Anderson JD, Clausen JM, et al. Keep it off: a phone-based intervention for long-term weight-loss maintenance. Contemp Clin Trials. 2011;32:551–60.
31. Sjostrom L, Lindroos AK, Peltonen M, Torgerson J, Bouchard C, Carlsson B, et al. Lifestyle, diabetes, and cardiovascular risk factors 10 years after bariatric surgery. N Engl J Med. 2004;351:2683–93.
32. Sjostrom L, Narbro K, Sjostrom CD, Karason K, Larsson B, Wedel H, et al. Swedish Obese Subjects Study. Effects of bariatric surgery on mortality in Swedish obese subjects. N Engl J Med. 2007;357:741–52.
33. Sarwer DB, Dilks RJ, West-Smith L. Dietary intake and eating behavior after bariatric surgery: threats to weight loss maintenance and strategies for success. Surg Obes Relat Dis. 2011;7(5):644–51.
34. Bond DS, Jakicic JM, Unick JL, Vithiananthan S, Pohl D, Roye GD. Pre- to postoperative physical activity changes in bariatric surgery patients: self report vs. objective measures. Obesity. 2010;18(12):2395–7.
35. Bond D, Thomas J, Ryder B, Vithiananthan S, Pohl D, Wing RR. Ecological momentary assessment of the relationship between intention and physical activity behavior in bariatric surgery patients. Int J Behav Med. 2013;20(1):82–7.
36. King W, Belle S, Eid G, Dakin GF, Inabnet WB, Mitchell JE, et al. Physical activity levels of patients undergoing bariatric surgery in the Longitudinal Assessment of Bariatric Surgery study. Surg Obes Relat Dis. 2008;4(6):721–8.
37. King W, Hsu J, Belle S, Courcoulas AP, Eid GM, Flum DR, et al. Pre-to postoperative changes in physical activity: report from the Longitudinal Assessment of Bariatric Surgery study. Surg Obes Relat Dis. 2011;7(6):548–57.
38. Bond D, Phelan S, Wolfe L, Evans RK, Meador JG, Kellum JM, et al. Becoming physically active after bariatric surgery is associated with improved weight loss and health-related quality of life. Obesity. 2009;17(1):78–83.
39. Shah M, Snell P, Rao S, Adams-Huet B, Quittner C, Livingston EH, et al. High-volume exercise program in obese bariatric surgery patients: a randomized, controlled trial. Obesity. 2011;19:1826–34.
40. Dixon J, Laurie C, Anderson M, Hayden MJ, Dixon ME, O'Brien PE. Motivation, readiness to change, and weight loss following adjustable gastric band surgery. Obesity. 2009;17:698–705.
41. Harper J, Madan AK, Ternovits CA, Tichansky DS. What happens to patients who do not follow-up after bariatric surgery? Am Surg. 2007;73:181–4.

42. Kaiser KA, Franks S, Smith A. Positive relationship between support group attendance and one-year postoperative weight loss in gastric banding patients. Obes Relat Dis. 2011;7(1):89–93.
43. Livhits M, Mercado C, Yermilov I, Parikh JA, Dutson E, Mehran A, Ko CY, Gibbons MM. Exercise following bariatric surgery: systematic review. Obes Surg. 2010;20(5):657–65.
44. Papalazarou A, Yannakoulia M, Kavouras SA, Komesidou V, Dimitriadis G, Papakonstantinou A, Sidossis LS. Lifestyle intervention favorably affects weight loss and maintenance following obesity surgery. Obesity. 2010;18(7):1348–53. Epub 2009 Oct 15.
45. Faria S, de Oliveira KE, Lins R, Faria O. Nutritional management of weight regain after bariatric surgery. Obes Surg. 2010;20:135–9.
46. Kalarchian MA, Marcus MD, Courcoulas AP, Cheng Y, Levine MD, Josbeno D. Optimizing long-term weight control after bariatric surgery: a pilot study. Surg Obes Relat Dis. 2012;8(6):710–5.
47. Sarwer DB, Moore RH, Spitzer JC, Wadden TA, Raper SE, Williams NN. A pilot study investigating the efficacy of postoperative dietary counseling to improve outcomes after bariatric surgery. Surg Obes Relat Dis. 2012;8(5):561–8.
48. Tate DF, Jackvony MPH, Wing RR. Effects of internet behavioral counseling on weight loss in adults at risk for type 2 diabetes: a randomized trial. J Am Med Assoc. 2003;289(14):1833–6. doi:10.1001/jama.289.14.1833.
49. Volpp KG, John LK, Troxel AB, Norton L, Fassbender J, Loewenstein G. Financial incentive-based approaches for weight loss: a randomized trial. J Am Med Assoc. 2008;300(22):2631–7.
50. West DS, DiLillo V, Bursac Z, Gore SA, Greene PG. Motivational interviewing improves weight loss in women with type 2 diabetes. Diabetes Care. 2007;30(5):1081–7. Epub 2007 Mar 2.
51. Hayes SC, Strosahl K, Wilson KG. Acceptance and commitment therapy: the process and practice of mindful change. 2nd ed. New York: Guilford Press; 2012.
52. Forman EM, Herbert JD. New directions in cognitive behavior therapy: acceptance-based therapies. In: O'Donohue W, Fisher JE, editors. General principles and empirically supported techniques in cognitive behavior therapy. Hoboken: Wiley; 2009. p. 77–101.
53. Forman EM, Hoffman K, McGrath KB, Herbert J, Brandsma L, Lowe MR. A comparison of acceptance- and control-based strategies for coping with food cravings: an analog study. Behav Res Ther. 2007;45(10):2372–86. Epub 2007 Apr 18.
54. Forman E, Hoffman K, Juarascio A, Butryn M, Herbert J. Comparison of acceptance-based and standard cognitive-based coping strategies for craving sweets in overweight and obese women. Eat Behav. 2013;14(1):64–8.
55. Lillis J, Hayes SC, Bunting K, Masuda A. Teaching acceptance and mindfulness to improve the lives of the obese: a preliminary test of a theoretical model. Ann Behav Med. 2009;37(1):58–69. Epub 2009 Feb 28.
56. Niemeier HM, Leahey T, Palm Reed K, Brown RA, Wing RR. An acceptance-based behavioral intervention for weight loss: a pilot study. Behav Ther. 2012;43(2):427–35. Epub 2011 Dec 1.
57. Forman EM, Butryn M, Hoffman KL, Herbert JD. An open trial of an acceptance-based behavioral treatment for weight loss. Cogn Behav Prac. 2009;16:223–35.
58. Sarwer DB, Wadden TA, Moore RH, Baker AW, Gibbons LM, Raper SE, et al. Reoperative eating behavior, postoperative dietary adherence, and weight loss after gastric bypass surgery. Surg Obes Relat Dis. 2008;4(5):640–6. Epub 2008 Jun 30.
59. Engstrom D. Eating mindfully and cultivating satisfaction: modifying eating patterns in a bariatric surgery patient. Bariat Nurs Surg Patient Care. 2007;2:245–50.
60. Leahey TM, Crowther JH, Irwin SR. A cognitive-behavioral mindfulness group therapy intervention for the treatment of binge eating in bariatric surgery patients. Cogn Behav Pract. 2008;15:364–75.
61. Weineland S, Arvidsson D, Kakoulidis TP, Dahl J. Acceptance and commitment therapy for bariatric surgery patients, a pilot RCT. Obes Res Clin Pract. 2012;6(1):e21–30.

Additional Readings

Bandura A. Social foundations of thought and action: a social cognitive theory. Englewood Cliffs: Prentice Hall; 1986.

Brolin RE, Kenler HA, Gorman RC, Cody RP. The dilemma of outcome assessment after operations for morbid obesity. Surgery. 1989;105:337–46.

Brownell KD. The LEARN program for weight management. Dallas: American Health Publishing; 2000.

Brownell KD, Horgen KB. Food fight: the inside story of America's obesity crisis and what we can do about it. Chicago: Contemporary Books; 2003.

Funnell MM, Anderson RM, Ahroni JH. Empowerment and self-management after weight loss surgery. Obes Surg. 2005;15:417–22.

Green BB, McAfee T, Hindmarsh M, Madsen L, Caplow M, Buist D. Effectiveness of telephone support in increasing physical activity in primary care patients. Am J Prev Med. 2002;22(3):177–83.

Hooper N, Sandoz EK, Ashton J, Clarke A, McHugh L. Comparing thought suppression and acceptance as coping techniques for food cravings. Eat Behav. 2012;13(1):62–4. Epub 2011 Oct 19.

Klem ML, Wing RR, McGuire MT, Seagle HM, Hill J. A descriptive study of individuals successful at long-term maintenance of substantial weight loss. Am J Clin Nutr. 1997;66:239–46.

Leventhal H, Cameron L. Behavioral theories and the problem of compliance. Patient Educ Couns. 1987;10:117–36.

Leventhal H, Zimmerman R, Gutmann M. Compliance: a self-regulation perspective, Handbook of Behavioral Medicine. New York: Pergamon; 1984.

National Heart, Lung, and Blood Institute (NHLBI) and the North American Association for the Study of Obesity (NAASO). The practical guide: identification, evaluation, and treatment of overweight and obesity in adults. Bethesda: National Institutes of Health; 2000.

Pontiroli AE, Fossati A, Vedani P, Fiorilli M, Folli F, Paganelli M, et al. Post-surgery adherence to scheduled visits and compliance, more than personality disorders, predict outcome of bariatric restrictive surgery in morbidly obese patients. Obes Surg. 2007;17:1492–7.

Poole NA, Atar AA, Kuhanendran D, Bidlake L, Fiennes A, MCluskey S, et al. Compliance with surgical after-care following bariatric surgery for morbid obesity: a retrospective study. Obes Surg. 2005;15:261–5.

Shen R, Dugay G, Rajaram K, Cabrera I, Siegel N, Ren CJ. Impact of patient follow-up on weight loss after bariatric surgery. Obes Surg. 2004;14:514–9.

Stevens VJ, Funk KL, Brantley PJ, Erlinger TP, Myers VH, Champagne CM, et al. Design and implementation of an interactive website to support long-term maintenance of weight loss. J Med Internet Res. 2008;10(1):e1.

Svetkey LP, Stevens VJ, Brantley PJ, Appel LJ, Hollis JF, Loria CM, et al. Comparison of strategies for sustaining weight loss: the weight loss maintenance randomized controlled trial. J Am Med Assoc. 2008;299(10):1139–48.

Tate DF, Wing RR, Winett RA. Using internet technology to deliver a behavioral weight loss program. J Am Med Assoc. 2001;285(9):1172–7.

U.S. Department of Agriculture, U.S. Department of Health and Human Services. Dietary Guidelines for Americans. Washington, DC (2005). Available from: http://www.health.gov/dietaryguidelines/dga2005/document/default.htm.

Wadden TA, Foster GD, Letizia KA, Mullen JL. Long-term effects of dieting on resting metabolic rate in obese outpatients. JAMA. 1990;264(6):707–11.

Wing RR, Jakicic J, Neiberg R, Lang W, Blair SN, Cooper L, Look AHEAD Research Group, et al. Fitness, fatness, and cardiovascular risk factors in type 2 diabetes: look ahead study. Med Sci Sports Exerc. 2007;39(12):2107–16.

Pharmacotherapy Management of Obesity

Amanda G. Powell and Caroline Apovian

Chapter Objectives

1. Define the indications for using pharmacotherapy to treat obesity.
2. Identify the medications available for the treatment of obesity and understand which patients are candidates for each type of treatment.
3. Understand the risks, benefits, and side effects of each of the treatment options.

Introduction

Obesity is a chronic disease and, as such, requires long-term, comprehensive treatment. It is important for healthcare professionals to view obesity as a disease, rather than assume it is a failure on the part of the patient. Fortunately, with growing research showing the complexity of energy regulation and balance, this formerly pervasive attitude has subsided. The interest in the field leads more practitioners to be ready to treat patients in the face of an obesity epidemic that has grown to encompass almost 70 % [1] of the US population and has become the second most preventable cause of death in North America [2]. Obesity needs to be treated both aggressively and chronically in order for patients to not only lose the weight, but to help them maintain it once they have achieved a specific goal. Defining success in obesity treatment needs to take into consideration not only a patient's ability to lose the weight, but also needs to incorporate the improvements in weight-related comorbidities.

The development of drugs for the treatment of obesity has historically been wrought with challenges. Some of the first medications used for the treatment of obesity included thyroid extract and subsequently dinitrophenol; however, both were discontinued due to serious side effects. In the 1930s, Benzedrine and amphetamines were introduced and their use increased over subsequent decades. However, the US Food and Drug Administration (FDA) banned the use of these agents in 1979 after an investigation revealed a number of drug-related deaths. In 1959, phentermine was approved for the treatment of obesity, and subsequently in 1973, it was combined with fenfluramine [3]. This combination, otherwise known as "fen-phen," was linked to both cardiac valvulopathy and pulmonary hypertension, and fenfluramine and its isomer, dexfenfluramine (Redux), were removed from the market in 1997. Phentermine alone was not deemed on its own to be a factor in cardiac valvulopathy, and it remained on the market. After the fen-phen debacle, the attitude towards drug treatment of obesity became one of skepticism among both the FDA and providers, and proving the safety and efficacy of the drugs used for obesity became paramount. The road for obesity treatment only became further challenged by the approval and subsequent removal of sibutramine, an anorectic agent used to control appetite. Although approved in 1997, in 2010 the FDA made the decision to withdraw sibutramine from the market due to concern regarding an increase in cardiovascular events revealed by the SCOUT trial [4].

In 2007, the FDA defined its criteria for approving any new weight loss medication. In order for a new weight loss drug to be considered effective, at least one of the following must be true after 1 year of treatment: the difference in mean weight loss between the active-product and placebo-treated groups is at least 5 % and is statistically significant or the proportion of subjects who lose greater than or equal to 5 %

A.G. Powell, MD (✉)
Department of Endocrinology, Diabetes, Nutrition and Weight Management, Boston Medical Center, 88 East Newton Street, Robinson Building, Suite 4400, Boston, MA 02118, USA
e-mail: Amanda.Powell@bmc.org

C. Apovian, MD, FACP, FACN
Department of Medicine, Boston University School of Medicine, 88 E. Newton Street, Robinson 4400, Boston, MA, USA

Nutrition and Support Service, Boston Medical Center, Boston, MA, USA
e-mail: caroline.apovian@bmc.org

of baseline body weight in the active-product group is at least 35 %, is approximately double the proportion in the placebo-treated group, and is statistically significant [5]. Until recently, there were only two classes of drugs approved for the treatment of obesity: pancreatic and gastric lipase inhibitors including orlistat and sympathomimetic agents, including phentermine. However, in 2012, two new drugs have been approved by the FDA for the first time in 13 years, and optimism is reinstituted for the future of pharmacotherapy for obesity.

Indications for Pharmacotherapy

Diet, exercise, and behavior modification should be the foundation of all treatments for obesity. However, pharmacological therapy can and should be used in the correct patient as an adjunctive treatment once a careful evaluation has been completed. The first step is to determine the patient's body mass index (BMI) and waist circumference and assess for any weight-related comorbidities, including hypertension, diabetes, hyperlipidemia, and obstructive sleep apnea. Pharmacotherapy can be appropriate for those patients with a body mass index (BMI) ≥30 kg/m2 or a BMI ≥27 with weight-related comorbidities and have failed to achieve weight loss goals through diet and exercise alone [6].

In addition to BMI, waist circumference is equally important in the initial evaluation of a patient. Regional fat distribution has been shown to be an independent predictor of cardiovascular risk, with central and visceral obesity displaying a higher risk for diabetes, coronary artery disease (CAD), and stroke [7] than fat distributed more peripherally. Moreover, the racial and ethnic background of a patient should be considered as there are certain patient populations with higher risk factors where BMI itself may be a poor reflection of their adiposity and cardiovascular risk. For example, Asian populations have more visceral fat at a much lower BMI than non-Hispanic whites [8], and as such, some nations have redefined obesity; the Japanese have defined obesity as any BMI greater than 25.

Contraindications for Pharmacotherapy

While each drug discussed in this chapter will have specific contraindications for use, the general contraindications include: pregnancy, breastfeeding, unstable cardiac disease, unstable severe systemic illness, history of anorexia nervosa, active severe psychiatric disorder, and/or drug-drug interactions. In addition, caution should be used in patients >65 years of age.

Goals of Pharmacotherapy

The first step prior to initiating treatment should be to set up a realistic weight loss goal and discuss this with the patient. Patients can achieve a significant reduction in their risk for both cardiovascular disease and diabetes with a weight loss of only 5–10 % [9]. Thus, one approach would be to set up an initial goal of losing 5–10 % of the baseline body weight over 6–12 months with shorter-term monthly targets to keep patients on track. In terms of measuring success with treatment, the weight should be considered as well as whether or not there is improvement in risk factors, including improved blood pressure, reduction in HbA1c, or lowering of triglycerides or low-density lipoprotein (LDL).

Further, it is well understood that once a drug is discontinued, the patient will likely regain the weight they have lost while on drug therapy. While there is no long-term data (>2 years) for many of the weight loss medications, a discussion should be made with the patient as to whether or not to continue treatment in order to maintain the weight lost. As with all other chronic medical conditions, obesity will require lifelong treatment in order to prevent weight regain.

Weight-Promoting Medications

In addition to initiating pharmacotherapy, the medical approach to treating obesity should include the avoidance of weight-promoting medications and optimizing treatment with weight-neutral alternatives. As discussed, overweight and obese patients suffer from a number of comorbid medical conditions including depression, cardiovascular disease, and diabetes, which are often treated with medications that may promote weight gain. There are often weight-neutral medications available and should be considered whenever possible (Table 16.1) [10–12].

Current FDA-Approved Drugs for the Treatment of Obesity (Table 16.2)

Orlistat (Xenical)

Orlistat is a gastrointestinal lipase inhibitor that reduces intestinal absorption of dietary fat by as much as 30 %. It was approved in 1997 for the treatment of both obese adults and adolescents. It is available both as a prescription at a dosage of 120 mg with meals and may also be purchased over the counter in some countries at a lower dose of 60 mg (Alli™). This medication is best prescribed with patients who are able

16 Pharmacotherapy Management of Obesity

Table 16.1 Weight-promoting versus weight-neutral medications

Weight-promoting medication	Weight-neutral alternatives
Hypoglycemics	Glucagon-like peptide analogues[a]
Insulin	Metformin[a], DPP-IV inhibitors
Thiazolidinediones	
Sulfonylureas	
Antipsychotics	Ziprasidone, aripiprazole
Clozapine, olanzapine	
Quetiapine, risperidone	
Antidepressants	Bupropion[a]
Tricyclics—amitriptyline	
Paroxetine	
Anticonvulsants/mood stabilizers	Topiramate[a], Lamictal, zonisamide
Valproate, carbamazepine	
Lithium	
Steroids	
Beta-blockers	
Antihistamines	Intranasal Flonase

[a]May induce weight loss

Table 16.2 Expected weight loss for currently approved weight loss medications

Medication	Drug treatment (kg)	Placebo (kg)	Net weight loss (kg)
Phentermine	6.8	2.8	4.0
Orlistat	7.3	3.5	3.0
Topiramate/phentermine	14.7	2.5	12.2
Lorcaserin	5.8	2.9	2.9

to comply with a diet in which fat calories are restricted to 30 % of total daily caloric intake. Data has shown that the average placebo adjusted weight loss at 1 year is 2.9 %.

Limitations of use include significant and undesirable gastrointestinal side effects. Namely, when a patient consumes a high-fat meal, the malabsorption of the fat can lead to abdominal cramping, flatulence, bloating, and steatorrhea. Patients often report having "accidents" due to unpredictable and urgent diarrhea or leakage.

This medication has few contraindications; however, it should be avoided in patients with known chronic malabsorption, cholestasis (due to a few documented cases of rare but fatal liver injury), or known hypersensitivity. In addition, it should be avoided in patients with a history of calcium oxalate stones as orlistat can increase levels of urinary oxalate. In addition, continued use can lead to altered levels of fat-soluble vitamins. Therefore, all patients who take orlistat should take a multivitamin at least 2 h before or after the administration of orlistat. Finally, there are some drug interactions to consider. Orlistat may enhance the anticoagulant effect of warfarin due to reduced absorption of the fat-soluble vitamin K. If a patient is taking levothyroxine, he or she should be advised to separate these medications by 4 h.

Phentermine/Diethylpropion (Also Known As Adipex, Fastin, Ionamin)

Phentermine stimulates the release of norepinephrine, which leads to early satiety and reduced food intake. Phentermine was approved in 1959 for the short-term treatment of obesity. It is available at doses of either 15 mg, 30 mg, or 37.5 mg by prescription only and is a schedule IV drug. In the longest study of 36 weeks of continuous treatment, subjects receiving phentermine 30 mg lost 12.2 kg versus 4.8 kg for placebo [13].

This medication should be used for patients who have difficulty controlling their appetite and only be used in conjunction with a structured diet and exercise program.

The most common adverse effects include xerostomia, insomnia, headache, overstimulation, palpitations, and constipation. Other common side effects include hypertension and tachycardia. In order to minimize the side effects, a patient should be treated with the lowest dose, and it can be titrated up if the patient tolerates it. Patients with uncontrolled hypertension should not use this medication, and all patients should be monitored closely for elevations in their blood pressure and heart rate. In addition, any patient with known structural heart disease, cardiomyopathy, cardiac arrhythmias, unstable coronary disease, hyperthyroidism, glaucoma, hypersensitivity to sympathetic medications, uncontrolled anxiety or panic disorder, or history of drug abuse should not be treated with phentermine. Finally, it is important to use with caution in patients with diabetes on antidiabetic agents, as the doses of the antidiabetic agents may need to be adjusted in the setting of caloric and carbohydrate restriction. This medication is contraindicated in pregnancy and during breastfeeding.

Phentermine Plus Topiramate

Qsymia™ is a newly approved weight loss drug that combines both phentermine and topiramate. Phentermine is a widely prescribed appetite suppressant described previously. Topiramate was originally approved for the treatment of epilepsy and migraine prophylaxis but was discovered to have a weight loss benefit. The combination produces weight loss via complementary mechanisms and allows for the use of each agent at a lower dose, thus potentially minimizing side effects and maximizing weight loss benefits. The drug is available in four strength combinations, which include phentermine mg/topiramate mg extended release (3.75 mg/23 mg, 7.5 mg/46 mg, 11.25 mg/69 mg, and 15 mg/92 mg). The medication should be initiated at the lowest dose and taken in the morning to avoid insomnia. The dose can be slowly titrated after 2 weeks if the patient tolerates it well. If patients fail to achieve significant weight loss at 12 weeks (at least 3 % of their total body weight), the dose can be further increased. However, if a patient fails to respond thereafter, the medication should be discontinued.

Data has shown that patients who take the highest dose of Qsymia (phentermine 15 mg/topiramate 92 mg) can achieve up to a 10.5 % weight loss after 2 years of treatment. In addition, a 10 % weight loss was achieved by >50 % of subjects in the treatment groups, whereas <12 % of placebo reached this goal [14]. In addition, treatment is associated with improvement in cardiometabolic parameters including improvements in both systolic and diastolic blood pressure, waist circumference, glucose, triglycerides, and high-density lipoprotein (HDL) and LDL cholesterol.

The most common side effects include paresthesias, dizziness, dry mouth, constipation, dysgeusia, and insomnia. In addition, Qsymia can cause cognitive dysfunction (e.g., impairment of concentration/attention, difficulty with memory, and speech or language problems, particularly word-finding difficulties).

Safety concerns include an increase in heart rate and elevation in blood pressure. Patients with a known history of cardiovascular disease, cerebrovascular disease, or uncontrolled hypertension should not be treated with this medication. In addition, routine monitoring of both blood pressure and heart rate should be initiated during treatment. There is also an increased incidence of oral cleft palate and/or cleft lip in babies of women taking topiramate during pregnancy. Therefore, it is important to screen patients of child-bearing potential with a urine pregnancy test prior to initiating treatment and subsequently counsel them to use an effective form of contraception. If a patient does become pregnant during therapy, the medication should be immediately discontinued.

Other contraindications include patients with a history of glaucoma and hyperthyroidism and patients receiving treatment or within 14 days following treatment with monoamine oxidase inhibitors (MAOIs).

There have been a few associated lab abnormalities associated with the use of Qsymia including a reduction in serum bicarbonate, elevated creatinine, and reduction in potassium. Routine lab monitoring of serum creatinine, bicarbonate, and potassium is recommended at baseline and periodically throughout treatment. If the acidosis persists, a reduction or discontinuation of the medication should be considered. Patients who are taking a non-potassium-sparing diuretic are at particular risk and should be monitored closely.

Lastly, weight loss may increase the risk of hypoglycemia in patients with type 2 diabetes mellitus treated with insulin or other secretagogues. These patients should be monitored closely and may require a reduction in their antidiabetic medications.

Lorcaserin

Lorcaserin became the first new weight loss drug to be approved by the FDA in 13 years and was approved in June 2012. Lorcaserin is a selective serotonin HT2C receptor agonist. The serotonin HT2C receptor is expressed in many areas of the brain, including the proopiomelanocortin (POMC) neurons of the hypothalamus, the major area involved in the control of appetite and metabolism. Activation of POMC neurons with lorcaserin is thought to promote appetite suppression and increased satiety. Previously, nonselective serotonergic agonists, including fenfluramine and dexfenfluramine, targeted not only the 2C receptor but also the 2B receptor, which is found in the cardiac valves. The medications, although effective for weight loss, were associated with a significant risk of cardiac valvulopathy. The increased selectivity towards the 2C receptor with lorcaserin has been shown to mitigate the risk of valvulopathy.

Lorcaserin will be available as a 10 mg tablet, and the recommended dose is 10 mg twice per day. Efficacy data has shown that almost 50 % of subjects treated with lorcaserin 10 mg twice daily achieved at least 5 % weight loss at 1 year (nearly double the placebo group) [15]. The mean change in body weight was −5.8 kg (versus: −2.9 kg for the placebo arm) add % weight loss. In addition to weight loss, lorcaserin has beneficial effects on cardiometabolic parameters, including blood pressure, heart rate, cholesterol, and glucose and insulin levels.

The most common side effects include headache, dizziness, fatigue, nausea, dry mouth, and constipation, and these are usually both mild and transient in severity. Certain patient populations should be cautioned with the use of this medication. Historically, nonselective serotonin agonists were associated with cardiac valvulopathy. However, clinical trials of lorcaserin included routine echocardiograms, which did not suggest an increase in valvulopathy. Any patient with congestive heart failure or known valvulopathy should likely avoid taking this medication. Patients taking other serotonergic or antidopaminergic agents should be monitored for the risk of serotonin syndrome or neuroleptic malignant syndrome. Patients with type 2 diabetes mellitus should be monitored closely for hypoglycemia, and their antidiabetic medications should be adjusted accordingly. This medication should be avoided in pregnancy or lactating women.

Drug Combination Pending Approval by the FDA

Bupropion Plus Naltrexone

Bupropion inhibits reuptake of 5-HT, dopamine, and norepinephrine and is approved for the treatment of depression and smoking cessation. Naltrexone is an opioid receptor antagonist. Bupropion has been shown to stimulate the hypothalamic POMC (proopiomelanocortin) neurons to release alpha-melanocyte-stimulating hormone (MSH) and B-endorphin. Alpha-MSH mediates the anorectic effect of POMC, whereas B-endorphin is responsible for the autoinhibitory feedback. Naltrexone blocks this negative feedback loop and facilitates a longer-lasting activation of POMC, amplifying the weight loss benefit of bupropion. Thus, bupropion acts as a catalyst for weight loss, while naltrexone has a complementary function to help maintain weight loss. The combination of bupropion plus naltrexone (Contrave™) has been investigated for approval as an anti-obesity treatment and was approved by the FDA Endocrinologic and Metabolic Drugs Advisory Committee in December 2010. However, the FDA has required long-term studies to demonstrate cardiovascular safety before final approval. The Light Study is an ongoing cardiovascular outcome study, which is investigating the long-term safety of Contrave.

Phase III trials have demonstrated that subjects treated for 1 year achieve a mean weight loss of 5 % for naltrexone 16 mg/bupropion SR 360 mg versus 6.1 % for naltrexone 32 mg/bupropion SR 360 mg versus 1.3 % for placebo. Significant side effects include headache, constipation, dizziness, vomiting, and dry mouth. If approved, it will likely be contraindicated in those patients for which bupropion is currently contraindicated, including patients with a history of seizures, severe depression, suicidal ideation, or suicide attempts.

Diabetes Medications Providing a Weight Loss Benefit (Table 16.3)

Metformin

Metformin is a peripherally acting antidiabetic drug that enhances insulin sensitivity and has been associated with a weight loss up to 2.5 % and is maintained during a 10-year period [9]. Although it is not a weight loss medication per se, it may be helpful in patients who are overweight or obese with impaired glucose tolerance or who are at risk for diabetes. In addition, studies have shown that metformin may be useful in conjunction with atypical antipsychotics to prevent weight gain. It is associated with gastrointestinal side effects, including diarrhea. However, it is a relatively inexpensive medication with no significant long-term adverse effects.

Table 16.3 Expected weight loss for currently approved diabetes medications

Metformin	0.6–2.7 kg
GLP-1 analogs	1.8–6.0 kg
Pramlintide	1.5 kg

GLP-1 Agonists

Liraglutide and exenatide are injectable medications currently approved for the treatment of type 2 diabetes. They act by mimicking the gastrointestinal incretin hormone glucagon-like peptide-1 (GLP-1), which is normally released in response to food intake. GLP-1 agonists enhance glucose-dependent insulin secretion, suppress inappropriate glucagon secretion, and slow gastric emptying, resulting in improved glycemic control, decreased energy intake, and weight loss [16]. Exenatide is dosed twice per day, 30–60 min prior to meals, whereas liraglutide has an extended half-life and can be injected as once-daily therapy. A once-weekly version of exenatide has been approved, allowing for simpler dosing regimens for patients. Studies have shown that patients receiving GLP-1 analogs achieve a reduction in HbA1c from 0.5 % to 1.5 % and a weight loss ranging from 1.8 to 6.0 kg [17].

Liraglutide has been investigated in obese nondiabetic patients at doses higher than what is currently approved [18]. Weight loss with the use of liraglutide 3.0 mg (currently approved dose is 0.6–1.8 mg) was 7.2 kg (versus 2.8 kg for placebo) after 20 weeks of treatment, and the weight loss was better maintained in a 2-year extension trial.

The most common side effects associated with GLP-1 agonists include mild to moderate nausea, which tends to be transient. Other side effects include diarrhea and injection site reactions. Patients to avoid the use of GLP-1 agonists are those with a history of pancreatitis and chronic kidney disease. Caution should be used with patients taking other antidiabetic medications, which can predispose them to hypoglycemia, including sulfonylureas. It is not recommended to use in conjunction with insulin. Dose adjustments may need to be made, and patients should be monitored closely.

Pramlintide

Pramlintide is a synthetic analog of amylin, which is a hormone co-secreted with insulin by the pancreatic beta cells, which acts to inhibit gastric emptying, food intake, and glucagon secretion. Pramlintide is approved for the use in both type 1 and type 2 diabetes in combination with insulin. It is administered via subcutaneous injection at doses of 60–120 μ(mu)g before meals. Pramlintide has been associated with modest weight loss of up to 1.5 % after 6 months of treatment [19].

Drugs Currently Under Investigation for the Treatment of Obesity

Zonisamide/Bupropion

Zonisamide is an antiepileptic drug approved for the treatment of partial seizures. Clinically, it has been shown to induce weight loss as a side effect [20]. The addition of bupropion to zonisamide as an obesity drug was designed to reduce the side effects and improve the efficacy compared to either drug when administered alone. More specifically, it was felt that bupropion might offset the sedative properties associated with zonisamide, while the latter might reduce the possibility of seizures, a known side effect of bupropion [21].

Patients treated with the combination zonisamide 360 mg plus bupropion 360 mg for 24 weeks resulted in a weight loss of 7.5 % [22], which was significantly superior to placebo (weight loss of 1.4 %). Both of these doses were significantly superior to placebo (1.4 % weight loss). The most common side effects include nausea, headache, and insomnia. Phase II studies have been completed.

Conclusion

Obesity is a chronic medical condition and, similar to other disease treatment paradigms, requires long-term management. Prior to initiation of treatment, patients should have a comprehensive evaluation to determine the appropriate risks and benefits of a particular therapy. Patients may differ in their response to a medication, and it is often difficult to determine who will respond. Therefore, it is important to start with a low dose of a single agent and titrate up as tolerated. A patient may require additional agents in order to achieve their goals. If a patient fails to respond to the agent after reaching the appropriate dose, the medication should be discontinued, and alternative options should be pursued. Importantly, if successful, treatment should be continued in order for the patient to maintain their weight loss and avoid weight regain.

Question and Answer Section

Questions

1. Which of the following medications does not contribute to weight gain?
   A. Atenolol
   B. Glyburide
   C. Lamictal
   D. Loratadine
2. Which of the following patients would not be a good candidate for the weight loss medication Qsymia?
   A. Forty-five-year-old male with BMI of 38 and hypertension controlled on two agents
   B. Fifty-two-year-old male with BMI of 44 and a history of stroke
   C. Thirty-four-year-old female with BMI 31 with polycystic ovarian syndrome
   D. Twenty-four-year-old male with a BMI of 29 and type II diabetes

Answers

1. Answer is **C**. Beta-blockers, sulfonylureas, and antihistamines can cause weight gain. Lamictal is a weight-neutral medication that can be used for seizure disorders and/or mood stabilization.
2. Answer is **B**. Patients with a history of stroke should not take Qsymia. Patient A is okay to use as long as the blood pressure is well controlled. Patient C is okay as long as you counsel her on the teratogenic risk and make sure she uses proper contraception. Patient D is okay because pharmacotherapy is indicated in patients with a BMI of 29 with comorbidities related to their weight (diabetes)

References

1. Flegal KM, Carroll MD, Kit BK, Ogden CL. Prevalence of obesity and trends in the distribution of body mass index among US adults, 1999–2010. JAMA. 2012;307(5):491–7.
2. Mokdad AH, Marks JS, Stroup DF, Gerberdine JL. Actual causes of death in the United States, 2000. JAMA. 2004;291(10):1238–45.
3. Colman E. Anorectics on trial: a half century of Federal Regulation of prescription appetite suppressants. Ann Intern Med. 2005;143(5):380–5.
4. Torp-Pedersen C, Caterson I, Coutinho W, Finer N, Van Gaal L, Maggioni A, SCOUT Investigators, et al. Cardiovascular responses to weight management and sibutramine in high-risk subjects: an analysis from the SCOUT trial. Eur Heart J. 2007;28(23):2915–23.
5. FDA 2007 Draft Guidance for Industry: developing products for weight management. http://www.fda.gov/downloads/AdvisoryCommittees/CommitteesMeetingMaterials/Drugs/EndocrinologicandMetabolicDrugsAdvisoryCommittee/UCM299133.pdf. Accessed 25 Feb 2013.

6. Yanovski SZ, Yanovski JA. Obesity. N Engl J Med. 2002;346:591–602.
7. Despres JP. Cardiovascular disease under the influence of excess visceral fat. Crit Pathw Cardiol. 2007;6(2):51–9.
8. Stevens J. Ethnic-specific cutpoints for obesity vs. country-specific guidelines for action. Int J Obes Relat Metab Disord. 2003;27(3):287–8.
9. Knowler WC, Barrett-Connor E, Fowler SE, Hamman RF, Lachin JM, Walker EA, et al. Diabetes Prevention Program Research Group. Reduction in the incidence of type 2 diabetes with lifestyle intervention or Metformin. N Engl J Med. 2002;346(6):393–403.
10. Cope MB, Nagy TR, Fernandez JR, Geary N, Casey DE, Allison DB. Antipsychotic drug-induced weight gain: development of an animal model. Int J Obes. 2005;29(6):607–14.
11. Lee P, Kengne AP, Greenfield JR, Day RO, Chalmers J, Ho KK. Metabolic sequelae of β-blocker therapy: weighing in on the obesity epidemic? Int J Obes. 2011;35(11):1395–403.
12. Zimmerman U, Kraus T, Himmerich H, Schuld A, Pollmacher T. Epidemiology, implications and mechanisms underlying drug-induced weight gain in psychiatric patients. J Psychiatry Res. 2003;37:193–220.
13. Munro JF, MacCuish AC, Wilson EM, Duncan LJ. Comparison of continuous and intermittent anorectic therapy in obesity. BMJ. 1968;1:352–4.
14. Garvey WT, Ryan DH, Look M, Gadde KM, Allison DB, Peterson CA, et al. Two-year sustained weight loss and metabolic benefits with controlled-release phentermine/topiramate in obese and overweight adults (SEQUEL): a randomized, placebo-controlled, phase 3 extension study. Am J Clin Nutr. 2012;95(2):297–308.
15. Fidler MC, Sandchez M, Raether B, Weissman NJ, Smith SR, Shanahan WR, et al. BLOSSOM Clinical Trial Group. A one-year randomized trial of lorcaserin for weight loss in obese and overweight adults: the BLOSSOM trial. J Clin Endocrinol Metab. 2011;96:3067–77.
16. Bray GA, Greenway FL. Pharmacological treatment of the overweight patient. Pharmacol Rev. 2007;59:151–84.
17. Siram AT, Yanagisawa R, Skamagas M. Weight management in type 2 diabetes mellitus. Mt Sinai J Med. 2010;77:533–48.
18. Astrup A, Rössner S, Van Gaal L, Rissanen A, Niskanen L, Al Hakim M, et al. Effects of liraglutide in the treatment of obesity: a randomized, double-blind, placebo-controlled study. Lancet. 2009;374(9701):1606–16.
19. Aronne LJ, Halseth AE, Burns CM, Miller S, Shen LZ. Enhanced weight loss following coadministration of pramlintide with sibutramine or phentermine in a multicenter trial. Obesity. 2010;18(9):1739–46.
20. Oommen KJ, Mathews S. Zonisamide, a new anti-epileptic drug. Clin Neuropharmacol. 1999;22:192–200.
21. Gadde KM, Yonish G, Foust MS, Wagner HR. Combination therapy of Zonisamide and Bupropion for weight reduction in obese women: a preliminary randomized open label study. J Clin Psychiatry. 2007;68:1226–9.
22. Fujioka K, Greenway F, Cowley M, Guttadauria M, Robinson J, Landbloom R, et al. The 24 week experience with a combination sustained release product of zonisamide and bupropion; evidence of an encouraging benefit: risk profile. Obesity. 2007;15 Suppl 1:A85.

Medical Preparation for Bariatric Surgery

Peter N. Benotti and Gregory Dalencourt

Chapter Objectives

1. To review current practices for medical preparation of the bariatric surgery patient
2. To identify medical factors that may affect risk and when to intervene to reduce risk
3. To identify and address those factors that may diminish the probability of successful long-term weight loss and nutritional safety

Introduction

Bariatric surgery has become the preferred treatment for patients with refractory extreme obesity associated with impaired health and quality of life. Since 1991 when bariatric surgery became an accepted treatment for severe obesity, these procedures have become widely recognized for their therapeutic potential and have become important service lines at most university and community medical centers throughout the country. An important component of the evolution of bariatric surgery has been the improvement in surgical outcomes during this period. In 1991, best practice mortality rates for bariatric surgery were 0.5–01.5 %. Present best practice mortality rates from large patient registries are 0.1–0.3 % [1]. Despite improved outcomes and increasing popularity, the number of bariatric procedures has recently plateaued after major increases. Possible explanations for this include the increased financial burden for society to support a procedure costing an estimated $25,000, limitations imposed by insurance providers for this treatment, and the failure to include obesity care as an essential health benefit for insurance coverage.

It is estimated that 5.7 % of the American population suffers from extreme obesity, which means that the patient pool eligible for this treatment approximates 17 million. A recent estimate for current bariatric surgical volume was about 250,000 bariatric procedures for 2012. This indicates that only 1.5 % of the eligible patient population has access to this treatment at present. In the midst of this major treatment access situation, it is also apparent that surgical mortalities still occur and that bariatric surgery is not always successful. Therefore, obesity treatment centers must continue to improve processes for patient preparation and selection for surgery, thereby improving the value of this treatment modality. This chapter will review current practices for medical preparation of the bariatric surgery patient. The overall objectives of the preoperative preparation for bariatric surgery are as follows:

- To confirm that bariatric surgery is indicated for the patient and that the benefits of bariatric surgery outweigh the risks
- To identify medical factors that may affect risk and intervene to reduce risk when necessary
- To identify and address those factors that may diminish the probability of successful long-term weight loss and nutritional safety

Physician Education

A large fraction of referrals for bariatric surgery are patient driven. Severely obese patients learn about the therapeutic efficacy of bariatric surgery from acquaintances who have achieved successful surgical weight loss, from the media, or from Internet research. Many community primary care providers have a lack of confidence in managing obesity. Several recent surveys of primary care physicians indicate that they perceive obesity care as frustrating, largely ineffective, and

P.N. Benotti, MD, FACS (✉)
Obesity Institute, Geisinger Medical Center, Danville, PA, USA
e-mail: pbenotti64@gmail.com

G. Dalencourt, MD
Faxton St. Luke's Healthcare, William A. Graber, MD, PC Weight Loss Surgery, New Hartford, NY, USA
e-mail: gdalencourt@hotmail.com

Table 17.1 Strategies to increase the involvement of primary care physicians in obesity management of patients

Strategies to involve primary care physicians in obesity management
Improve communications between referring providers and obesity treatment programs
Implement regional and national CME programs for primary care providers to disseminate current information regarding indications, outcomes, risk-benefit, and complications of bariatric surgery
Involve interested primary care providers in the preoperative and postoperative management of bariatric patients
Encourage participation of interested primary care physicians as bariatricians in multidisciplinary obesity centers

CME continuing medical education

Table 17.2 Criteria for patient eligibility for bariatric surgery

Eligibility criteria for bariatric surgery
Body mass index (BMI) ≥ 40 kg/m^2 or ≥ 35 kg/m^2 with comorbid illness
Failure of medical weight-loss treatments
Absence of major contraindication for surgery

Table 17.3 Topics for the appropriate education of bariatric surgery candidates

Information for bariatric surgery candidates
Success and failure rates of the different operative procedures
The proven health benefits of bariatric surgery
The risks and outcomes of open versus laparoscopic procedures
The importance of physical activity and exercise on surgical weight-loss success

poorly reimbursed. Many are reluctant to prescribe medications for weight loss or to refer patients for bariatric surgery. Others lack the office equipment to effectively examine extremely obese patients. Bariatric treatment centers need to be aware of the important role of the primary care physician in obesity care and do a better job of involving the primary care physician in the management of patients. Possible strategies to bring this about are listed in Table 17.1.

Improved collaboration between obesity treatment centers and primary care physicians will increase the primary care physician's comfort level with obesity care and enhance referrals for bariatric surgery. It will reduce the travel burden for surgical patients as more of the preoperative workup and the postoperative follow-up can occur in the community.

Patient Education

Bariatric surgery is unique among surgical procedures in that it does not eradicate a disease, is non-curative, and requires patient participation in the form of changes in lifestyle and behavior for long-term successful weight control. The fact that 10–25 % of patients who undergo bariatric procedures will struggle and ultimately fail in achieving long-term successful weight control is likely related to poor patient compliance with necessary lifestyle and behavioral changes. The ultimate success of bariatric surgery may well depend on the quality of patient education and the ability of the patient to understand and comply with diet and nutritional expectations. Prospective patients should be familiar with the rationale for surgical treatment of severe obesity including the major health risks and poor quality of life that are associated with extreme obesity as well as the lack of success with nonsurgical weight-loss treatments.

Candidates for bariatric surgery should be aware of the eligibility criteria and the clinical indications for this surgery (Table 17.2), as well as the variability among insurance providers in regard to requirements for coverage.

Candidates must understand that the patient education process as well as the medical and behavioral evaluations will each provide the surgical team with information that will influence the program's decision to offer bariatric surgery. Prospective patients should be made aware of the different surgical procedures that are offered, as well as the anticipated weight-loss results and complications of each procedure. The advantages and disadvantages of each procedure should be discussed. Because patients often have unrealistic expectations about weight loss after bariatric surgery, they should be made aware of the collective weight-loss results of the patients in the program or published literature and the risk of weight-loss failure. In addition, the evaluating team should make the patient aware of the potential impact of existing comorbid medical, psychological, and/or behavioral factors on anticipated weight loss. The individual procedure complication rates, both early and late, as well as risk of mortality should be shared with patients. Finally, the importance of follow-up, patient networks, and participation in support groups should be emphasized. Additional topics for the appropriate education of bariatric surgery candidates are listed in Table 17.3.

It is apparent that the process of patient education for bariatric surgery is labor intense and time consuming. Most successful bariatric surgery programs have developed teaching modules, collected patient education information on Web sites, and integrated successful patients in the patient education process.

Recent observational studies suggest that factors such as income, socioeconomic status, race, level of insurance coverage, and access to educational resources such as the Internet may influence the level of patient comprehension regarding bariatric surgery as well as early weight-loss outcomes. If bariatric surgery is to be offered to a greater fraction of the eligible patient pool, increased time and resources should be directed to the patient education process and efforts to monitor patient understanding.

Patient Informed Consent

The uniqueness of bariatric surgery justifies a comprehensive informed consent process, which is complimentary to the patient education process and may provide information for patient selection. Much of the information conveyed to patients in the education sessions should be summarized in the informed consent document, which the patient must read, understand, and sign prior to surgery. Many programs hold prospective patients accountable for the information involved in education and informed consent by administering some form of examination before surgery. This is an important aspect of patient selection for surgery as significant cognitive impairment is felt to be a contraindication for surgery. The assessment of the degree of patient learning in the form of a preoperative examination will provide programs with direct feedback regarding the efficacy of the patient education process.

Initial Patient Assessment

Severely obese patients are often victims of discrimination, and treatment centers should be mindful of this in the creation of a supportive environment, which acknowledges the limitations of the extremely obese. Office resources should include nearby parking, oversized wheelchairs, furniture, gowns, and blood pressure cuffs, accessible exam tables, and a scale in a private area. A detailed weight history should be obtained including weights at different times of life, highest weight, family history of obesity, and success with weight-loss efforts. Previous success with prior weight loss and weight maintenance indicates the potential to make some lifestyle changes and diminish food intake for a sustained period. In this discussion, providers should attempt to understand the potential barriers to successful weight loss as well as the extent of patient motivation. A young mother who contemplates bariatric surgery in order to be there for her grandchildren has a more rational motivation than the same individual who wishes to lose weight in order to improve her sex appeal. The major incentive for patients seeking bariatric surgery should be to improve health. A detailed diet history, which includes an assessment of eating behavior, food preferences, and meal size, will, on occasion, provide information that may be of importance in selecting the optimal surgical procedure. An assessment of the amount of preparation, research, and inquiry done by the patient in advance of the consultation will provide information about motivation and intellectual capacity—important factors in patient selection.

The medical history should focus on those conditions that may increase surgical risk or cause complications during weight loss. Surgical risk factors include a history of thromboembolism, unstable coronary artery disease, active congestive heart failure, smoking, obstructive sleep apnea, obesity hypoventilation, chronic liver disease, and superobesity (body mass index [BMI] > 50 kg/m^2). Additional information in the patient history should include information about alcohol consumption and drug use as well as details of the home environment. The extent of patient support in the home environment is felt to be an important factor in patient selection.

Some assessment of the level of physical activity is an important part of the patient history. Increases in physical activity should be a recognized component of any comprehensive weight control program and is increasingly recognized as an important behavior adaptation necessary for optimal results following bariatric surgery, as well as preservation of muscle and bone mass during surgical weight loss. In addition, aerobic fitness may be a predictor of surgical risk [2]. A recent study of bariatric surgery candidates using activity diaries and accelerometers indicated that BMI is inversely related to the amount and intensity of daily exercise—that 20 % of bariatric surgery candidates are sedentary and that 20 % are quite active [3]. Additional studies of preoperative and postoperative physical activity levels are necessary to determine if activity levels are truly predictors of surgical risk and weight-loss outcome.

The physical examination of the patient with extreme obesity is limited by the extent and thickness of subcutaneous adipose tissue, which makes it difficult to detect neck vein distension, the intensity of heart sounds, adventitious heart sounds, and the clinical assessment of liver size. Nevertheless, certain aspects of the exam are important. These include an accurate blood pressure, heart rate, patient height, weight, and BMI calculation. Resting pulse rates in extreme obesity may be surprisingly high. Recognition of this will assist in the interpretation of tachycardia occurring after surgery. Careful cardiopulmonary assessment and a search for signs of Cushing's disease are important in the exam. The presence of leg edema is very common in extreme obesity, and often the clinical exam will not provide clues as to the etiology.

The routine laboratory assessment will assist in assessing organ function, degree of metabolic disturbance associated with obesity, nutritional status, and possible causes of obesity. Table 17.4 lists the recommended laboratory tests for bariatric surgery candidates [4].

Behavioral Assessment

It is now generally accepted that those patients with the best health outcomes after bariatric surgery are those who are able to implement changes in behavior, which include adherence to a regular nutritional and exercise plan and the acquisition of coping skills that eliminate the reliance on food in response to emotional stress. Failure to make the necessary behavioral changes can lead to weight-loss failure, nutritional complications, and major depression after bariatric surgery.

Table 17.4 Recommended laboratory tests for bariatric surgery candidates

Routine laboratory testing for bariatric surgery
Fasting blood glucose
Lipids Studies: cholesterol, triglycerides, HDL cholesterol, LDL cholesterol
Chemistry profile: renal function and liver function
Complete blood count
Ferritin, vitamin B12 levels
TSH
25-Hydroxyvitamin D
Fat-soluble vitamins (if a malabsorptive procedure is a consideration)
Screen for Cushing's syndrome when indicated

Adapted from Collazo-Clavel et al. [4]
HDL high-density lipoprotein, *LDL* low-density lipoprotein, *TSH* thyroid-stimulating hormone

Recognition of the importance of behavioral change has increased the role of the behavior/psychological assessment in the patient evaluation/selection process. Although a psychological evaluation has been a best practice recommendation since the inception of bariatric surgery and is now a part of patient evaluation in most bariatric surgery centers, there are no accepted guidelines for assessment procedures. The reader is referred to recent reviews, which outline the published structured interviews available [4].

The behavioral evaluation should consist of an assessment of those factors considered important for weight-loss success and a psychological assessment to look for psychopathology. Factors known to influence outcome include social support systems, interpersonal relationships, marital satisfaction, past diet success, or other evidence of behavioral change and an understanding of risks, benefits, and requirements for success in bariatric surgery. In addition, the assessment should include an evaluation of cognitive ability—an area of increasing importance in patient selection.

Bariatric surgery candidates have a greater prevalence of psychopathology than that of the general population. The more common conditions encountered are depression and binge eating disorders. Other conditions found less frequently include anxiety disorders, substance abuse, psychosis, and inability to provide informed consent. In a review of 459 bariatric surgery candidates, Pawlow et al. found that 81.5 % were referred for immediate surgery with no psychological contraindications. For 15.8 %, surgery was deferred for psychological or psychiatric treatment, and for 2.7 %, surgery was contraindicated for mental health reasons [5]. A survey of bariatric programs from the University of Virginia revealed that the common mental health conditions recognized as contraindications for bariatric surgery included active drug and alcohol abuse, uncontrolled schizophrenia, severe mental retardation, lack of knowledge about surgery, and evidence of poor compliance [6]. Other generally accepted behavioral contraindications to bariatric surgery include recent suicide attempts, active psychosis, and borderline personality. Behavioral issues, which may mandate additional preoperative counseling or treatment and/or postoperative adjuvant behavioral treatment, include suboptimal control of a mental illness, moderate to severe binge eating disorder, and inadequate home support system.

Another area of importance in the mental health evaluation is related to possible patient benefits of obesity. Surprising numbers of patients with severe obesity have a childhood history of sexual abuse. For these patients, obesity may be protective from emotional trauma and surgical weight loss may activate major emotional stress. Preliminary evidence indicates that these patients should be identified and considered for mental health treatment as an adjunct to bariatric surgery.

Unfortunately, little is known about how psychological and behavioral factors influence long-term surgical outcomes. Those who have tried to manage the postoperative bariatric surgery patient with noncompliant eating behavior know how labor intense and frustrating this can be. Improved methods to recognize these patients in advance of surgery are badly needed as well as better strategies for behavioral and mental health management in the perioperative period.

Comprehensive Medical Evaluation

Extreme obesity is associated with many comorbid conditions that increase the risk of cardiovascular disability and death. This cardiovascular risk increases with increasing BMI. The following are clinical findings of concern and indications for additional preoperative cardiopulmonary workup [7]:
- History or evidence of atherosclerotic cardiovascular disease
- Congestive heart failure
- Hypertension
- Pulmonary hypertension
- Cardiac arrhythmia
- Thromboembolism
- Limited exercise capacity

These conditions are more likely to be present in those with superobesity and older patients with extreme obesity of longer duration.

Respiratory

Respiratory problems and respiratory symptoms are common in patients with extreme obesity. Limited exercise tolerance, especially when breathlessness is the limiting factor, is common and a nonspecific finding because of the many respiratory abnormalities and deconditioning associated

Table 17.5 Changes in lung function that are associated with obesity

Alterations in pulmonary function associated with obesity
Reduced compliance of the lungs and chest wall
Increased respiratory resistance
Increased work of breathing
Reduced lung volumes

with extreme obesity. Many sedentary obese patients have significant impairment of pulmonary function in the absence of symptoms. The physiologic changes in lung function associated with obesity are listed in Table 17.5.

In general, these alterations in pulmonary function are related to BMI, and many patients with high BMI may have significant reductions in lung volume in the absence of symptoms. The reduction in lung volume found in obese patients is clinically important because of its association with small airway closure and atelectasis resulting in ventilation/perfusion (V/Q) mismatch and resting hypoxemia in some patients—especially in the recumbent position. Preoperative pulmonary function tests are indicated for those bariatric surgery candidates with documented pulmonary conditions, those with limited exercise tolerance because of dyspnea, for patients with a history of heavy smoking, and those with BMI ≥ 60. Since pulmonary function is significantly reduced in the first few days following open or laparoscopic upper abdominal surgery, preoperative pulmonary function testing will identify those patients at highest risk for hypoxemia and respiratory failure. Perioperative hypoxemia is frequent in postoperative bariatric surgery patients and correlates with reduced perioperative tissue oxygenation, which has been recently documented following bariatric surgery [8]. Tissue hypoxia will adversely affect tissue resistance to infection as well as anastomotic and wound healing.

Obesity hypoventilation is also a common occurrence in bariatric surgery candidates. An elevation of the bicarbonate level on the electrolyte panel may be a clue to this. For those patients deemed at risk, preoperative pulmonary function studies and arterial blood gas analysis will provide information for planning perioperative respiratory care and use of supplemental positive pressure ventilator support.

Sleep disordered breathing, like hypoventilation, is common among bariatric surgery candidates and should be considered in any patient with polycythemia or a history of regular snoring, nocturnal gasping or choking, witnessed apnea episodes, or daytime sleepiness. Obstructive sleep apnea (OSA) with its associated hypoxia is an important cause of pulmonary hypertension and right heart failure, major risk factors for bariatric surgery. Detection of pulmonary hypertension and right heart failure in patients with extreme obesity is difficult as symptoms are nonspecific, ankle and leg edema are common in extreme obesity, and clues like neck vein distension and hepatojugular reflux are obscured by subcutaneous fat. Patients suspected of having obstructive sleep apnea should have this diagnosed by sleep study and treated by nocturnal continuous positive airway pressure (CPAP) via nasal mask. This treatment will improve nocturnal hypoxia and pulmonary vasoconstriction, which will improve right ventricular working conditions.

Common causes of pulmonary hypertension in extreme obesity include left ventricular failure, chronic thromboembolism, and obstructive sleep apnea. Clinical and electrocardiogram (ECG) evidence of right heart failure occurring may not be present, even though significant pulmonary hypertension is diagnosed by right heart catheterization.

The proven surgical risks associated with long-standing heavy smoking are well known to surgeons. Chronic nicotine use is associated with vasoconstriction and tissue hypoxia, the mechanism for the increase in surgical site infections for heavy smokers. Most bariatric surgery programs insist on cessation of smoking as the smoking risks decline with eight weeks of abstinence. A recent National Surgical Quality Improvement Program (NSQIP) study in a bariatric Veterans' Affairs (VA) population documents smoking as a risk factor for surgical complications and postoperative ventilator dependence [9]. Patients currently nonsmoking with histories of heavy smoking may also be at increased risk. These patients should be considered for preoperative pulmonary function studies and pulmonary consultation in order to optimize lung function before surgery.

Cardiac

Extreme obesity is associated with potentially harmful changes in cardiac structure and function, a process called maladaptive remodeling [10]. Obesity is associated with increased metabolic demands, increased cardiac work, increased blood volume, and increased cardiac output. In response to this increased circulatory demand, cardiac chambers begin to dilate, which increases wall tension. In order to compensate for an increased wall stress, myocardial mass increases resulting in ventricular hypertrophy. Systemic hypertension, common in severe obesity, is an added stimulus to ventricular hypertrophy. Autopsy studies in the severely obese demonstrate that cardiac weight is directly proportional to BMI. With longer durations of severe obesity, the hypertrophied heart commonly demonstrates impaired diastolic and also, less commonly, impaired systolic function, which may progress to congestive heart failure. When the process of maladaptive cardiac remodeling eventually progresses to congestive heart failure, the diagnosis of obese cardiomyopathy is established. The risk of obese cardiomyopathy and heart failure rises steeply after 10 years of extreme obesity. The impact of bariatric surgery on cardiac physiology is exciting and an area of intense interest as

Table 17.6 Cardiac risk factors following surgery

Risk factors for cardiovascular complications following surgery
Major surgery (abdominal, thoracic, vascular)
History of coronary artery disease (MI, chest pain, previous coronary revascularization)
History or clinical findings of congestive heart failure
History of cerebrovascular disease
Preoperative treatment with insulin
Preoperative creatinine level >2 mg/dl

Adapted from Lee et al. [12]
MI myocardial infarction

Table 17.7 Changes in cardiovascular physiology in extreme obesity

Cardiovascular physiology in extreme obesity	
Heart rate at rest	↑
Cardiac output at rest	↑
Stroke volume at rest	↑
Ventricular wall thickness	↑
Maximal exercise O_2 consumption	↓

post-bariatric surgery weight loss has been shown to result in reduction in ventricular wall thickness and chamber size as well as improvements in systolic and diastolic function. This process has been termed "reverse remodeling" [11].

Atherosclerotic cardiovascular disease is also frequent in extreme obesity. This risk is influenced by common comorbid conditions including diabetes, hyperlipidemia, chronic inflammation, and a prothrombotic state. Diagnosed or occult coronary artery disease will increase the risk in bariatric surgery. The exact prevalence of coronary disease in bariatric surgery candidates is unknown, but acute cardiac complications following bariatric surgery are well known and occur in 0.7–1.5 % of patients [9]. The Revised Cardiac Risk Index [12] identifies risk factors for perioperative complications in the general population as specific predictors for cardiovascular complications after surgery. These risk factors are listed in Table 17.6.

These risk factors are derived from studies of large numbers of patients undergoing elective noncardiac surgical procedures. The risk of a cardiovascular complication increases with the number of risk factors present. Although such an index has not as yet been established for patients with extreme obesity, it is likely that these risk factors should be used in decision-making regarding the need for additional cardiovascular studies. It is quite likely that young patients who are not superobese and who have no risk factors do not need routine detailed cardiovascular testing. In bariatric patients with multiple risk factors, additional cardiovascular testing is indicated in order to initiate treatments to reduce risk and to better prepare for perioperative management and resource allocation.

There are no guidelines for the necessity of additional noninvasive cardiovascular testing in severe obesity. Recommendations are derived from the published guidelines for cardiac evaluation for noncardiac surgery [12]. A functional assessment of exercise capacity is an essential part of the evaluation. A series of questions should be asked to assess the individual's capacity to perform common daily tasks ranging from self-care tasks to housework, climbing one or two flights of stairs, walking 1–2 blocks at 4 mph up to jogging. A patient with known coronary artery disease and on treatment in a regular physical exercise program may be of less cardiovascular concern than a patient with risk factors who has a very limited functional capacity. Aerobic exercise capacity has been studied in bariatric surgery candidates and the findings are striking in that aerobic fitness levels in extreme obesity are similar to those seen in patients with varying degrees of heart failure [13]. Exercise testing is also a possible predictor of major postoperative complications as they appear to cluster in patients with major limitations in maximal oxygen consumption [2]. Cardiovascular physiologic changes associated with extreme obesity are summarized in Table 17.7.

Exercise testing is an important component of noninvasive cardiac testing, because it may demonstrate symptoms and signs of ischemia in patients with occult and asymptomatic disease that is clinically significant. As many bariatric surgery candidates are not able to exercise because of extreme obesity, dobutamine may be substituted for exercise to produce cardiovascular stress. A stress test using ECG is usually of little value because of difficulties obtaining adequate tracings. Stress echocardiography is a more accurate method of assessing cardiac structure and function in extreme obesity. When external ultrasound quality is limited by echocardiography windows and adequate images, consideration should be given to transesophageal ultrasound with stress administered to achieve an adequate heart rate. The accuracy of thallium scanning is reduced in patients with extreme obesity and is of little value.

Thrombosis

Obesity is also a risk factor for arterial and venous thrombosis through a variety of mechanisms involving substances secreted by adipose tissue, direct effects on the coagulation factors, oxidative stress, and the association with chronic inflammation. Adipose tissue substances that stimulate thrombosis include leptin, resistin, tumor necrosis factor-α(alpha) (TNF-α[alpha]), and interleukin 6. Coagulation factors known to be elevated in obesity include plasminogen activator inhibitor-1 (PAI-1), fibrinogen, tissue factor, factor VII, and factor VIII. The chronic inflammatory state associated by obesity is driven by inflammatory cytokines interleukin 6 and TNF-α(alpha) and is associated with a prothrombotic state. Obesity is associated with increased production of pro-oxidant substances that promote endothelial dysfunction and platelet aggregation, which promotes thrombosis. The prothrombotic conditions associated with obesity contribute to the cardiovascular risks in obesity and the cardiovascular complications following bariatric surgery. These metabolic changes form the rationale for aggressive pharmacotherapy for thrombosis prevention during the perioperative period. The prothrombotic tendencies in obesity improve with weight loss, another exciting area in bariatric surgery outcomes [14].

Many bariatric surgery candidates are taking oral agents for long-term anticoagulation for indications related to cardiovascular disease treatment or prevention. Patients with chronic atrial fibrillation or prosthetic heart valves will require anticoagulation during the preoperative period, transition to heparin or low-molecular-weight heparin before surgery, and aggressive perioperative prophylaxis with heparin or low-molecular-weight heparin with transition to full anticoagulation while under close surveillance. Heparin and low-molecular-weight heparin should be dosed on the basis of patient body weight.

Risk-Benefit Analysis

The decision to offer bariatric surgery, when to proceed with surgery, and which operation to offer should be driven by the preoperative comprehensive assessment. Risk issues to be carefully considered include the operative risks based on patient health factors and an analysis of predictors of a successful long-term weight-loss result. For a high-risk patient who does not appear motivated and capable of the necessary lifestyle changes, the surgical risks may be deemed greater than the anticipated benefit.

The advent of institutional and administrative databases as well as clinical registries have allowed for the identification of patient factors that increase the surgical risks of bariatric surgery. Proven risk factors for surgery include older age, high BMI, male gender, congestive heart failure, chronic liver disease, pulmonary hypertension, and severe sleep apnea with hypoventilation. There are several bariatric risk scoring tools that are now available to assist bariatric programs in identifying high-risk patients. DeMaria et al. developed the Obesity Surgery Mortality Risk Score for Gastric Bypass [15] from a multivariate analysis of a single institution experience with 2,075 open and laparoscopic gastric bypass patients and 31 fatalities with a 30-day mortality of 1.5 %. Risk factors identified included male gender, a BMI ≥ 50 kg/m^2, hypertension, thromboembolism risk, and age ≥ 45 years. Each of these risk factors contributed to a single point in the risk score. This risk score was subsequently validated in a study of 4,431 patients [16].

Turner et al. developed a nomogram for predicting surgical complications using data from the NSQIP database in a study of 32,426 patients. Risk factors identified included low serum albumin, high BMI, older age, and functional dependence [17]. Most recently, a mortality risk calculator was developed by Ramanan et al. using NSQIP data from 21,891 patients. Identified risk factors included higher age, BMI, dyspnea at rest, previous percutaneous coronary intervention, a history of peripheral vascular disease requiring revascularization or amputation, and chronic corticosteroid use. This risk calculator was validated in 10,998 patients [18].

The ability to identify high-risk patients during the preoperative preparation allows for more intense focus and attention to these patients as they proceed through the evaluation phase, better decision-making regarding fitness for surgery, and better preparation for surgery and the necessary resources for the perioperative period. Close collaboration between the surgeon, the bariatric physician, and specialists is essential for patient selection and optimal outcomes.

Risk Reduction Strategies

Opportunities to reduce risk relate to the patient's comorbid disease burden and to behavioral, educational, or social factors that may be barriers to long-term weight-loss and health success. The study of the efficacy of bariatric risk reduction during the preoperative period is a new and important area of study in bariatric surgery. Little is known regarding the effects of intensive psychological counseling, behavioral treatment, or patient education, used either before surgery, or as an adjuvant treatment. Additional studies are needed to see if patients with behavioral or mental health conditions that reduce the likelihood of a successful weight-loss result can be improved with more intensive mental health treatment.

Supervised weight loss in the preoperative period has been used as a method of risk reduction by bariatric programs. The catabolism associated with the use of hypocaloric diets or very low calorie diets does not contribute to nutritional or wound healing problems affecting surgical outcomes. A recent study of 881 patients from Geisinger Medical Center [19], where supervised preoperative weight loss is strongly encouraged during the 6-month preoperative program, found that 67 % of the patients were able to lose more than 5 % of excess body weight and 48 % were able to lose more than 10 % of excess body weight. Weight loss of this magnitude in extreme obesity will improve physiology by lowering blood pressure, improving glucose control, inducing spontaneous diuresis in those with expanded extracellular fluid volume, and improving pulmonary gas exchange. Additional beneficial effects of preoperative weight loss include an increase in mobility and exercise tolerance, a reduction in liver size, and an opportunity for the bariatric program to confirm the patient's ability to change behavior.

The effects of preoperative weight loss on outcomes in bariatric surgery have been studied in a number of small observational studies with inconclusive results. In the largest study of 881 patients, Still et al. demonstrated that preoperative weight loss was associated with a shorter hospital length of stay [19]. Benotti et al. subsequently reviewed the same patient cohort and demonstrated that preoperative weight loss was associated with reduced surgical complications [20]. The favorable effect of preoperative weight loss on 30-day complication rates was recently demonstrated in a multicenter, randomized controlled trial of 273 patients comparing a 2-week very low calorie diet with usual diet [21]. Additional controlled studies investigating the beneficial effects of preoperative weight loss and its effect on patient physiology and surgical complications are needed. Short-term preoperative weight loss is achievable in bariatric surgical candidates using hypocaloric diets, very low calorie diets, pharmacotherapy, less invasive endoscopic procedures, or various combinations of these therapies. The ability to identify high-risk bariatric candidates and to intensify risk reduction treatments should favorably influence surgical results.

Conclusion

Bariatric surgeons have made great progress since the introduction of minimally invasive bariatric surgery. Major complication rates following bariatric surgery are similar to complication rates following cholecystectomy. In the era of expanding bariatric surgery treatment to more of the population who may benefit from this treatment, bariatric programs need to refine and reformat preoperative patient assessment techniques and treatments in order to identify early patients who are at risk for early surgical complications and later struggles with health and weight loss. Early identification of these patients will increase the program focus on these patients and the development of risk reduction strategies. The unique knowledge and skill of the experienced bariatric surgeon, the close collaboration with the multidisciplinary bariatric program personnel, and strategic input from consultants should be components of the important task of patient selection for surgery.

Many are called, but few are chosen. Matthew 22:14

Question and Answer Section

Questions

1. The following are risk factors for operative mortality after bariatric surgery except:
   A. Older age
   B. High BMI
   C. Congestive heart failure
   D. Female gender
   E. Limited exercise capacity
2. In a patient with extreme obesity for 20 years, surgeons can expect diminished cardiac reserve related to structural and functional changes in the heart.
   A. True
   B. False
3. Which patient requesting bariatric surgery is least likely to be successful in achieving long-term weight loss after bariatric surgery?
   A. A 54-year-old college professor with syndrome X, depression, and a BMI of 51.
   B. A 35-year-old with a BMI of 54, hypertension, and compulsive eating behavior
   C. A 35-year-old single mother of 4, with a BMI of 50, receiving disability from Medicare, who admits to using marijuana and other recreational drugs
   D. A 45-year-old female with a BMI of 56, type II diabetes, hypertension, and binge eating disorder

Answers

1. Answer **D**. Female gender is not a known risk factor.
2. Answer **A**. True.
3. Answer is **C**. Substance abuse is a contraindication to bariatric surgery.

References

1. Finks JF, Kole KL, Yenumula PR, English WJ, Krause KR, Carlin AM, et al. Predicting risk for serious complications with bariatric surgery: results from the Michigan Bariatric Surgery Collaborative. Ann Surg. 2011;254(4):633–40.
2. McCullough P, Gallagher M, DeJong A, Sandberg KR, Trivax JE, Alexander D, et al. Cardiorespiratory fitness and short-term complications after bariatric surgery. Chest. 2006;130:517–25.
3. King W, Belle S, Eid G, Dakin GF, Inabnet WB, Mitchell JE, et al. Physical activity levels of patients in the longitudinal assessment of bariatric surgery study. Surg Obes Relat Dis. 2008;4:721–8.
4. Collazo-Clavel M, Clark M, McAlpine D, Jensen MD. Assessment and preparation of patients for bariatric surgery. Mayo Clin Proc. 2006;81(10 suppl):S11–7.
5. Pawlow L, O'Neil P, White M, et al. Findings and outcomes of psychological evaluations of gastric bypass applicants. Surg Obes Relat Dis. 2005;1:523–9.
6. Bauchowitz A, Gonder-Frederick L, Olbrisch M, Azarbad L, Ryee MY, Woodson M, et al. Psychological evaluation of bariatric surgery candidates: a survey of present practices. Psychosom Med. 2005;67:825–32.
7. Poirier P, Alpert M, Fleisher L, Thompson PD, Sugerman HJ, Burke LE, American Heart Association Obesity Committee of Council on Nutrition, Physical Activity and Metabolism, Council on Cardiopulmonary Perioperative and Critical Care, Council on Cardiovascular Surgery and Anesthesia Council on Cardiovas, et al. Cardiovascular evaluation and management of severely obese

patients undergoing surgery: a science advisory from the American Heart Association. Circulation. 2009;120:86–95.
8. Kabon B, Nagele A, Reddy D, Eagon C, Fleshman JW, Sessler DI, et al. Obesity decreases tissue oxygenation. Anesthesiology. 2004;100:274–80.
9. Livingston E, Arterburn D, Schifftner T, Henderson WG, DePalma RG. National quality improvement program analysis of bariatric operations: modifiable risk factors contribute to bariatric surgical adverse outcomes. J Am Coll Surg. 2006;203:625–33.
10. Ashrafian H, Athanasiou T, le Roux C. Heart remodeling and obesity. Heart. 2011;97:171–2.
11. Ashrafian H, le Roux CW, Darzi A, Athanasiou T. Effects of bariatric surgery on cardiovascular function. Circulation. 2008;118:2091–102.
12. Lee T, Mercantonio E, Mangione C, Thomas EJ, Polanczyk CA, Cook EF, et al. Derivation and prospective validation of a simple index for prediction of cardiac risk of major noncardiac surgery. Circulation. 1999;100:1043–9.
13. Gallagher M, Franklin B, Ehrman J, Keteyian SJ, Brawner CA, de Jong AT, et al. Comparative impact of morbid obesity vs heart failure on cardiorespiratory fitness. Chest. 2005;127:2197–203.
14. Darvall KA, Sam RC, Silverman SH, Bradbury AW, Adam DJ. Obesity and thrombosis. Eur J Vasc Endovasc Surg. 2007;33(2):223–33.
15. DeMaria EJ, Portenier D, Wolfe L. Obesity surgery mortality risk score: proposal for a clinically useful score to predict mortality risk in patients undergoing gastric bypass. Surg Obes Relat Dis. 2007;3(2):134–40.
16. DeMaria EJ, Murr M, Byrne TK, Blackstone R, Grant JP, Budak A, et al. Validation of the obesity surgery mortality risk score in a multicenter study proves it stratifies mortality risk in patients undergoing gastric bypass for morbid obesity. Ann Surg. 2007;246(4):578–82; discussion 583–4.
17. Turner P, Saager L, Dalton J, Abd-Elsayed A, Roberman D, Melara P, et al. A nomogram for predicting surgical complications in bariatric surgery patients. Obes Surg. 2011;21:655–62.
18. Ramanan B, Gupta P, Gupta H, Fang X, Forse RA. Development and validation of a bariatric surgery mortality risk calculator. J Am Coll Surg. 2012;214:892–900.
19. Still C, Benotti P, Wood C, Gerhard GS, Petrick A, Reed M, et al. Outcomes of preoperative weight loss in high risk patients undergoing gastric bypass surgery. Arch Surg. 2007;142:994–8.
20. Benotti P, Still C, Wood C, Akmal Y, King H, El Arousy H, et al. Preoperative weight loss before bariatric surgery. Arch Surg. 2009;144:1150–5.
21. Van Nieuwenhove Y, Dambrauskas Z, Campillo-Soto A, van Dielen F, Wiezer R, Janssen I, et al. Preoperative very low-calorie diet and operative outcome after laparoscopic gastric bypass: a randomized multicenter study. Arch Surg. 2011;146:1300–5.

The Perioperative and Postoperative Medical Management of the Bariatric Surgery Patient

Christopher Still, Nadia Boulghassoul-Pietrzykowska, and Jennifer Franceschelli

Chapter Objectives

1. Summarize the strategies for risk reduction in the bariatric surgery preoperative period.
2. Describe postoperative medication administration considerations after bariatric surgery.
3. Summarize postoperative medical management including medication adjustments and common complications associated with bariatric surgery.

Introduction

The disease of obesity, and its associated comorbid medical problems, is a major public health concern that has reached epidemic proportions. To date, bariatric surgery remains the only safe and long-term treatment modality for the chronic and relapsing disease of obesity. Although sustained weight loss is important, the surgery's ability to resolve chronic comorbid medical problems such as diabetes mellitus, obstructive sleep apnea, fatty liver disease, and lipid dyscrasias arguably makes the weight loss itself secondary to its profound medical benefits. It stands to reason then that bariatric surgery patients presenting for surgery have a high incidence of comorbid medical problems. In a published large cohort of bariatric surgery comorbidities, approximately 36 % of patients were diabetic, 30 % had obstructive sleep apnea, 25 % had fatty liver disease, and 12 % had cardiovascular disease [1]. This chapter will review perioperative and postoperative medical management of the bariatric surgery patients with an emphasis on practical clinical care.

Preoperative Risk Reduction Strategies

Two controversial risk reduction strategies include pre-op weight loss and smoking cessation. Drs. Benotti and Dalencourt outlined the benefits of preoperative weight loss nicely in the previous chapter (Chap. 17). Like preoperative weight loss, preoperative smoking cessation remains controversial. It has been well known that smoking cessation has a number of detrimental effects on microvascular surgery. It can damage a large number of organ systems including endothelial cells. With regard to bariatric procedures creating anastomosis, several studies cite smoking as a significant risk factor for marginal ulcers and strictures by increasing platelet adhesion and its effect on endothelial cells [2, 3]. In addition to increased marginal ulcers and strictures, smoking has been associated with increased postoperative morbidity with regard to increased nausea, poor wound healing, and suboptimal nutrient intake [4].

Smoking cessation can be confirmed by a negative urine cotinine level. On average, 6 weeks of abstinence is required for a negative test. Confounding agents like nicotine replacement patches or E-cigarettes can give a "false" positive for active smoking. Therefore, a serum cotinine test may be necessary to differentiate replacement products versus continued active nicotine use.

Despite the significant amount of cited literature detailing the negative effects of continued smoking use following bariatric surgery, Nguyen et al. showed in a prospective study of 150 consecutive laparoscopic gastric bypass patients performed by a single surgeon that smoking had no statistical association with operative outcomes [5].

Patients who continue to smoke or use nonsteroidal anti-inflammatory drugs (NSAIDs) are at high risk for marginal ulcers. Wilson et al. concluded that 12 months of

C. Still, DO, FACN, FACP (✉) • J. Franceschelli, DO
Department of GI and Nutrition, Geisinger Obesity Institute, Geisinger Medical Center, Danville, PA, USA
e-mail: CSTILL@Geisinger.edu

N. Boulghassoul-Pietrzykowska, MD, FACP
Center for Medical Weight Management, Nutrition, Fitness and Lifestyle, Weight & Life MD, 1901 N. Olden Ave Ext., Suite 29, Ewing, NJ 08618, USA
e-mail: npietrzykowksa@weightlifemd.com

postoperative proton pump inhibitors (PPI) therapy was protective against marginal ulcers in these high-risk patients [6].

Preoperative Liquid Diets

Fatty liver disease is a major, and often overlooked, comorbid medical problem affecting approximately 35–50 % of all bariatric surgery patients. Steatosis, primarily due to glycogen accumulation with resulting hepatomegaly, is common. This fatty infiltration commonly limits the surgeon's view of the gastroesophageal area, requiring retraction of the enlarged and often vascular left caudal lobe. In order to reduce liver size prior to surgery, a short-term, 7–10 days, liquid diet is often prescribed. Fris demonstrated a highly significant reduction in liver size in patients consuming a 2-week, low-energy liquid diet prior to bariatric surgery [7]. Colles et al. similarly described and recommended a 2-week preoperative low-energy-density liquid diet to achieve significant reduction in liver mass and 6 weeks to achieve significant reduction in visceral adipose tissue without compromising patient compliance and acceptability [8]. In diabetic individuals for whom you are prescribing preoperative low-energy-density liquid diets, adjustments in their insulin requirements and oral hypoglycemic medications may be necessary to prevent hypoglycemia.

Preoperative Colonic Preparations

By and large, routine preoperative colon cleansing is not indicated nor warranted. In the superobese patient (body mass index [BMI] greater than 70), chronic constipation and colonic distention can be problematic. This chronic constipation is further exacerbated by anesthesia, narcotics for pain control, and postoperative high-protein liquid diets. These patients can develop a megacolon-like picture with colonic distention and significant fecal impaction. A regular bowel regimen with isotonic polyethylene glycol solution may be beneficial prior to surgery and postoperatively as needed [9]. Caution should be taken with the use of oral sodium phosphate preparations for they may cause electrolyte abnormalities and, among other things, may precipitate acquired QT interval prolongation, which could cause life-threatening cardiac arrhythmias in predisposed patients with obesity and metabolic syndrome [10].

Preoperative Medication Adjustments

Although there is a paucity of level 1 evidence of preoperative medication adjustments prior to bariatric surgery, best practice outcomes have *recommended* various medication adjustments or cessation prior to surgery.

Diabetic Medications

If preoperative low-energy-density liquid diets are recommended, consider decreasing the dose of insulin and oral agents to avoid hypoglycemia since insulin requirements decrease. Insulin sensitizers such as the biguanides and thiazolidinediones should not cause hypoglycemia and may not need dose adjustments. However, stopping metformin 48 h prior to surgery may be beneficial in patients at risk for acute kidney injury following bariatric surgery.

NSAIDs/Aspirin/Antiplatelet Medications

Due to the increased risk of bleeding, most surgeons recommend holding aspirin and nonsteroidal anti-inflammatory medications for 5–7 days prior to surgery. Although not specifically evaluated in bariatric surgery patients, the American College of Cardiology recommends holding antiplatelet medications such as clopidogrel for at least 5 days prior to coronary artery bypass graft (CABG) surgery based on multicenter analysis [11].

ACE Inhibitors

The common comorbid medical problems of obesity including diabetes, hyperlipidemia, hypertension, and heart failure can predispose patients to postoperative acute kidney injury (AKI). In addition, medications, anesthesia, postoperative dehydration, and increased protein consumption can further precipitate that risk. Risk factors identified with increased frequency of AKI include hyperlipidemia, preoperative use of angiotensin-converting enzyme inhibitors (ACE inhibitors) and angiotensin II receptor blockers (ARBs), intraoperative hypotension, and high BMI with ACE inhibitor and ARBs being independently associated with AKI [12]. For that reason, consideration for holding ACE inhibitors and ARBs as well as metformin and nonessential diuretic medications for 48 h prior to surgery may be beneficial in at-risk patients as outlined previously.

Preoperative Pulmonary Training

Postoperative atelectasis in the bariatric surgery patient is common and can lead to pneumonic processes and hypoxemia. Anesthesia, pain causing splinting, and somnolence can all exacerbate this process. Early aggressive pulmonary toilet, mobilization, and lung expansion maneuvers are critical to maintain normal respiratory function and decrease postoperative pulmonary complications [13]. However, pain, somnolence from anesthesia, and inadequate pain control can interfere with proper teaching of incentive spirometry devices in the immediate postoperative period. To alleviate this, providing the patient with an incentive spirometer device with instruction at the surgical history and physical outpatient visit can allow the patient to familiarize themselves with the device and provide inspiratory muscle training prior to surgery.

Perioperative Hospital Stay

Day of Surgery

For the morning of surgery, most centers have set guidelines for what medication in general should be taken versus held. For the bariatric surgery patient specifically, there are no concrete recommendations. A reasonable recommendation would be to continue prescribed beta blockers, anti-reflux medications, thyroid replacements, arrhythmic medication, psychiatric medications, and inhalers, which should be safe to be taken the morning of surgery. Depending on the surgical start time, holding or modifying the dose of antidiabetic medications may be warranted.

Intraoperatively

From a medical standpoint, an important factor influencing postoperative morbidity and length of stay is perioperative glycemic control. Obese diabetics, and even obese nondiabetics, require higher insulin requirements than expected. This is compounded with the "stress" of surgery. Anesthesiologists and surgeons are understandably cautious about treating hyperglycemia in patients with or without a diagnosis of diabetes using standardized protocols due to ensuing adverse hypoglycemic effect. Continuous insulin infusion (CII) has been proven to decrease morbidity and mortality in surgical critical care patients but has not been vastly studied in individuals with type II diabetes undergoing bariatric surgery. Blackstone et al. demonstrated that continuous insulin infusion can be administered safely to diabetic patients undergoing bariatric surgery [14]. Moreover, there was a decreased number of postoperative cholecystectomies in the CII group; however, there was no effect on the stricter rate. Of note, there was an increased number of patients with postoperative port site infections that received CII with no plausible explanation. Continuous insulin infusion protocols are available for a wide variety of patients with varying degrees of insulin infusions.

Early ambulation is critical for thromboembolic prevention and should be encouraged the night of the surgery. If the patient is unable to get out of bed and ambulate that evening, sitting up over the side of the bed for a bedside dangle is beneficial in preventing venostasis. Low molecular weight heparin should be continued per surgical protocols.

Obstructive Sleep Apnea Management

From a medical standpoint, an important issue that is often controversial is the immediate postoperative use of noninvasive positive pressure devices such as continuous positive airway pressure (CPAP) or bi-level positive airway pressure (BiPAP). The primary concern by some surgeons with initiating CPAP in the immediate postoperative period is the increase in staple line disruption and frequent nausea and vomiting. Vasquez et al. published case studies showing significant bowel distension and subsequent anastomotic leaks documented after BiPAP use [15]. However, Ramirez et al. retrospectively reviewed 310 patients who underwent laparoscopic Roux-en-Y gastric bypass (RYGB) from the completion of surgery until 2 weeks postoperatively [16]. They concluded that the use of CPAP after laparoscopic RYGB did not result in increased morbidity in the immediate postoperative period compared to patients who did not require CPAP. Moreover, Meng analyzed more than 350 patients requiring CPAP postoperatively and found no increased risk of postoperative nausea and vomiting compared to patients without CPAP use [17].

Interestingly, Jensen reported that postoperative CPAP/BiPAP use can be safely omitted in laparoscopic RYGB patients with known obstructive sleep apnea provided they are observed in a monitored setting and their pulmonary status is optimized by aggressive incentive spirometry and early ambulation [18]. Although they reported men having greater CPAP/BiPAP dependency, none of the apnea/hypoxia ratios were provided to determine the severity of the obstructive sleep apnea in study patients.

In summary, obstructive sleep apnea is a common comorbid medical problem in the bariatric surgery population. Many of these patients require noninvasive positive pressure devices for varying severities of obstructive sleep apnea. In the postoperative period, hypoventilation and hypoxemia with hypercarbia are not uncommon due to residual influence of general anesthesia, postoperative atelectasis, postoperative analgesia, and pain. For this reason, in the studies outlined above, when warranted, postoperative CPAP or BiPAP should be continued unless otherwise recommended by the bariatric surgeon.

After surgery, continued CPAP is recommended but adherence may be difficult for some patients. As weight loss ensues, patients often complain of ill-fitting masks and pressure settings too powerful. If available, "autoPAP" noninvasive positive pressure delivery devices regulate pressures to patients in real-time requirements, alleviating the problem with overpressure. If patients are able to continue their CPAP device after surgery, knowing when it is safe for patients to discontinue the CPAP is highly variable and not well studied to date. Varela et al. followed 29 patients requiring CPAP for obstructive sleep apnea postoperatively and concluded, based on the Epworth Sleepiness Score, that only four (14 %) patients required CPAP at 3 months and none required CPAP at 9 months [19]. Although this study is encouraging, no postoperative polysomnogram studies were performed to definitively determine that CPAP was not recommended based on objective study criteria. Marti-Valeri et al. followed 105 patients with respiratory conditions, which included obstructive sleep apnea, chronic obstructive pulmonary disease (COPD), and obesity hypoventilation syndrome [20]. Thirty patients required noninvasive ventilation preoperatively. At 1 year, polysomnogram, arterial blood gas (ABG), and pulmonary function tests were reported on all patients. Not surprisingly, significant improvement was seen in arterial hypertension with less hypoxemia, hypercapnia, and improvement in spirometry. Of the 30 patients requiring noninvasive ventilation devices, all but four patients had their devices withdrawn. This was with a mean weight loss of 34 %. Since patients have varying degrees of obstructive sleep apnea and the rate of weight loss differs between patients, no clear-cut timeframe from surgery or specific weight loss thresholds should negate the need for a follow-up polysomnogram on average of 7–10 months postoperatively.

DVT Prevention

As you have read in previous chapters, pulmonary embolism accounts for a majority of the mortality among bariatric surgery patients. It stands to reason that bariatric surgery patients are prone to thromboembolism episodes due to increased blood viscosity, deceased concentration of antithrombin III in the obese, increased concentration of fibrinogen and plasma activation inhibitor-1 (PAI-1) produced by adipose tissue along with sedentary lifestyle, venous stasis, and pulmonary hypertension, which all augment the risk. Culminating at the time of surgery with endothelial injury completes Virchow's triad, increasing the thromboembolic risk even further. The American Society of Metabolic and Bariatric Surgery (ASMBS) has suggested that all patients have early postoperative mobilization and perioperative use of sequential compression devices and recommends that chemoprophylaxis be utilized unless otherwise contraindicated. Reasonable contraindications include known medication allergy or adverse reaction, heparin-induced thrombocytopenia, coagulation disturbance, the presence of active bleeding, or clinic concern for high risk of bleeding. The most important may be early ambulation as discussed previously.

With greater than 90 % of all bariatric surgeries performed laparoscopically, improved clinical pathways, and center of excellent institutions, length of stay has dropped dramatically with the average being approximately 2.1 days. Although there are recommendations for prolonged thromboprophylaxis in major abdominal, pelvic, orthopaedic, and trauma patients [20–22] the important question, which has not been well studied to date, is the duration of thromboprophylaxis following bariatric surgery. Borkgren-Okonek et al. carried out a prospective open trial of 223 patients who were assigned to two doses of enoxaparin (depending on body mass index) twice daily while hospitalized and once daily for 10 days after discharge [24]. They concluded BMI-stratified, extended enoxaparin dosing regimen provided well tolerated, effective prophylaxis against venous thromboembolism in patients undergoing gastric bypass surgery.

Postoperative Medication Administration Considerations After Bariatric Surgery

Following bariatric surgery, proper medication adjustments are crucial to adequately dose patients without under- or overdosing based on their new altered anatomy. Which surgical procedure is performed will dictate how much, if any, medication adjustment is required. A purely restrictive procedure, like the adjustable gastric band, may not require any medication adjustment, whereas Roux-en-Y gastric bypass or duodenal switch procedures, based on their altered anatomy, do require administration considerations following bariatric surgery. This is due to nearly all oral agents being maximally absorbed in the small intestine, which is bypassed in several bariatric procedures. Delayed gastric emptying, diminished opportunity for mucosal exposure, and changes in drug dissolution and solubility resulting from alterations in intestinal pH are additional factors that may potentially impair drug absorption [25]. Despite the growing number of bariatric surgeries being performed in the United States, with Roux-en-Y gastric bypass being the most frequently performed, there is a paucity of pharmacokinetic studies of drug absorption following bariatric surgery. A concise review of 26 studies and case reports were summarized by Padwal et al. who found varying degrees of reduced drug absorption that appeared drug specific [26]. Inherently, with the altered anatomy following bariatric surgery, reduced and augmented absorption is not surprising. From a clinician's standpoint, however, there were no citations found or prescribing recommendations of disease-specific medications following bariatric surgery. To that end, the following discussed specific recommendations are class three—expert recommendations and not necessarily consensus:

Diabetic Medications

Bariatric surgery, specifically the Roux-en-Y gastric bypass, has shown to be safe and effective treatment for patients suffering from type 2 diabetes. For reasons not clearly understood, improvement of insulin sensitivity and glycemic control ensues immediately after RYGB before any appreciable weight loss has occurred. Continued administration of pre-op diabetic medication without adjustment usually results in unwarranted hypoglycemia. Following RYGB, most insulin-requiring diabetics' daily insulin regimens can be held and replaced with sliding scale coverage. Since PO intake is reduced both in volume and time of consumption, regular Humulin coverage may be better tolerated than the fast-acting Humalog. Like insulin requirements, significant reduction in oral medication dose is common; a significant proportion of patients controlled only with oral agent preoperatively will require little if any medication administration, especially in the immediate post-op period (7–10 days).

If the patient does require resumption of oral medications, regular release and crushed or liquid rather than sustained release/extended release formulation are recommended in order to maximize absorption. The newly created 15–30 cc pouch in RYGB patients has reduced surface area and reduced parietal cell mass and change in pH among other factors [25]. Not surprisingly, metformin, at least in the immediate postoperative period, is not well tolerated due to gastrointestinal (GI) intolerance and should be held. The thioglitazones may be better tolerated than metformin, but because of their propensity to cause weight gain or retard weight loss as well as increase total body water, they are usually not recommended.

In individuals undergoing a laparoscopic adjustable gastric band (LAGB), the immediate improvement in insulin sensitivity and glycemic control is not usually apparent. Therefore, continuing 75 % of their preoperative diabetic medication is usually required. Reduction in the amount of medication in the LAGB patient is predicated on weight loss itself. Moreover, changing to regular release and slower acting insulin coverage is usually not necessary.

Antihypertensive Medications

For a variety of reasons, blood pressure routinely is decreased in the immediate postoperative period in patients undergoing RYGB. This, in turn, necessitates reduced doses of antihypertensive medications. Usually, medication dosages can be cut in half, and ACE inhibitors that had been held 48 h prior to surgery can be restarted postoperatively at a reduced dose. Diuretics for blood pressure control can usually be held. As discussed previously, medications that are prescribed should be in the regular release and crushed/liquid formulation in order to ensure maximum absorption in the immediate postoperative period.

Antidepressant/Mood-Altering Medications

Due to the potential withdrawal effect with abruptly stopping these medications, they should be continued postoperatively. For the reasons already discussed, medications should be prescribed in the regular release, crushed/liquid form. Capsules can be opened and mixed with sugar-free pudding or taken with warm water to expedite disintegration. Due to the propensity to cause weight gain, alternative medication to the tricyclic antidepressants and Remeron specifically may be warranted if possible.

Dyslipidemic Medications

Although not as immediate as the improvement of insulin sensitivity/glycemic control, lipid profiles have been shown to significantly improve from 3 to 12 months after surgery [27]. Coupled with propensity of statins causing nausea in the immediate postoperative period and the fact that with rapid weight loss elevation in transaminases can occur, consideration for holding dyslipidemic medications for the first 12 weeks after surgery and reevaluating their need may outweigh the risk of restarting it in the immediate postoperative period. If, however, a patient with known cardiovascular disease is prescribed statins for primary or secondary prevention of acute coronary events, the statins should be prescribed in the regular release formulation upon discharge.

Aspirin and Ibuprofen Products

Due to the increased risk of ulcers, strictures, and bleeding, the chronic use of aspirin and anti-inflammatory products should be avoided. Numerous studies have demonstrated increased complications, especially with concomitant tobacco use. If chronic anti-inflammatory use cannot be avoided, consideration for more of a restrictive type of procedure may be in the patient's best interest. Short courses of anti-inflammatory therapy (3–5 days) for acute issues like gout attacks, migraine headaches, and acute musculoskeletal strain are usually well tolerated but should be taken with food and in its liquid form if possible so as not to cause direct mucosal irritation. Patients requiring aspirin therapy for antiplatelet cardioprotection should chew the 81 mg doses up to the prescribed amount.

Warfarin and Antiplatelet Medication

As discussed earlier, warfarin and antiplatelet therapy such as clopidogrel bisulfate should be held 7–10 days prior to surgery. Surgeon preference should dictate when these medications should be restarted. If there were no complicating surgical issues, warfarin can usually be restarted safely on the evening of postoperative day 1 and bridged with low molecular weight heparin therapy until therapeutic levels of warfarin are achieved. Preoperative warfarin dosage may need to be adjusted due to altered anatomy and changes in diet postoperatively. Similarly, if no surgical issues occur, antiplatelet therapy can usually be safely restarted on the day of discharge from the hospital. If patients are discharged home on prolonged thromboprophylaxis, providers should be cognizant of their potential additive effects.

Oral Contraceptive Agents

For reasons probably similar to improvement in insulin sensitivity immediately after bariatric surgery, ovulatory rates improve soon after RYGB surgery despite little, if any, weight loss. However, for many reasons, pregnancy is not recommended for at least 12 months after surgery [28]. Like with other medications, oral contraceptive absorption is inconsistent, and therefore an alternative barrier method of birth control should be recommended. This becomes an important issue to discuss with patients, for many of them suffered from polycystic ovarian syndrome or amenorrhea with resultant infertility for many years and are under the impression that they will not be able to conceive. Since this is contrary to the truth, patient education and adherence to alternative barrier method of birth control is important in addition to their regular formulation of their oral contraceptive [29].

Medication such as Depo-Provera injections may be effective to prevent pregnancy but also can inhibit weight loss after surgery so should be avoided if possible. Also some patches and barrier methods for contraception are not recommended in women with a BMI greater than 40 kg/m^2.

Postoperative Medical Management

Anastomotic Leak Detection

With 90 % of all bariatric surgeries being performed laparoscopically, the average length of stay is approximately 2.1 days. Although the incidence of anastomotic leak is less than 1 % when performed within a center of excellence, the usual time to detect anastomotic leak is 2–7 days postoperatively. To this end, although clearly a surgical issue, medical professionals should be cognizant of the signs and symptoms of an anastomotic leak so that appropriate communication and transfer to the surgical facility can be expedited.

Patients presenting to your office with a suspected anastomotic leak can have a wide variety of signs and symptoms. Patients can complain of vague abdominal discomfort, malaise, and low-grade fever. Two important signs and symptoms are shoulder pain (often left-sided referred pain) and tachycardia greater than 120 beats per minute. Any bariatric surgery patients presenting with tachycardia greater than 120 beats per minute should have a high index of suspicion for an anastomotic leak until proven otherwise. If an anastomotic leak is suspected and the patient is clinically stable, communication with the bariatric surgeon performing the procedure should be undertaken. He or she will recommend and facilitate transfer to the appropriate institution if warranted. The usual workup for a suspected anastomotic leak includes complete blood count (CBC) with differential, comprehensive medical panel, computed tomography (CT) scan of the abdomen with oral contrast, and a PA and lateral chest X-ray. Time is of importance in diagnosing an anastomotic leak, because, if detected early enough, patients can usually be managed conservatively without necessitating re-exploration.

Nausea and Vomiting

Postoperative nausea and vomiting is not uncommon and therefore practitioners should be familiar with common etiologies and treatment options. Dehydration in and of itself can cause nausea in a subgroup of individuals. Often just aggressive hydration even without the need of antiemetic medication will suffice for amelioration. If pharmacotherapy is warranted, a scopolamine patch behind the ear every 3 days along with increased hydration is often effective.

Pain medications and also PO vitamin supplementation can also cause nausea. Most postoperative protein supplements/meal replacements are fortified with vitamins/minerals, and therefore additional MVI supplementation, at least in the early postoperative period, may not be needed. Eating too much or too quickly or not chewing food adequately can also cause nausea. To this end, preoperative education on the importance of chewing food adequately and slowly as well as not drinking liquids for 20–30 min after eating is important to alleviate postoperative nausea and vomiting.

Small Pouch Syndrome

There is a small subgroup of patients who, for unclear reasons, are unable to tolerate much, if any, liquids or solids by mouth after surgery. Anatomically there are no strictures or abnormalities seen on the upper GI; however, these individuals are very nauseous and vomit much of what is taken in. This is obviously frustrating for the patient and physician alike. Intravenous (IV) fluids with multiple vitamins, thiamine, and antiemetic medications are often needed for an extended period of time. Moreover, parenteral nutrition may be warranted in some individuals as well. A speculative etiology is poor protein intake, and supplementation with IV fluids, multiple vitamin, and thiamine, as well as salt-poor albumin may help these individuals. Another potential etiology is once a small pouch is created during surgery, the nausea and vomiting sensor in their hypothalamus becomes hyperactive to liquids and solids in their newly created pouch. In addition to IV fluids and/or total parenteral nutrition and antiemetics, the use of Remeron (mirtazapine) may prove beneficial. This medication helps with appetite, mood, and sleep, which all can be affected by this "small pouch syndrome" for a lack of a better term. Even the most symptomatic patients resolve their symptoms in 4–6 weeks and then continue with a "normal postoperative course."

Thiamine Deficiency

Fortunately there are few "nutritional emergencies" seen in patients undergoing bariatric surgery. However, thiamine deficiency is one of them. Thiamine (B_1) is a water-soluble vitamin absorbed mostly in the jejunum. It is a key coenzyme in carbohydrate metabolism. Severe thiamine deficiency (beriberi) results in a spectrum of neuropsychiatric, cardiac, and gastrointestinal symptoms. There are four clinical presentations of beriberi. Neuropsychiatric beriberi (Wernicke's disease) that classically presents as a classic triad of symptoms including ocular abnormalities, gait ataxia, and mental status changes. Neurologic or "dry beriberi" presents with seizures or numbness, pain, and weakness in the extremities. Cardiovascular or "wet beriberi" presents as high-output heart failure. And lastly, gastrointestinal beriberi manifests with delayed emptying of the stomach. In patients who underwent RYGB, thiamine becomes easily depleted, and aggressive and timely repletion is necessary.

For patients undergoing gastric banding, sleeve gastrectomy, or even RYGB, diarrhea is unusual, but common causes usually are "easily" identified. Depending on the surgical procedure and institutional rates, one should have a high index of suspicion for *Clostridium difficile* colitis. If patients complain of watery diarrhea for greater than 24 h, *C. difficile* toxin should be considered. Of all the common causes, *C. difficile* colitis poses the most morbidity. The other causes of diarrhea include occult ingestion of sucrose in medications (OTC/RX) or food. A careful history of medications, especially in the liquid form, should be obtained.

It is not uncommon for patients to complain of "lactose intolerance" after undergoing a gastric bypass procedure. In reality, their symptoms most likely represent an intolerance to lactose sugar rather than a lactase deficiency for there is no pancreatic manipulation during surgery to account for a true lactose deficiency. The most common cause of postoperative diarrhea seen in at least gastric bypass patients is dumping syndrome. Dumping syndrome is a constellation of gastrointestinal and vasomotor symptoms including nausea, cramping, diarrhea, sweating, palpitations, and lightheadedness. It may present early or late in the digestion process. Early dumping syndrome occurs within 15–30 min of a meal when the contents of the stomach empty too quickly into the small intestine. The partially digested food draws excess fluid into the small intestine causing these unpleasant symptoms. Dumping usually occurs after the consumption of too much simple or refined sugar in a patient who underwent gastric bypass surgery. Dietary compliance with avoidance of refined sugars and high glycemic carbohydrates is the primary treatment. Late dumping occurs 1–3 h after a meal. It is thought to be related to the early development of hyperinsulinemic (reactive) hypoglycemia. An initially high concentration of carbohydrates in the proximal small bowel results in a rapid absorption of glucose, which is countered by a hyperinsulinemic response. The high insulin levels are responsible for the subsequent hypoglycemia. The symptoms include sweating, shaking, loss of concentration, hunger, and fainting. If late dumping persists despite dietary compliance, it may be treated with a small amount of sugar about 1 h after a meal, which may prevent its occurrence. Acarbose or somatostatin may also be helpful. If symptoms are resistant to medical management, the rare possibility of an insulinoma or nesidioblastosis of the pancreas should be considered.

Conclusion: Disease Management

As stated at the beginning of this chapter, the primary reason for considering bariatric surgery is for the reduction of comorbid medical problems—weight loss is secondary. To that end, continued diligence of monitoring blood sugar, blood pressure, sleep apnea, fatty liver disease, and dyslipidemia is important for 9–12 months after surgery. Medication recommendation immediately postoperatively may need to be adjusted to meet metabolic needs.

Question and Answer Section

Questions

1. Which of the following is the **MOST** sensitive sign indicating an anastomotic leak following gastric bypass surgery?
   A. Persistent nausea/vomiting
   B. Tachycardia >120 beats per minute
   C. Low-grade fever
   D. Shoulder pain
   E. Low urine output

2. Your local bariatric surgeon asks you to evaluate a 54-year-old white male, with a BMI of 56 kg/m2 and PMH of OSA requiring nocturnal CPAP, who is in postoperative day #1 of an uncomplicated laparoscopic gastric bypass. Overall he is doing well and tolerating sugar-free clear liquids. Vitals: BP 146/96, HR 102, RR 16. Which of the following recommendations is **NOT** recommended?
   A. Aggressive pulmonary toilet/incentive spirometry
   B. Early ambulation
   C. SCDs/impulse boots while in bed
   D. Metoprolol 5 mg intravenous now then 50 mg PO crushed twice a day
   E. Continue CPAP with naps and Q HS at the same pressure setting at home

3. Which of the following is a **FALSE** statement regarding postoperative medication adjustments following gastric bypass surgery?
   A. Diuretic medications should be held or dosage reduced for at least 7–10 days following gastric bypass surgery to prevent dehydration or hypotension.
   B. Extended release medications should be changed to regular release formulation and be crushed or in the liquid form for maximum absorption following gastric bypass surgery.
   C. Insulin requirements are significantly reduced immediately following gastric banding surgery.
   D. Hypertensive medication requirements may be significantly reduced immediately following gastric bypass surgery.
   E. NSAID should be avoided whenever possible postoperatively in patients following gastric bypass since they can significantly increase the incidence of strictures and ulcers.

Answers

1. Answer **B**. Tachycardia greater than 120 beats per minute is an indicator of a possible anastomotic leak.
2. Answer **D**. Metoprolol is not recommended.
3. Answer **C**. Typically, gastric banding does not cause an immediate improvement in insulin sensitivity and glycemic control. Therefore, continuing 75 % of the preoperative diabetic medication is usually required.

References

1. Wood GC, Chu X, Manney C, Strodel W, Petrick A, Gabrielsen J, et al. An electronic health record-enabled obesity database. BMC Med Inform Decis Mak. 2012;12:45. doi:10.1186/1472-6947-12-45.
2. Tosun Z, Karabekmez FE, Duymaz A, Ozkan A, Keskin M, Avunduk MC. Preventing negative effects of smoking on microarterial anastomosis. Ann Plast Surg. 2010;65(1):91–5.
3. Avunduk MC. Preventing negative effects of smoking on microarterial anastomosis. Ann Plast Surg. 2010;65(1):91–5.
4. Warner DO. Tobacco dependence in surgical patients. Curr Opin Anaesthesiol. 2007;20:279–83.
5. Nguyen NT, Rivers R, Wolfe BM. Factors associated with operative outcomes in laparoscopic gastric bypass. J Am Coll Surg. 2003;197(4):548–55.
6. Wilson JA, Romagnuolo J, Byrne TK, Morgan K, Wilson FA. Predictors of endoscopic findings after Roux-en-Y gastric bypass. Am J Gastroenterol. 2006;101(10):2194–9.
7. Fris RJ. Preoperative low energy diet diminishes liver size. Obes Surg. 2004;14(9):1165–70.
8. Colles SL, Dixon JB, Marks P, Strauss BJ, O'Brien PE. Preoperative weight loss with a very-low-energy diet: quantitation of changes in liver and abdominal fat by serial imaging. Am J Clin Nutr. 2006;84(2):304–11.
9. Corazziari E, Badiali D, Bazzocchi G, Bassotti G, Roselli P, Mastropaolo G, et al. Long term efficacy, safety, and tolerability of low daily doses of isosmotic polyethylene glycol electrolyte balanced solution (PMF-100) in the treatment of functional chronic constipation. Gut. 2000;46(4):522–6.
10. Hanci V, Yurtlu S, Aydin M, Bilir S, Erdogan G, Okyay RD, et al. Preoperative abnormal P and QTc dispersion intervals in patients with metabolic syndrome. Anesth Analg. 2011;112(4):824–7.
11. Berger JS, Frye CB, Harshaw Q, Edwards FH, Steinhubl SR, Becker RC. Impact of clopidogrel in patients with acute coronary syndromes requiring coronary artery bypass surgery: a multicenter analysis. J Am Coll Cardiol. 2008;52(21):1693–701.
12. Thakar CV, Kharat V, Blanck S, Leonard AC. Acute kidney injury after gastric bypass surgery. Clin J Am Soc Nephrol. 2007;2(3):426–30.
13. Duggan M, Kavanagh BP. Perioperative modifications of respiratory function. Best Pract Res Clin Anaesthesiol. 2010;24(2):145–55.
14. Blackstone R, Kieran J, Davis M, Rivera L. Continuous perioperative insulin infusion therapy for patients with type 2 diabetes undergoing bariatric surgery. Surg Endosc. 2007;21(8):1316–22.
15. Vasquez TL, Hoddinott K. A potential complication of bi-level positive airway pressure after gastric bypass surgery. Obes Surg. 2004;14(2):282–4.
16. Ramirez A, Lalor PF, Szomstein S, Rosenthal RJ. Continuous positive airway pressure in immediate postoperative period after laparoscopic Roux-en-Y gastric bypass: is it safe? Surg Obes Relat Dis. 2009;5(5):544–6.
17. Meng L. Postoperative nausea and vomiting with application of postoperative continuous positive airway pressure after laparoscopic gastric bypass. Obes Surg. 2010;20(7):876–80.
18. Jensen C, Tejirian T, Lewis C, Yadegar J, Dutson E, Mehran A. Postoperative CPAP and BiPAP use can be safely omitted after laparoscopic Roux-en-Y gastric bypass. Surg Obes Relat Dis. 2008;4(4):512–4.
19. Varela JE, Hinojosa MW, Nguyen NT. Resolution of obstructive sleep apnea after laparoscopic gastric bypass. Obes Surg. 2007;17(10):1279–82.
20. Marti-Valeri C, Sabate A, Masdevall C, Dalmau A. Improvement of associated respiratory problems in morbidly obese patients after open Roux-en-Y gastric bypass. Obes Surg. 2007;17(8):1102–10.
21. Rasmussen MS, Jorgensen LN, Wille-Jorgensen P. Prolonged thromboprophylaxis with low molecular weight heparin for abdominal or pelvic surgery. Cochrane Database Syst Rev. 2009;(1):CD004318.
22. Geerts WH, Bergqvist D, Pineo GF, Heit JA, Samama CM, Lassen MR, et al. Prevention of venous thromboembolism: American College of Chest Physicians Evidence-Based Clinical Practice Guidelines (8th Edition). Chest. 2008;133(6 Suppl):381S–453.

23. Huo MH, Muntz J. Extended thromboprophylaxis with low-molecular-weight heparins after hospital discharge in high-risk surgical and medical patients: a review. Clin Ther. 2009;31(6):1129–41.
24. Borkgren-Okonek MJ, Hart RW, Pantano JE, Rantis Jr PC, Guske PJ, Kane Jr JM, et al. Enoxaparin thromboprophylaxis in gastric bypass patients: extended duration, dose stratification, and antifactor Xa activity. Surg Obes Relat Dis. 2008;4(5):625–31.
25. Miller AD, Smith KM. Medication and nutrient administration considerations after bariatric surgery. Am J Health Syst Pharm. 2006;63(19):1852–7.
26. Padwal R, Brocks D, Sharma AM. A systemic review of drug absorption following bariatric surgery and its theoretical implications. Obes Rev. 2010;11(1):41–50.
27. McDonnell ME, Apovian CM, Hess Jr DT. Medical management of the patient after gastric bypass surgery. In: Farraye RA, Forse RA, editors. Bariatric surgery: a primer for your medical practice. Thorafare: SLACK Inc; 2006. p. 157–81.
28. Edwards JE. Pregnancy after bariatric surgery. AWHONN Lifelines. 2005;9(5):388–93.
29. Woodward CB. Pregnancy following bariatric surgery. J Perinat Neonatal Nurs. 2004;18(4):329–40.

The Importance of a Multidisciplinary Team Approach

19

Tracy Martinez

Chapter Objectives

1. Outline the need for the multidisciplinary team approach in bariatric and metabolic surgery.
2. Explain each individual's role in the multidisciplinary team, i.e., necessary training, education, and long-term follow-up.
3. Explain the importance and goals of an effective patient support group.

Introduction

The role of the multidisciplinary team has been acknowledged as a vital component in the care of the individual affected with clinically severe obesity undergoing bariatric surgery [1–3]. The Integrated Health team approach in bariatric surgery was officially recognized in the 1991 National Institutes of Health (NIH) Consensus Development Statement and reemphasized in 2000 by both the American College of Surgeons (ACS) and the American Society for Bariatric Surgery/Society of American Gastrointestinal and Endoscopic Surgeons (ASBS/SAGES) recommendations for bariatric surgery practices. Building on this momentum, accreditation programs were developed by both the American Society for Metabolic and Bariatric Surgery (ASMBS) and ACS in order to ensure that all aspects of the multidisciplinary team are implemented to create a well-trained, safe, and effective environment for the complex medical patient in the ongoing clinical pathway of bariatric surgery.

The disease of *morbid obesity* has been described as a lifelong, chronic, multifactorial disease. The complexities of this disease commonly impact an individual physically, medically, psychologically, and economically. It affects nearly every organ system in the human body [4]. The consequences of these considerations are staggering. Bariatric surgery has been around since the early 1950s. Currently, bariatric surgery remains the only proven treatment for sustained resolution of weight loss and related health conditions [5]. Surgery is always most effective when the patient is in the care of a skilled surgeon and a well-trained and committed multidisciplinary team who are prepared to care for the patient acutely and long term.

Obesity and morbid obesity rates continue to rise with enormous economic consequences in the United States and worldwide health-care spending. In 2008, US medical costs associated with these diseases were estimated at 147 billion [6]. In 2010, type II diabetes mellitus (T2DM) alone cost an estimated 376 billion dollars worldwide, with as many as 23 % of patients also suffering from morbid obesity [7]. The sobering statistics of the growing epidemic of morbid obesity, metabolic disorders, and escalating health-care economic stress [8] reinforces the importance of delivering effective, quality, safe, and comprehensive care to the surgical bariatric patient. In-depth knowledge in the multidisciplinary delivery of care is required for optimal clinical outcomes [9].

Building the Team

When assembling a bariatric multidisciplinary team, it is important that those who choose to work in this specialty are committed to clinical competence as well as compassion (Fig. 19.1). Individuals who suffer from this disease commonly present with significant complex medical comorbidities [7]. Although the goal is to medically optimize their health state, it is not uncommon that these patients are still very ill even while being transported to the operating room. Therefore a heightened awareness of the need for astute assessment skills is important. Equally important, each team member must be sensitive to the bias endured by this patient population.

T. Martinez, RN, BSN, CBN (✉)
Wittgrove Bariatric Center, La Jolla,
9834 Genessee Ave, Suite 328, La Jolla, CA 90237, USA
e-mail: TMartinezRN@lapbypass.com

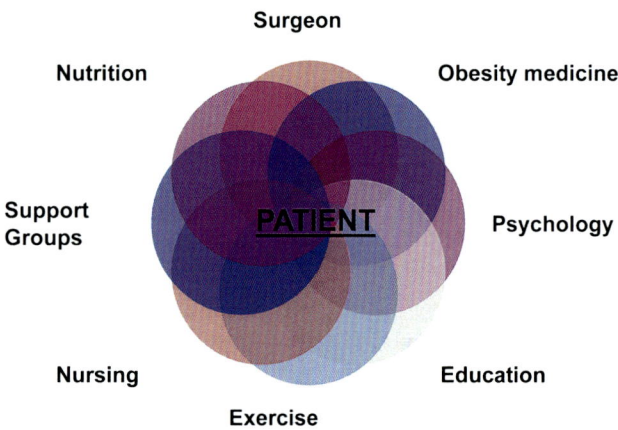

Fig. 19.1 The Integrated Health team approach combines a spectrum of disciplines to support the short- and long-term health goals of bariatric surgery patients. The multidisciplinary approach has been recognized by the National Institutes of Health (*NIH*), the American College of Surgeons (*ACS*), and the American Society for Bariatric Surgery/Society of American Gastrointestinal and Endoscopic Surgeons (*ASBS/SAGES*)

It appears that societal prejudice forms very early in human development [10]. This bias leads to patients often having endured a lifetime of discrimination. Alarmingly, the healthcare field is not immune to conveying their own bias toward those who suffer with morbid obesity. A study of nursing attitudes toward an individual with obesity reported that nurses believed that the obese person most likely had issues with anger and were lazy and overindulgent [11]. Simple supportive behavior such as a caring touch on the arm, direct eye contact, and conveying a nonjudgmental attitude can make tremendous difference in the patient's comfort and hospital experience.

Specialized Nursing

Perioperative nursing care following bariatric and metabolic surgery entails diligent, prudent, and specific assessment skills. The numerous comorbidities associated with severe obesity significantly increase the risk for postoperative complications [12]. Because of the complexity of this disease, it is imperative that the clinical nursing staff is educated and sufficiently trained to care for this patient population. This clinical competence includes psychological support, astute clinical assessment, complication recognition, and physical safety and comfort.

The nurse must possess in-depth knowledge of potential complications and the training and experience to quickly recognize and effectively manage these complications [13]. Often, the signs and symptoms of emergent complications can be quite subtle, yet even brief delays in perceptive assessment and intervention may well lead to the demise of the surgical patient [14]. The clinic nurse must possess a broad base of knowledge for safe and optimal short- and long-term outcomes. The importance of the diverse roles fulfilled by specialized nurses in achieving a comprehensive continuum of care was recognized in 2007 when the ASMBS initiated the Certified Bariatric Nurse (CBN) examination [15]. To date there are more than 1,100 certified bariatric nurses.

Registered Dietitian

The role of the specialized registered dietitian is invaluable [16]. Preoperative comprehensive nutritional assessment is extremely helpful in implementing a nutritional plan of care based on evidence-based nutrition guidelines specific to bariatric and metabolic surgery. Postoperative nutrition education should begin preoperatively. Nutrition assessment and ongoing dietary surveillance have been shown to be an important correlate with success [17]. Postoperatively, rapid weight loss commonly occurs. It is essential that the patient consumes adequate protein to protect lean muscle mass and augment thermogenesis during this phase [18]. All patients undergoing bariatric and metabolic surgery are at risk of vitamin and mineral deficiencies [19]. Therefore, ongoing nutritional assessment and specific biochemical monitoring is important to help prevent surgery-specific vitamin and mineral deficiencies. Appropriate supplementation counseling and advice is essential [20]. Lifestyle changes including disciplined and mindful eating is essential for long-term weight maintenance. The specialized registered dietician can be a great educator in this important behavioral adherence.

Behavioral Health Specialist

Behavioral health specialists fulfill a critical role in promoting successful bariatric surgery outcomes. The preoperative assessment provides a means by which the team can evaluate the patient's cognitive understanding, affective status, and relational behaviors. This allows a more objective determination of the patient's readiness for surgery and it gives insight as to possible barriers to postoperative success [21]. If specific postoperative psychological disorders are identified such as eating disorders, substance abuse, and body image challenges, a specific and focused therapeutic environment is valuable. Additionally, the behavioral health specialist can provide individual, family, and group support. This is a great asset not only to the patient but to the team as well.

Exercise Specialist

Increasing evidence supports the role of habitual physical activity (PA) in optimizing bariatric surgery outcomes [22, 23]. However, research employing objective PA assessments indicates that a vast majority of patients do not engage in habitual PA and are highly sedentary preoperatively [24, 25]. Many patients have barriers to regular exercise including hesitation to exercise in public places, frustration with recommended exercises, and musculoskeletal problems that hinder mobility and activity. Physical activity is recommended postoperatively for improving general health, weight loss, and weight loss maintenance. Given considerable difficulties that patients face in adopting and/or maintaining habitual PA [26], there is a clear role for the exercise specialist to deliver appropriate counseling, training, and support in the context of a multidisciplinary surgical treatment program aimed at achieving long-term weight loss, resolution of comorbidities, and improved health-related quality of life [27].

Obesity Medicine

Currently, the specialty of obesity medicine physicians is relatively small; however, the awareness of the need is growing [28]. This specialty brings a comprehensive understanding of the treatment of obesity, incorporating genetic [29], environmental, social, and behavioral factors of obesity [30]. An obesity medicine specialist can make a significant impact in the preoperative and postoperative care of the patient. Their role in medical readiness for surgery and postoperative surveillance of comorbidities is beneficial [31].

The Team

It is widely recognized that the integrated team is vital to the management and success of the bariatric patient. Both early and long-term follow-up is imperative for optimal outcomes and safety. Unfortunately, there still remains a high prevalence of bias, stigmas, and misconceptions about severe obesity within health professionals [32]. Research strongly supports this fact [33]. Therefore, it makes sense that those taking care of this patient population have empathy, understanding, and a desire to work in this field.

Working together as a dedicated team that is patient-focused can enhance patients' short- and long-term outcomes while improving quality, reducing costs, and improving efficiency [34]. Program policies and procedures as well as clinical pathways will maintain consistency of care and clarity to both the patient and team members of the preoperative and postoperative continuum care plan. All team members should adhere to a unified patient clinical pathway. Clinical pathways should be designed by the team to ensure best practice, optimal patient outcomes, and decreased legal liability [13, 35].

Clinical excellence and working collaboratively should be the core requirement for each team member.

Long-term patient follow-up results in better patient outcomes. Therefore, the program should have an infrastructure to support comprehensive, collaborative longitudinal care following bariatric surgery.

Regularly scheduled team meetings will encourage collaboration, communication, quality improvement, and program development. Early on as a new program gets started, team meetings can keep individuals accountable for the development of the program. This includes everything from equipment needs, education requirements, staff development, policy and procedure implementation, and patient education protocols.

Bariatric team meetings should include professionals who represent disciplines and departments that the patient normally interacts with during their operative experience. These members often include: medical director, program director or coordinator, clinical unit manager, behavioral health, nutritionist or registered dietician, exercise coordinator, administration representative, quality assurance coordinator, and a nursing educator.

The benefit of regularly scheduled team meetings in a mature program is to allow a timely and efficient response when issues arise. Ongoing team meetings must encourage evaluation of current program practices, protocols, pathways, and policies and assess a need for change if necessary. Quality improvement should be based on both the individual program outcome data and published studies.

Always keep the team focused on patient satisfaction, patient safety, and optimal outcomes. Ongoing quality assessment and improvement will help identify real or potential risks and implement a plan to minimize risk and adverse outcomes.

Detailed minutes with a list of agreed upon action items and assigned responsibility for follow-up will promote ongoing positive development and momentum of the program.

Staff Development and Education

Surgeons performing bariatric and metabolic surgery today are expected to have specific surgical training. It is also true that each multidisciplinary team professional achieves the same. Each team member must be specifically trained to support the patient pre-, peri-, and postoperatively.

Currently, there are no certification programs for team members other than nursing (CBN). However, this will most likely evolve in time. The current expectation, both publically and professionally, is that each of the integrated team members acquires in-depth expertise beyond their basic professional education requirements prior to caring for this clinically challenging patient population. All team members are obliged to understand and be fully competent in their scope of practice. Equally important is understanding and conveying, within each team member specialty, the essential causative factors that contribute to a patient's optimal outcome. Possessing in-depth knowledge of the disease of morbid obesity and surgical intervention, clinical assessment skills, lab surveillance, competence in both long-term and short-term complication recognition, and compassion will help the patient through a safe surgical intervention and beyond.

Beginning in the late 1980s, the Joint Commission on Accreditation of Healthcare Organizations (JCAHO) mandated that staff be assessed for competency. The components of competency include three critical domains. These domains are "cognitive skills," which means the ability to analyze and utilize critical thinking; psychomotor skills that demonstrate the ability to perform physical tasks necessary to do the job—in other words "technical skills"; and lastly "interpersonal skills," which demonstrate the ability to work as an integral part of an interdisciplinary team.

Implementing Nursing Competencies

Competencies are a relatively new program that hospitals have initiated to demonstrate the knowledge, skills, and attitudes considered by the organization to be essential to do the job of a bariatric nurse. Competency assessment is the process of understanding an individual's potential knowledge and skills. Competency assignment is a process that continually verifies the individual's ability to perform and apply his or her knowledge and skills [36]. Currently, more hospitals who perform bariatric surgery are implementing bariatric nursing competencies. Competencies for bariatric nurses should address the unique knowledge base that a bariatric nurse should possess. These include:
- In-depth knowledge of the disease of morbid obesity
- Comorbidities and how they may increase the risk of complications
- In-depth anatomical changes following the bariatric procedures performed at their specific institution
- Symptoms of complications (both the obvious and subtle)
- Nutritional support and guidelines
- Long-term expected results and complications
- Last, but not least, empathy awareness

There is not one way to assess competency. Testing methods can vary. These include true/false test questions, multiple choice questions, and case studies with priority action questions.

Patient Education

The goal of each team member should be their commitment to utilize their expertise within their discipline to optimize patient outcomes. This goal is achieved through patient selection and preoperative preparation and astute clinical assessment preoperatively and in long-term postoperative follow-up. The patient must also play an active role in this process.

Educating bariatric surgical patients is the obligation of the multidisciplinary staff. The purpose of education is to maximize the patient's success potential while decreasing stress from lack of knowledge. Patient education should be a mandatory component of all bariatric programs. Many practitioners in the field describe bariatric surgery as a "tool." Teaching the patient to use his or her "tool" adequately to his or her best advantage is the professional obligation of the multidisciplinary team. Education is a team effort. Each member of the team should be dedicated to convey his or her expertise to the bariatric patient. Each patient needs to understand that morbid obesity is a chronic disease, one for which we have no cure. It is equally important that the patient has a clear understanding that lifelong treatment and lifelong follow-up are required. Assuming the patient has no surgical complication, technical or otherwise, the patient's success or failure depends on his or her acceptance of surgery as a tool. Learning to utilize the tool appropriately can help them change their relationship with food, exercise, and improving overall health. Severe obesity is a chronic disease. Unfortunately there is no cure today. Like any chronic disease, lifelong attention and ongoing effort is imperative to keep morbid obesity under control with weight loss and weight maintenance. Therefore, lifelong commitment should be the responsibility of the patient and the program's multidisciplinary team. Preoperative consultation and informed consent should include the patient's responsibilities and obligations. Lifelong follow-up and education, including support group attendance, should be verbalized well in advance of the patient's surgery.

Education begins with the first patient contact. This could be a consultation or patient information session. All team members should standardize education objectives and document that it has been done. An education policy and procedure manual can ensure accuracy and consistency. Education can be conducted one-on-one or in a group setting. Often group classes can be more stimulating for the patient as they interact with others as well as efficient for the staff. Individuals all learn and retain information differently. Therefore visual (PowerPoint), verbal (classroom lecture), and written (patient education manual) should be considered to meet the vast majority of the individual's unique

Table 19.1 Bariatric surgical patients' education checklist

Preoperative education
    All aspects of procedure-specific informed consent (risks, benefits, alternatives, outcomes)
    Pre-op diet (liver reduction)
    Bowel preparation (if ordered)
    Admitting pre-op processes, IV access, premedication, Foley catheter, head cover, gown
    Pain management
    Transfer to OR/waking up in PACU
    Any routine drains
    Introduction of fluids and diet progression
    DVT prevention—anticoagulants, compression devices, early ambulation
    Incentive spirometer demonstration
    Procedure-specific diet supplementation and protein requirements, dietary advancement stages
    Any routine postoperative tests—upper GI series, for example
    Follow-up requirements
Discharge education
    Dietary advancement guidelines
    Any medication to be restarted or held
    Necessary monitoring—blood sugars, blood pressure
    Importance of ambulation—DVT precautions/preventions
    Wound observation/care
    Need to call surgeon—temperature, increased pain, abnormal wound discharge, vomiting, shortness of breath
    Contact number for concerns or emergency
    Follow-up appointments
Postoperative education
    Anatomical surgical changes
    Dietary advancement by month
    Protein requirements and importance of muscle mass protection
    Procedure-specific vitamin supplementation
    Importance of exercise for long-term success
    Importance of hydration
    Specific instructions based on procedure—NSAIDS, alcohol intake, contraception, smoking
    Required blood surveillance
    Importance of support group and long-term follow-up

IV intravenous, *OR* operating room, *PACU* postanesthesia care unit, *DVT* deep vein thrombosis, *GI* gastrointestinal, *NSAIDs* nonsteroidal anti-inflammatory drugs

learning capabilities. It is essential that patients not only understand what to do but also understand why it is important (Table 19.1).

For example, a patient must understand that after undergoing gastric bypass, B12 supplementation is required for life. They must also be educated that noncompliance with B12 supplementation can lead to neuropathy that may be permanent. Therefore, lifetime lab surveillance is necessary (ASMBS nutritional guidelines). Empowering the patient through education also encourages self-responsibility.

Support Group

One of the many misunderstandings about those who suffer from the disease of morbid obesity is that they have an excessive percentage of psychological illness. On the contrary, studies of severely overweight persons conducted before seeking treatment have shown that there is no single personality type that characterizes the severely obese [37]. Often society shows the ignorant belief that if a patient ate less and exercised more, then they could control their weight. In other words, patients "choose" to be obese. The fact is that morbid obesity is a multifactorial disease, but a strong genetic predisposition contributes to an individual's clinically severe obesity. Nonsurgical weight management does not demonstrate sustained weight loss long-term in those suffering from severe obesity [38]. Twin studies show that two-thirds of the variation in body weight can be attributed to genetic factors [39].

The psychological aspects due to the bias of this disease are as important as the more publicized major medical comorbid conditions when one considers the quality of life of the severely obese [40].

Successful support groups should provide ongoing education and support for this unique peer group. In addition, most importantly, support group meetings should create a safe and empathetic environment to help individuals through their journey. If your support group is created with this in mind, your patients will be more likely to return and successfully continue along their postoperative path while maximizing their own success potential.

The Purpose of a Support Group

Patients who attend a support group regularly have better postoperative success [41]. There are numerous reasons why support groups are conducted in bariatric programs. One is to educate the prospective patient on the postoperative lifestyle as they interact with postoperative patients. The preoperative patient who attends a support group prior to surgery may have a significant advantage because they are in a less stressful environment to absorb information. They gain knowledge at a more leisurely pace than a postoperative patient who may be in the "buyer's remorse" state of mind (that some patients experience immediately postoperatively). Seeing, interacting, and listening to actual patients who have already undergone bariatric surgery may diminish anxiety for the pre-op patient. Having patients attend support groups preoperatively is another aspect of the numerous ways in which informed consent may be provided. This is in addition to the traditional consultation and written informed consent. For this reason, some programs make attendance mandatory for the preoperative patient. Secondarily, many patients with severe obesity present to the program with a sense of shame and guilt from years of failed dieting. Many individuals have damaged self-esteem as well as limited friends. It is not uncommon for this population to put their needs on hold—commonly doing for others to gain acceptance while neglecting their own requirements. A successful support group should provide an environment of understanding of these common traits: demonstrating empathy for the patients in today's society and creating an environment that facilitates a sense of belonging, therefore reducing stress and enhancing self-image. This environment can facilitate learning if the patient feels understood and comfortable.

Education is an extremely important goal of a support group. As previously mentioned, many practitioners in the field of bariatrics call bariatric surgery a "tool": teaching the patient to utilize their "tool" to maximize their individual postoperative success. This is achieved best in a compassionate environment. The educational opportunities offered in a support group gives patients the knowledge they need to take ownership of their decision to have surgery to treat their obesity and enables them to take ownership of their necessary lifestyle changes. Being immersed in a group of peers with common life struggles, with the chronic disease of morbid obesity, creates an environment of knowledge, empowerment, and self-responsibility. All of these are necessary for long-term success.

Thirdly, educational needs change from the acute postoperative patient (0–12 months) to the more advanced patient of 12 months or longer.

Commonly seen needs of the acute patient are food advancement and intolerances and the importance of protein intake and vitamin supplementation. Other educational needs include mobility and the role of exercise (in particular resistance training for prevention of muscle mass loss), body image challenges, hair loss, and criticism from others for the decision to have surgery. Commonly, patients express a fear that surgery will not be successful, having failed at every other attempt at weight loss.

After approximately 1 year after bariatric surgery, education and support needs change. Because of the distinct difference in needs of the acute patient versus the over 1 year patient, one might consider having two separate support group meetings (0–12 months and over 12 months) in order to meet the needs of the patients in the two postoperative phases. The vast concerns and issues previously mentioned demonstrate the value in the multidisciplinary approach in a support group.

Another goal of a support group is to facilitate a social environment. As discussed earlier, numerous patients have isolated themselves from society. Many patients have limited friends, dating is less common, and there is research documenting employment discriminations as well as reduced acceptance to major colleges [42]. A successful support group can, for the first time in a patient's life, create a feeling of belonging and acceptance, as well as a sense of not being alone. The burden of failure and shame is lightened, therefore, creating an environment that potentiates self-confidence and self-worth.

Another purpose for a support group is for the long-term postoperative patient to get "back on track." As mentioned numerous times, there is no known cure for the chronic disease of morbid obesity. Sometimes postoperative patients feel bulletproof for 1, 2, and even 3 years, only to rediscover that surgery really is only a powerful tool. When a patient returns to the program with the chief complaint of weight gain, it is important to reemphasize the postoperative guidelines of nutrition, vitamin supplementation, and the role of exercise and education. All of which should be achieved in a support group. Encouraging these patients to return to a support group can be very effective at helping them lose their regained weight and reestablish the importance of ongoing follow-up. The patient must accept the fact that maintaining weight loss is an ongoing, lifetime commitment and effort. Patients should be congratulated on taking responsibility for reaching out for the necessary support. The program should provide the opportunity to get them back on track in the continuum of care pathway.

The facilitator plays a crucial role in support group success. Thoughtful selection of the group facilitator is imperative. It is essential that the facilitator be a well-trained professional who represents the surgeon and the program with a unified mission, in other words, an arm of the program. The leader should have training or experience in group facilitation and be capable of creating a constant format for the meeting—providing a compassionate and empathetic environment that enables the patient to feel comfortable. The leader should be knowledgeable of and aim for the program's goals and mission statement. The group facilitator can be successfully fulfilled by a variety of professionals within the program's multidisciplinary team. The psychologist, registered nurse, registered dietician, and surgeon can be equally successful and effective. However, they should possess basic characteristics of a qualified group facilitator.

The Four Phases

There are some common characteristics observed in bariatric patients, in my experience. The support group facilitator should have some insight into these phases in order to best understand the group dynamics. I break them up into four phases commonly exhibited in various stages from the preoperative period and years after surgery:

1. *The "Hope Phase"*
   This phase consists of patients who decided to have surgery and are preparing for it. They are extremely optimistic and are commonly full of questions for the group participants. They are, often for the first time in their life, surrounded by a group of individuals who understand their plight, sense of guilt, defeat, and hopelessness. The veterans in the group will eagerly share their experiences and give advice and encouragement. It is important the facilitator not allow the patient to monopolize the meeting, allowing others to speak and voice their questions, concerns, and opinions. Sometimes the patient has a knowledge deficit. This is when it would be appropriate to encourage that patient to attend an informal seminar or consult in order to gain basic knowledge about surgery. It is important for preoperative patients to have the opportunity to interact with postoperative patients as part of the in-depth and multifaceted consent.

2. *The "Honeymoon Phase"*
   This phase often occurs in month 1 through 12 following bariatric surgery. This is the time when patients often, for the first time, experience a sense of satiety. Commonly, depending on the type of procedure performed, patients may even experience minimal to no hunger. The scale continues to move downward, often with little effort on the patient's part. You will hear words like "unbelievable" and "it's a miracle." Reinforcement that this sensation is commonly experienced early on following surgery is important. In addition, stressing that compliance with the program guidelines including nutrition, supplementation and physical exercise is imperative. Equally important is stressing that lifestyle changes are imperative for long-term control of severe obesity and resolved related medical conditions.

3. *The "Reality Phase"*
   This occurs between the sixth and eighth month. One of the most common and fearful experiences shared by patients in this phase is when active hunger returns and dietary consumption increases. Patients often fear that their "tool" is not going to work for them. They can obsess about every food eaten, often weighing themselves several times a day. Commonly, this group of patients requires reassurance that their sensations have been experienced by others. It is appropriate to assure the patient that this is common. Postoperative patients will add their experiences of going through this phase as well. Any symptoms of maladaptive behavior in this phase, or at any time, may need further investigation and treatment. Depending on the symptoms exhibited, further evaluation with the appropriate team member may be needed, including the surgeon, obesity medicine physician, program nurse, registered dietician, or behavioral health specialist.

4. *The "Maintenance Phase"*
   The last phase commonly occurs from the twelfth month on. This phase I call the "maintenance phase." Although there is often a decline in support group attendance in this patient population, support group meetings are extremely beneficial for several reasons. They continually remind and reinforce the idea that surgery is a "tool" not a cure, and therefore constant and consistent lifestyle changes are needed for weight maintenance. This is the key for success. Often patients want to be "normal" and want to distance themselves from the memory of having had bariatric surgery at all. This attitude can be dangerous because weight gain as well as vitamin deficiencies can occur with noncompliance. For this reason, reinforcement of long-term follow-up and support group attendance should be taught and reinforced both preoperatively and postoperatively by a dedicated multidisciplinary, integrated team. This phase is when the patient learns they are not "bulletproof" and that surgery is not the "magic pill" that it seemed to be in the first months after surgery. Offering a multidisciplinary approach in a support group will help patients maintain a healthy lifestyle emotionally, as well as medically. The reinforcement that they need to assume self-responsibility is beneficial. Directing patients to the appropriate discipline, within the program, can be extremely helpful when a specific need is

Table 19.2 Special equipment needs for providers of bariatric surgery

Clinic/office/admitting areas
Wide doorways (48 in. in width or >)[a]
Wide wheelchair accessible[a]
Wide, weight-safe seating (30 in. in width or >)[a]
Scales to 500 lb
Large gowns
Large blood pressure cuffs
Weight-safe exam tables
Floor-mounted toilet seats with guardrails

Bariatric unit
Bariatric beds (appropriate weight limit, width)
Large gowns
Large sequential compression devices
Large blood pressure cuffs
Weight-appropriate transfer devices
Floor-mounted toilet seats with guardrails
Wide wheelchairs and walkers
Wide shower stalls and shower chairs

Operating room
Dedicated bariatric trays
Dedicated special needs intubation cart
Weight-bearing OR tables
Large monitor blood pressure cuffs

[a]Source: Facility Guidelines Institute 2010 (FGI), American Institute of Architects (AIA)

identified. This period can be extremely complex because patients have undergone a dramatic transformation medically, physically, and emotionally. Resolution of comorbidities are shared and celebrated. Relationships and body image challenges are commonly presented.

Bariatric surgical patients go through dramatic transformations both physically, medically, and emotionally. Often the program support groups are the only interaction available to individuals to discuss the disease and lifestyle changes preoperatively, as well as the unique experiences postoperatively. Support groups should be considered a priority in all bariatric programs.

Equipment and Environment Considerations

If you can imagine yourself 100 lb heavier than you are, the environment most likely would look very intimidating, uninviting, and quite frightening. Many of our patients have, all too often, had to worry about their size preventing them from sitting in a chair, fitting through a narrow doorway, or fitting in a patient gown. Hospitals performing bariatric surgery should anticipate the patients' needs long before the first case is scheduled. Any institution providing this specialty should provide all the special equipment and other needs for patients seeking treatment (Table 19.2). Walking the same pathway a patient would, from admission through discharge, highlights vulnerable, unsafe areas. Prudent programs will continually check to make sure the appropriate equipment, with manufacturer's specifications of weight limitations, is offered in all relevant departments.

Conclusion

The significance of an integrated multidisciplinary team in bariatric and metabolic surgery is well accepted throughout the United States and beyond. Being part of this team can be immensely challenging but rewarding. Individuals with severe obesity commonly present with a myriad of medical, physical, nutritional, and psychological complexities. In-depth knowledge and expertise is imperative for optimal outcomes. Treating each patient with competence, safety, and compassion should be the main objective for each provider. The team should be well coordinated and committed to clinical excellence from the initial consultation through long-term engagement and follow-up.

Question and Answer Section

Questions

1. The role of the integrated team is imperative for optimal short- and long-term outcomes. All of the following requirements are necessary for each team member except:
   A. Clinical expertise and excellence
   B. Ability to work collaboratively
   C. Specialized certification as a specialist in their discipline
   D. Dedicated to providing long-term follow-up
2. Which of the following statements are true regarding surgical complications following bariatric surgery?
   A. Signs and symptoms of life-threatening complications can be subtle.
   B. Assessing for complications following a bariatric operation is like any other abdominal surgical assessment.
   C. Life-threatening surgical complications can happen post-op days 1–3 only.
   D. Delay in recognition of a serious complication is a common cause contributing to malpractice lawsuits.

Answers

1. Answer **C**. Specialized training and competency is an expectation for each team member caring for the bariatric and metabolic surgical patient. To date, only obesity

medicine and registered nurses (CBN) have a certification in the field of bariatric, metabolic, and obesity medicine.
2. Answers **A** and **D**. Surgical complications can occur in even the most experienced surgeon's hands. Therefore, it is important to continuously monitor the patient's vital signs, urine output, pain scale, and lab results. However, aggravation of associated comorbidities can mask classic signs and symptoms, resulting in more subtle symptom presentation. Serious complications typically occur within days after surgery, but it is important for the patient and family to be educated on signs and symptoms that can occur weeks following discharge. Research has shown that a common reason for a lawsuit is not because of a surgical complication but a delay in recognition and treatment of the complication.

References

1. American College of Surgeons. Continuing quality improvement. Bariatric Surgery Center Network Program. http://www.facs.org/cqi/bscn/index.html. Accessed 2009.
2. Gastrointestinal Surgery for Severe Obesity.NIH consensus statement online, 25–27 Mar 1991. http://www.ncbi.nlm.nih.gov/books/bv.fcg?rid=hstat4.chapter.9282. 1991.
3. American Society for Bariatric Surgery, Society for American Gastrointestinal Endoscopic Surgeons. Guidelines for laparoscopic and open surgical treatment for morbid obesity. Obes Surg. 2000;10:378–9.
4. Sugerrman H. Pathophysiology of severe obesity. Surg Obes Relat Dis. 2005;1(2):109–19.
5. Kendrick M, Clark M, et al. Multidisciplinary team in a bariatric surgery program. In: Buchwald H, Cowan G, editors. Surgical management of obesity. Philadelphia: Saunders/Elsevier; 2007.
6. CDC.gov/obesity/data/adult.html. Accessed 2012.
7. Hofso D, Jennsen T, et al. Fasting plasma glucose in the screening of type II diabetes in morbid obese subjects. Obes Surg. 2010;20:302–7.
8. Finkelstein E, Trogdon JG, et al. Annual medical spending attributable to obesity: Payor-and service-specific estimates. Health Aff. 2009;28(5):w822–31.
9. Lehman Center Weight Loss Surgery Expert Panel. Commonwealth of Massachusetts Betsy Lehman center for patient safety and medical error reduction expert panel on weight loss surgery; executive report. Obes Res. 2005;13:205–26.
10. Al Z, Zoon CK, Klein HW, et al. Psychiatric aspects of childhood and adolescent obesity: a review of the past 10 years. J Am Acad Child Adolesc Psychiatry. 2004;43(2):134–50, 151–3.
11. Maronet D, Golub S. Nurses attitudes toward obese persons and certain ethnic groups. Percept Mot Skills. 1992;75:387–91.
12. De Maria EJ, Portenier D, et al. Obesity surgery mortality risk score: proposal for a clinically useful score to predict mortality risk in patients undergoing gastric bypass. Surg Obes Relat Dis. 2007;3:134–40.
13. Cottam D, Lord J, et al. Medicolegal analysis of 100 malpractice claims against bariatric surgeons. Surg Obes Relat Dis. 2007;3(1):60–6.
14. Livingston E. Complications of bariatric surgery. Surg Clin N Am. 2005;85:853–68.
15. Berger N, Callahan J, et al. Path to bariatric nurse certification: the practice analysis. Surg Obes Relat Dis. 2010;6(4):399–407.
16. Kushner R, Neff L. Bariatric surgery: a key role for registered dieticians. Jour Diet Assoc. 2010;110(4):524–6.
17. Aills L, Blankenship J, et al. Bariatric nutrition: suggestions for the surgical weight loss patient. Surg Obes Relat Dis. 2008;4:S73–108.
18. Krieger JW, Sitrens HS, et al. Effects of variation in protein and carbohydrate intake on body mass and composition during energy restriction: meta-regression. Am J Clin Nutr. 2006;83:260–74.
19. Zielegler O, Sirveaux MA, et al. Metical follow up after bariatric surgery: nutritional and drug issues general recommendation for prevention and treatment of nutritional deficiencies. Diabetes Metab. 2009;35:544–57.
20. Sarwer DB, Wadden TA, et al. Pre operative eating behavior, post operative dietary adherence, and weight loss after gastric bypass surgery. Surg Obes Relat Dis. 2008;4(5):640–6.
21. Wadden TA, Sarwer DB. Psychological and behavioral status of patients undergoing bariatric surgery; what to expect after surgery. Med Clin North Am. 2007;91(3):451–69.
22. Jacobe D, Ciangura C, et al. Physical activity and weight loss following bariatric surgery. Obes Rev. 2011;12:366–77.
23. King WC, Bond DS. The importance of preoperative and post operative physical activity counseling in bariatric surgery. Exerc Sport Sci Rev. 2013;41:26–35.
24. Bond DS, Jakicic JM, et al. Objective quantification of physical activity in bariatric surgery candidates and normal weight controls. Surg Obes Relat Dis. 2010;6:72–8.
25. Bond DS, Thomas JG, et al. Self reported and objectively measured sedentary behaviors in bariatric surgery candidates. Surg Obes Relat Dis. 2013;9:123–8.
26. McMahon MM, Sarr M, et al. Clinical management after bariatric surgery: value of a multidisciplinary approach. Mayo Clin Proc. 2006;81(10 suppl):s34–45.
27. Bond D, Phelan S, et al. Becoming physically active after bariatric surgery is associated with improved weight loss and health- related quality of life. Obesity. 2009;17(1):78–83.
28. Presutti RJ, Gorman RS. Primary care perspective on bariatric surgery. Mayo Clin Proc. 2004;79(9):1158–66.
29. Bell C, Walley AJ, et al. The genetics of human obesity. Genetics. 2005;6:221–34.
30. Cdc.gov/obesity/adult/causes/index.html. Accessed Jan 2013.
31. Still C. Before and after surgery: the team approach to management. J Fam Prac. 2005.
32. My P, Tarrant M. Obesity: attitudes of undergraduate student nurses and registered nurses. J Clin Nurs. 2009;18(16):2355–65.
33. Schwartz M, Chammbliss H, et al. Weight bias among healthcare professionals specializing in obesity. Obes Res. 2003;11:1033–77.
34. Funnell M. The organization of multidisciplinary care team: modeling internal and external influences on care quality. J Nat Cancer Ins Monog. 2010;2010(40):72–80.
35. Kaufman A, McNelis J, et al. Bariatric surgery claims- a medicolegal perspective. Obes Surg. 2006;16:1555–58.
36. D'Alfonso J. Designing competencies that count. Denver: Certified Boards Inc.; 2004.
37. Ryden A, Sullivan M. Severe obesity and personality: a comparative controlled study of personality traits. Int J Obes Relat Metab Disord. 2003;27(12):1534–40.
38. Klein S. Medical management of obesity. Surg Clin N Am. 2001;81:1025–38.
39. Stunkard AJ, Froch TT, et al. A twin study on human obesity. JAMA. 1986;265:51–4.
40. Latner JD, Stunkard AJ, et al. Stigmatized students: age, sex, and ethnicity effects in stigmatization of obesity. Obes Res. 2005;13:1226–31.
41. Song Z, Reinhardt K, et al. Association between support group attendance and weight loss after Roux-en-Y gastric bypass. Surg Obes Relat Dis. 2008;4:100–3.
42. Brownell KD, Puhl R, Schwartz MB, Rudd L, editors. Weight bias: nature, consequences, and remedies. New York: Guilford Publications; 2005.

Genomic and Clinical Predictors Associated with Long-Term Success After Bariatric Surgery

Glenn S. Gerhard and G. Craig Wood

Chapter Objectives

1. Discuss the known variables, clinical and biological, that are associated with differential weight loss outcomes following Roux-en-Y gastric bypass (RYGB) surgery.

Introduction

Obesity, commonly defined as a body mass index (BMI) greater than 30 kg/m^2, is associated with an increased risk for a number of metabolic derangements including type 2 diabetes mellitus (T2DM), hypertension, dyslipidemia, as well as cardiovascular disease and overall mortality. Class 3 obesity (BMI >40 kg/m^2), which afflicts a growing segment of the US population, further increases disease burden and risk of mortality. Weight loss is effective at decreasing these risks, as well as ameliorating disease severity; thus, reducing body weight in the morbidly obese is a major clinical goal. Currently available dietary and pharmacological modalities can produce small to moderate levels of weight loss, which can have significant impact on comorbidities, but are difficult to achieve or sustain in many patients. Bariatric surgery has thus emerged as a highly effective therapy for long-term weight loss in morbidly obese patients, and more recently as a surgical therapy for the potential cure of type 2 diabetes. However, the degree of weight loss and improvement in specific comorbid conditions is variable. The clinical, biological, and genetic determinants of surgical weight loss in the morbidly obese are thus not well defined.

This scenario is further complicated by the clinical options available to patients and the definition of weight loss success. Thresholds for defining successful weight loss following bariatric surgery range from 40 to 70 % of excess body weight lost, with some degree of long-term weight regain occurring in many patients. The main classes of surgical procedures currently in general use, including the two most commonly performed operations, the Roux-en-Y gastric bypass (RYGB) and laparoscopic adjustable gastric banding (LAGB), also continue to evolve. Roux-en-Y gastric bypass creates a small gastric pouch to restrict the size of the stomach to cause early satiety, as well as a bypass of the proximal small intestine to decrease nutrient absorption. This procedure in the morbidly obese usually induces about 65–70 % excess body weight loss (EBWL), although weight loss plateaus at 1–2 years, often with some regain, and a subgroup of patients remain resistant to weight loss. Gastric banding creates a pouch and a small stoma using a band high on the stomach. It is the least invasive and the safest, but also the least effective bariatric procedure, with weight loss at about 50 % of EBWL commonly followed by some regain. Analysis of variables associated with weight loss following these procedures has shown little consistency; thus, long-term sustained weight loss may depend upon as yet unidentified factors [1]. The purpose of this chapter is to discuss the known variables, clinical and biological, that are associated with differential weight loss outcomes following Roux-en-Y gastric bypass surgery.

Published Clinical Predictors

A systematic review of preoperative predictors of weight loss following bariatric surgery analyzed a large number of previously published studies (between 1988 and April 2010) in which one or more clinical variables were associated with either greater postoperative weight loss, no appreciable

---

G.S. Gerhard, MD (✉)
Institute for Personalized Medicine, Pennsylvania State University,
College of Medicine, 500 University Drive,
Hershey, PA 17033, USA
e-mail: ggerhard@hmc.psu.edu

G.C. Wood, MS
Geisinger Health System, Geisinger Obesity Institute,
100 North Academy Ave., Danville, PA 17822, USA
e-mail: cwood@geisinger.edu

effect on postoperative weight loss, or less postoperative weight loss regarded as a poorer outcome [2]. The variables analyzed for association with postoperative weight loss were preoperative BMI, preoperative weight loss, and the presence of eating disorders or related psychiatric disorders including substance abuse. A total of 115 studies were found in which data on variables with potential association with weight loss following bariatric surgery were reported. Suggestive evidence was found for preoperative BMI (negative association), preoperative weight loss (positive association), and personality disorders (negative association). Patients with maladaptive personality disorders are generally excluded from many bariatric surgery programs so are not discussed here. Unclear or no evidence was found to support previous weight loss attempts, binge eating, sweet eating, hunger, other maladaptive eating habits, emotional eating, depression, anxiety, sexual abuse, self-esteem, alcohol use/abuse, or other psychiatric disorders, which are also not discussed.

Preoperative BMI

A number of studies have reported that preoperative BMI was significantly associated with less weight loss generally using multivariate regression approaches. This is reflected in a meta-analysis in which the majority of studies reported a negative association with postoperative weight loss with follow-up times that ranged from 6 to 144 months [2]. Studies that reported a negative association were more likely to be based on RYGB in contrast to LAGB procedures, with the reverse the case for studies that reported no or a positive association studies. The majority of studies reporting a negative or no association calculated weight loss outcomes via %EWL and not in absolute terms of pounds or BMI units, while most studies that found a positive association used absolute weight loss as the outcome, usually as BMI units or kilograms lost.

The studies generally reported follow-up times between 1 and 2 years and a variety of outcome measures such as an odds ratio of poorer %EBWL below a certain threshold at a certain postoperative time, expressing %EBWL as a continuous variable at a specific postoperative time point, and dichotomizing patients into good and poor outcome groups based on various thresholds of %EBWL (e.g., $\geq 60\%$). Based on these studies, preoperative BMI is perhaps the clinical variable most widely and strongly reported to be associated with postoperative weight loss, especially for studies on RYGB that report %EBWL.

Interestingly, more than 30 studies reported on just under 14,000 patients with a preoperative BMI >50 kg/m^2, defined as "super-obesity." Pooling data for meta-analysis from more than ten of these studies on more than 3,000 patients with a mean follow-up time of 30 months found that the super-obese group lost significantly less %EWL postoperatively compared to the non-super-obese. However, a subgroup meta-analysis of only those studies reporting on RYGB (i.e., excluding the lap band and other bariatric procedures) found no significant association.

The degree and direction of the association of preoperative BMI with postoperative weight loss depends upon how weight loss is measured. If a relative measure is used, such as %EBWL or percent excess BMI, then higher preoperative BMI has been found to be associated with poorer weight loss outcomes. i.e., less postoperative weight loss. This is the case for most studies reported thus far. If an absolute outcome measure is used, such as change in body weight (pounds) or BMI units, then the higher the initial BMI the greater the weight loss. This makes sense since the heavier the person, the more weight there is to lose. The %EBWL as the measure of postoperative weight loss has been recommended as the standard metric [3], despite the fact that %EBWL is a relative measure that diminishes the significance of the absolute amount of weight lost, i.e., two patients who have lost the same number of pounds will have different %EBWL depending upon their initial BMIs. While the absolute amount of weight lost may be an important factor in the degree of improvement in a variety of comorbid conditions, BMI is directly correlated with health risks, thus the lower the BMI, the less the risk. In addition, the strength of the association of higher initial BMI to weight loss over an extended follow-up period is not known. The disparity between %EBWL and other weight loss measures may be magnified by the length of postoperative follow-up; the relatively short lengths of follow-up (i.e., 12 months) of many studies may not allow sufficient time for patients with higher BMIs to shed sufficient number of pounds to reach their weight nadir. The short length of follow-up may also explain that although larger patients have more absolute weight to lose, they would have to lose their weight at a faster rate than lighter patients in order to achieve the same percent of excess body weight lost. Ideally, studies should have sufficient length of follow-up to allow all patients to reach their weight loss nadirs.

Another factor that has not yet been fully explored, but suggested by some data, is that the poorer weight loss outcomes in patients with higher initial BMIs may be due to distinct biological characteristics of these patients. The higher initial BMI may be due to a more severe underlying biological mechanism underlying the severe obesity that may be resistant to the strong effects of bariatric surgical interventions. Initial BMI is also a generally crude predictor since many patients with such severe obesity do very well after bariatric surgery. More research is needed to define what variables are associated with poor weight loss outcomes in patients with higher BMIs.

Preoperative Weight Loss

Modest preoperative weight loss has been used to minimize the effects of obesity-related comorbid disease on the perioperative complications and outcomes related to bariatric surgery. For example, a preoperative low-calorie diet appears to decrease liver size, presumably by depleting liver triglycerides and/or glycogen. The smaller liver increases visualization of the surgical region, which decreases the complexity and length of the procedure. Two systematic review articles have evaluated the effect of preoperative weight loss on bariatric surgery outcomes [2, 4]. The results of each are discussed below.

Preoperative weight loss as an outcome was reported in 14 studies comprising more than 3,000 patients who had undergone preoperative weight loss [2]. The most common preoperative weight loss goals were either between 5 and 10 % or >10 % EBWL. About half of the studies found a positive correlation between preoperative and postoperative weight loss, although not surprisingly there was a large variation in the length of follow-up and the amount of postoperative weight loss reported across the studies. Most reported at least 12 months of follow-up with about 50–75 % EBWL at 12 months.

Another systematic analysis evaluated the effect of preoperative weight loss using data from 27 published studies from more than 6,000 patients on postoperative weight loss, operative time, length of stay, and/or complication rates [4]. The association with postoperative weight loss was reported in 24 of the 27 studies, with nine reporting significant improvement in postoperative weight loss. In five studies of laparoscopic RYGB patients, the operative time was 12.5 min shorter in patients with preoperative weight loss. The mean length of stay of RYGB patients was found to be 0.64 day shorter in those with preoperative weight loss. Finally, of 11 studies reporting on perioperative complications, two concluded a positive association with preoperative weight loss. However, regardless of the outcome under evaluation, the methods used to quantify preoperative and postoperative weight loss varied, the amount of follow-up time ranged from 3 months to 3 years, and the procedure types varied, further complicating the interpretation of these results.

Preoperative weight loss effects are difficult to compare across studies because of the wide variation in weight loss approaches. For example, in some programs formal nutrition consults are made, low-calorie and/or liquid diets are used, and the degree to which ongoing behavioral support and exercise and nutritional counseling are provided can vary substantially. The interpretation of such results is also problematic. Preoperative weight loss may merely be a surrogate for increased postoperative compliance and/or indicate greater motivation to lose weight.

Other Clinical Variables

Most studies of preoperative clinical variables associated with postoperative weight loss have analyzed only one or a few of many potential variables, often in relatively small cohorts of patients, from up to 20 variables in up to 300 patients [2, 5]. Such studies have also reported on relatively short lengths of follow-up, usually 12 months. Few studies have analyzed more than 1,000 patients longer than 2 years following RYGB. One used mixed linear modeling up to 36 months on 1,168 patients to assess associations with gender, anastomotic technique, age, race, initial weight, height, and institution—with gender and initial weight as the two variables associated with weight loss [6]. Three other studies analyzed more than 300 RYGB patients and evaluated the association between a range of preoperative clinical characteristics with postoperative weight loss [7–9]. Presence of diabetes was significantly associated with less postoperative weight loss for each of these studies. Other items that were associated with less weight loss in at least one of these three studies included older age, male gender, higher body weight, larger pouch size, and higher BMI.

Geisinger RYGB Predictors Project

We have been working to identify the clinical, biological, and genetic predictors of weight loss outcomes following RYGB surgery [10–16]. To do so, we have converted the Bariatric Surgery Program at the Geisinger Center for Nutrition and Weight Management into a research-based clinic. All patients undergo a standardized program during which data collected for clinical care is obtained for research. Consent has been obtained from more than 3,000 patients since initiating the study in late 2004. The average age is ~47 years, the average BMI is ~50 kg/m^2, about 80 % are female, and ~97 % are Caucasian. Exclusions for the program include active substance abuse, psychiatric disorders including borderline personality disorder, schizophrenia, active severe depression, binge-type eating disorder, and defined noncompliance.

RYGB Program

Most of the clinical data collected were obtained as part of standard of care during the preoperative and postoperative program. These include careful and standardized ascertainment of medical history and current medications, a variety of laboratory tests, questionnaires, intraoperative liver biopsy, and questionnaire/survey data. Research items collected in addition to these standard of care items include additional

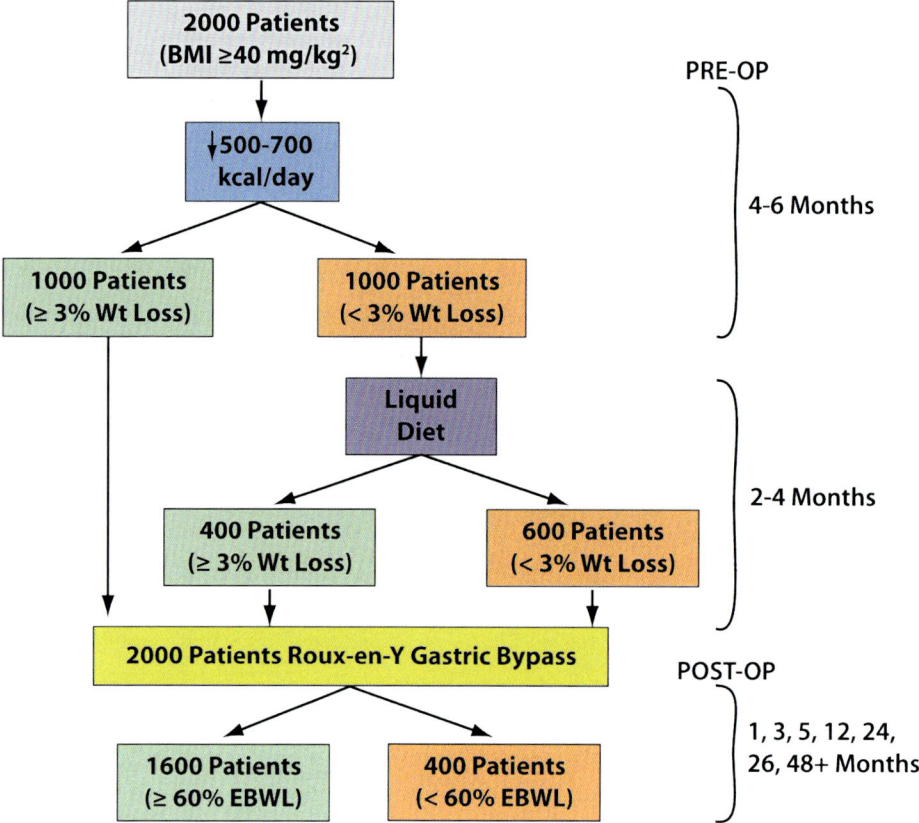

Fig. 20.1 Schema of preoperative and postoperative weight loss program with approximate numbers of patients based on a population of 2000

blood sample for DNA isolation; serum samples for biomarker studies; and liver, fat, and intestinal tissue obtained intraoperatively. All of the extensive clinical data, such as weight measurement and physical findings, comorbidities, medical history, laboratory measures, behavioral and social surveys, and medication use, were extracted from the electronic health record and entered in a research database. The clinical program has been optimized, with much attention paid to maintaining the highest quality of care, to obtain clinical data with research grade quality requirements in mind.

Our multidisciplinary bariatric surgery program instituted the recommendation of a preoperative weight loss goal as a requirement for undergoing RYGB surgery since the inception of the program in 2001. The hypocaloric dietary intervention has been designed to produce a weight loss of at least 3 % with a target of 10 % without the use of a weight loss medication (Fig. 20.1). Patients were placed on a diet with a 500–700 kcal deficit with support that includes individual and group sessions with monthly meetings and sessions of nutrition and physical activity education and social support for 4 months. Clinical staff run the meetings and follow the patients. Patients' specific comorbidities and general health care were also managed during the preoperative program. In this program, a large percentage of patients can and do lose a meaningful amount of weight in the preoperative period. For example, fewer than 10 % of the patients gained more than 5 % excess body weight during the preoperative period, and about 10 % of the patients gained less than 5 % excess body weight, while about 15 % experienced up to 5 % EBWL, about 20 % had a 6–10 % EBWL, and about half had a greater than 10 % EBWL.

We examined whether there were differences among those who lost more preoperative weight. We stratified by %EBWL and examined the groups for differences in demographic characteristics and comorbidities. A small statistically significant but clinically insignificant difference in age was found. Initial weight and BMI were lower in the group that experienced a gain of more than 5 % excess body weight in the preoperative period. The frequency of a variety of comorbidities and the sex distribution were not significantly different among the preoperative weight loss groups.

We then used Kaplan-Meier analyses to identify a significant association between preoperative and postoperative weight loss. Patients who experienced the most %EBWL before surgery reached their weight loss goal sooner than patients who had less %EBWL, or weight gain, prior to surgery. This effect was not BMI dependent, with similar results found for a baseline preoperative BMI <50 or >50 kg/m^2. We also used Cox regression to estimate hazard ratios for

Table 20.1 Clinical factors associated with weight loss 24 months after RYGB surgery

	Difference from reference	SE	p-value
Baseline BMI			
35–39.9	32.3	2.9	<0.0001
40–49.9	17.8	2.1	<0.0001
50–59.9	3.5	2.2	<0.0001
60+	Reference		
Diabetes group			
Any diabetes medication	−4.6	1.3	0.0004
Age and surgical access			
Age <50 with laparoscopic surgery	Reference		
Age <50 with open surgery	−0.3	1.8	0.886
Age 50+ with laparoscopic surgery	−2.1	1.7	0.209
Age 50+ with open surgery	−9.7	1.8	<0.0001
Liver pathology and baseline BMI			
No fibrosis	Reference		
Any fibrosis with baseline BMI <50	−14.1	3.8	0.0003
Any fibrosis with baseline BMI 50+	−3.0	3.8	0.429
Iron deficiency			
Low serum iron (<45 men, <35 women)	−7.6	3.5	0.0330
Time from baseline visit to surgery			
>2 years	−5.3	2.7	0.045
Gender			
Male	−4.6	1.7	0.0059

achieving a desired weight loss goal of more than 70 % EBWL. The amount of preoperative EBWL was used as the primary predictor variable (controlling for age, sex, and comorbidities) and was significant in all models. Those patients who achieved more than a 10 % preoperative excess body weight loss were more than twice as likely to achieve 70 % postoperative EBWL than those patients who had a 0–5 % excess body weight loss prior to surgery. Unfortunately this association was only present for those achieving a greater than 10 % %EWL.

Statistical Modeling

We have conducted an analysis of more than 350 variables on a cohort of 1,380 patients who underwent RYGB surgery on whom 24-month weight loss data was available. The group as a whole had a 62.5 % EBWL at 24 months. The clinical variables that were associated with less than 24-month weight loss (Table 20.1) were higher baseline BMI, use of diabetes medication prior to surgery, older age and type of surgical access, fibrosis of the liver by pathology (if BMI >50 kg/m^2), iron deficiency (defined as low serum iron), long preoperative period (>2 years in program), and male gender. A male patient over the age of 50 who is diabetic and iron deficient whose BMI is greater than 60 and undergoes an open RYGB procedure can expect to achieve about half of the %EBWL than a younger nondiabetic iron-replete woman who undergoes a laparoscopic procedure. A need for clinical practice is more robust information on weight loss outcomes tailored to the specific characteristics of patients.

Genetic Factors

Based upon heritability and linkage studies, genetic variation plays a strong role in obesity and related comorbid conditions. Genome-wide association studies (GWAS) have identified single nucleotide polymorphisms (SNPs) in or near dozens of genes that are related to increased BMI and associated comorbid conditions. Few have been studied in the context of morbid obesity. In addition, the relatively small effect of these and other individual GWAS SNPs suggests that multiple SNPs may act in combination to influence disease susceptibility. To date, only a few candidate genes have been evaluated in small studies in relation to diet and surgical weight loss. We have previously analyzed weight loss [16], as well as GWAS SNPs related to obesity, diabetes, and cardiovascular disease [17, 18], in a cohort of morbidly obese patients from a comprehensive obesity research program that provides access to clinical data, DNA samples, and dietary and surgical treatment outcomes. Our approach parallels pharmacogenomic analysis of medication use in obesity and diabetes [19, 20], which we have termed "surgicogenomics" [17].

Genetics and Obesity

The regulation of body weight and energy homeostasis is subject to complex regulatory mechanisms that maintain balance between energy intake, energy expenditure, and energy stores. Genetic factors play an important role in this regulation as well as in the development of obesity as shown in studies estimating the heritability of obesity. Based on the current knowledge of the pathogenesis of obesity, the level of involvement of genetic factors in the development of obesity is estimated to be 30–70 %. The last edition of the *Human Obesity Gene Map* from October 2005 reported more than 600 loci from single-gene mutations in mouse models of obesity, non-syndromic human obesity cases due to single-gene mutations, obesity-related Mendelian disorders, loci from genome-wide scans, and genes or markers that have been shown to be associated or linked with an obesity phenotype [21].

Genetics and Weight Loss

Clinical observation documents the wide variation in the ability of obese subjects to lose weight in response to the same negative energy balance. Genetics and heritable factors appear to contribute to the ability to lose weight with potentially high levels of heritability similar to obesity [22]. For example, degree of weight loss is more similar within pairs of overweight identical twins in response to a negative energy balance than between pairs. Also paralleling studies on obesity are reports of associations between weight loss and a number of polymorphisms in candidate genes. Candidate genes that have been replicated in more than one study include LEP, LEPR, HTR, NMB, PLIN, PPARG2, ADRB2, ADRB3, UCP1, UCP2, UCP3, IL6, IRS, CYP1, COMT, PNMT, and GNB3 [22]. However, lack of homogeneity of the study groups, ethnic differences, and/or small sample sizes may contribute to the failure to replicate more broadly.

Genes and Response to Bariatric Surgery

Several candidate genes have been studied in relation to bariatric surgery. Weight loss at the 6-month follow-up after laparoscopic gastric banding was related to polymorphisms in the interleukin 6 (IL6) and uncoupling protein 2 (UCP2) genes. UCP2 SNPs were also related to weight loss outcomes following gastric banding and gastric bypass. Neither a UCP3 promoter nor a tumor necrosis factor (TNF) alpha polymorphism was related to weight loss outcomes 1 year after biliopancreatic diversion. Similarly, SNPs in GNB3 and GNAS1 were not related to weight loss following gastric banding.

Obesity GWAS SNPs

Several dozen SNPs found through GWAS have now been reported to be associated with BMI/obesity [23–27]. The insulin signaling protein type 2 (INSIG2) gene was perhaps the first obesity gene variant identified through GWAS. INSIG2 is involved with lipid and cholesterol metabolism and has been linked to obesity in rodents. In a meta-analysis of nine cohorts drawn from eight different populations and including a total of almost 17,000 individuals revealed significant independent validation of the association of the SNP with BMI, but with likely population heterogeneity. Other studies have also failed to find an association with BMI. However, studies of populations with higher BMIs tend to have positive associations [28], including our own [15].

One of the most robust GWAS SNPs initially found resides within the FTO (fat mass and obesity associated) gene. The FTO obesity SNP was first found to be associated with type 2 diabetes in a genome-wide association study that compared almost 2,000 type 2 diabetes patients and about 3,000 population controls for almost 500,000 SNPs. The FTO gene region on chromosome 16 was strongly associated with type 2 diabetes that was replicated in another large population of type 2 diabetes cases and nondiabetic controls. However, reanalysis of the data with adjustment for BMI abolished the association with type 2 diabetes, demonstrating that the diabetes-risk alleles at FTO were strongly associated with increased BMI. Independently, another SNP within the first intron of the FTO gene was also strongly associated with BMI. Meta-analysis and other studies have confirmed this strong association [27, 29]. Thus, the initial observation of association with type 2 diabetes was actually reflective of the increased BMI of the patients with diabetes relative to the lower BMIs of the nondiabetic control population.

Homozygosity for the INSIG2 obesity GWAS allele has been associated with increased weight loss [30] or no effect upon a lifestyle intervention [31] in adults, while homozygosity for both INSIG2 and FTO was found to retard weight loss in a pediatric cohort [32]. Mechanistic studies on these obesity SNPs relating to food intake, nutrient density, and physical activity have also recently been reported [33–36].

Another large-scale meta-analysis of genome-wide association data available for almost 17,000 individuals phenotyped for adult BMI based upon a European population demonstrated that a cluster of SNPs mapped nearby the coding sequence of melanocortin receptor 4 (MC4R) [26]. MC4R represents a compelling biological candidate, as rare coding mutations in the gene are a leading cause of monogenic obesity in humans.

Table 20.2 SNPs associated with weight loss 12 or 24 months after RYGB surgery

	12-month follow-up			24-month follow-up		
	N	Mean (SD)	p-value	N	Mean (SD)	p-value
INSIG2			0.21[a]			0.11[a]
Homozygous obese	110	65.4 % (21.8)		67	63.1 % (26.9)	
Heterozygous	385	68.8 % (22.7)		226	69.9 % (22.1)	
Homozygous normal	397	69.0 % (23.1)		223	69.9 % (25.9)	
FTO			0.33[a]			0.20[a]
Homozygous obese	202	66.7 % (23.0)		116	65.6 % (22.3)	
Heterozygous	432	68.6 % (22.2)		246	70.5 % (24.5)	
Homozygous normal	258	69.8 % (23.5)		154	69.2 % (26.0)	
MC4R			0.99[a]			0.78[a]
Homozygous obese	71	68.7 % (22.6)		39	70.0 % (29.6)	
Heterozygous	332	68.6 % (22.7)		187	68.0 % (23.1)	
Homozygous normal	489	68.4 % (22.9)		290	69.5 % (24.7)	
PCSK1			0.45[a]			0.73[a]
Homozygous obese	74	65.6 % (17.2)		38	66.2 % (19.4)	
Heterozygous	344	68.2 % (23.2)		200	69.7 % (24.7)	
Homozygous normal	474	69.1 % (23.3)		278	68.9 % (25.0)	
# of homozygous obese genotypes			0.065[b]			0.043[b]
0	519	69.6 % (23.3)		306	70.9 % (24.6)	
1	294	67.5 % (22.3)		163	67.3 % (24.0)	
2+	79	64.5 % (20.9)		47	63.1 % (25.2)	
# of obesity alleles			0.032[b]			0.0084[b]
0	33	74.5 % (21.1)		22	79.7 % (32.4)	
1–2	377	69.2 % (23.9)		222	69.4 % (25.0)	
3–4	400	68.0 % (22.3)		221	68.9 % (23.2)	
5+	82	64.8 % (20.4)		51	63.3 % (23.3)	

**12-month follow-up was defined as the weight occurring closest to 12 months from surgery but between 9 and 18 months postsurgery
**24-month follow-up was defined as the weight occurring closest to 24 months from surgery but between 19 and 30 months postsurgery
[a]One-way ANOVA
[b]Linear regression

Mutations in the proprotein convertase subtilisin/kexin type 1 (PCSK1) gene also cause monogenic obesity, and an SNP producing a nonsynonymous variant was associated with obesity in adults and children of European ancestry [37].

Surgicogenomics of Weight Loss

We have genotyped patients who had undergone RYGB for the INSIG2, FTO, MC4R, and PCSK1 obesity SNPs. Patients were categorized as homozygous obese if they were homozygous for the obesity risk allele for each SNP, heterozygous obese if they were carriers of the obesity risk allele, and homozygous non-obese if they were homozygous for the low-risk allele. Patients were also classified by number of homozygous SNP genotypes and by the total number of obesity risk alleles they possessed whether in the homozygous or heterozygous configuration. Approximately 10 % of the population had either two or more homozygous obesity genotypes or carried five or more obesity risk alleles.

Association with Postoperative Weight Loss

Genotype data was analyzed using weight loss data (obtained at 12 and 24 months following Roux-en-Y gastric bypass surgery) calculated as %EBWL—an estimate of fat mass used for assessing weight loss that is based upon an idealized BMI of 25 kg/m^2. Patients were stratified by genotype based upon total number of FTO, INSIG2, MC4R, and/or PCSK1 obesity SNPs they carried, thus patients had from 0 to 8 SNPs. The data was also analyzed by regrouping based on the number of homozygous SNPs carried, thus patients had from 0 to 4 homozygous genotypes. No individual SNP was statistically associated with weight loss (Table 20.2). However, an association between decreasing %EBWL at 24 months and an increasing number of obesity SNP alleles was present, which was also seen for the number of homozygous SNPs that patients carried: patients who carried at least five alleles versus those who carried four or less. Patients with five or more alleles lost significantly less weight at both 12 and 24 months following gastric bypass surgery.

We also analyzed available clinical data on comorbidities, laboratory results, medication use, and survey data to identify nongenetic factors that could account for differences between the super obese and morbidly obese. No variables with expected clinical relevance were identified.

Question and Answer Section

Questions

1. Suggestive evidence for potential association with weight loss following bariatric surgery has been found for the following variables:
   A. Previous weight loss attempts
   B. Binge eating
   C. Preoperative BMI
   D. Depression
2. Preoperative weight loss effects are difficult to compare across studies because of the wide variation in weight loss approaches.
   A. True
   B. False
3. Genes found through GWAS reported to be associated with BMI/obesity include all of the following except:
   A. MC4R (melanocortin receptor 4)
   B. TNF (tumor necrosis factor)
   C. FTO (fat mass and obesity associated)
   D. PCSK1 (proprotein convertase subtilisin/kexin type1)

Answers

1. Answer **C**. In a number of studies, preoperative BMI has been associated with less weight loss following bariatric surgery.
2. Answer **A**. True
3. Answer **B**. TNF (tumor necrosis factor)

References

1. Lanyon RI, Maxwell BM. Predictors of outcome after gastric bypass surgery. Obes Surg. 2007;17(3):321–8.
2. Livhits M, Mercado C, Yermilov I, Parikh JA, Dutson E, Mehran A, et al. Preoperative predictors of weight loss following bariatric surgery: systematic review. Obes Surg. 2012;22(1):70–89 [Research Support, Non-U.S. Gov't Review].
3. Bray GA, Bouchard C, Church TS, Cefalu WT, Greenway FL, Gupta AK, et al. Is it time to change the way we report and discuss weight loss? Obesity (Silver Spring). 2009;17(4):619–21.
4. Cassie S, Menezes C, Birch DW, Shi X, Karmali S. Effect of preoperative weight loss in bariatric surgical patients: a systematic review. Surg Obes Relat Dis. 2011;7(6):760–7 [Review].
5. Hatoum IJ, Stein HK, Merrifield BF, Kaplan LM. Capacity for physical activity predicts weight loss after roux-en-y gastric bypass. Obesity (Silver Spring). 2009;17(1):92–9 [Research Support, N.I.H., Extramural].
6. Dallal RM, Quebbemann BB, Hunt LH, Braitman LE. Analysis of weight loss after bariatric surgery using mixed-effects linear modeling. Obes Surg. 2009;19(6):732–7 [Multicenter Study].
7. Melton GB, Steele KE, Schweitzer MA, Lidor AO, Magnuson TH. Suboptimal weight loss after gastric bypass surgery: correlation of demographics, comorbidities, and insurance status with outcomes. J Gastrointest Surg. 2008;12(2):250–5.
8. Campos GM, Rabl C, Mulligan K, Posselt A, Rogers SJ, Westphalen AC, et al. Factors associated with weight loss after gastric bypass. Arch Surg. 2008;143(9):877–83; discussion 884 [Research Support, N.I.H., Extramural].
9. Ma Y, Pagoto SL, Olendzki BC, Hafner AR, Perugini RA, Mason R, et al. Predictors of weight status following laparoscopic gastric bypass. Obes Surg. 2006;16(9):1227–31.
10. Wood GC, Chu X, Manney C, Strodel W, Petrick A, Gabrielsen J, et al. An electronic health record-enabled obesity database. BMC Med Inform Decis Making. 2012;12(1):45.
11. Matzko ME, Argyropoulos G, Wood GC, Chu X, McCarter RJ, Still CD, et al. Association of ghrelin receptor promoter polymorphisms with weight loss following roux-en-y gastric bypass surgery. Obes Surg. 2012;22(5):783–90 [Research Support, N.I.H., Extramural Research Support, Non-U.S. Gov't].
12. Mirshahi UL, Still CD, Masker KK, Gerhard GS, Carey DJ, Mirshahi T. The mc4r(i251l) allele is associated with better metabolic status and more weight loss after gastric bypass surgery. J Clin Endocrinol Metab. 2011;96(12):E2088–96 [Research Support, N.I.H., Extramural Research Support, Non-U.S. Gov't].
13. Still CD, Wood GC, Chu X, Erdman R, Manney CH, Benotti PN, et al. High allelic burden of four obesity snps is associated with poorer weight loss outcomes following gastric bypass surgery. Obesity (Silver Spring). 2011;19(8):1676–83 [Research Support, Non-U.S. Gov't].
14. Benotti PN, Still CD, Wood GC, Akmal Y, King H, El Arousy H, et al. Preoperative weight loss before bariatric surgery. Arch Surg. 2009;144(12):1150–5.
15. Chu X, Erdman R, Susek M, Gerst H, Derr K, Al-Agha M, et al. Association of morbid obesity with FTO and INSIG2 allelic variants. Arch Surg. 2008;143(3):235–40; discussion 241 [Research Support, Non-U.S. Gov't].
16. Still CD, Benotti P, Wood GC, Gerhard GS, Petrick A, Reed M, et al. Outcomes of preoperative weight loss in high-risk patients undergoing gastric bypass surgery. Arch Surg. 2007;142(10):994–8; discussion 999.
17. Chu X, Erdman R, Susek M, Gerst H, Derr K, Al-Agha M, et al. Morbid obesity is associated with two obesity gene variants (FTO and INSIG2). Arch Surg. 2008;143(3):235–40; discussion 241.
18. Wood GC, Still CD, Chu X, Susek M, Erdman R, Hartman C, et al. Association of chromosome 9p21 snps with cardiovascular phenotypes in morbid obesity using electronic health record data. Genom Med. 2008;2(1–2):33–43.
19. Adamo KB, Tesson F. Genotype-specific weight loss treatment advice: how close are we? Appl Physiol Nutr Metab. 2007;32(3):351–66.
20. Gable D, Sanderson SC, Humphries SE. Genotypes, obesity and type 2 diabetes–can genetic information motivate weight loss? A review. Clin Chem Lab Med. 2007;45(3):301–8.
21. Rankinen T, Zuberi A, Chagnon YC, Weisnagel SJ, Argyropoulos G, Walts B, et al. The human obesity gene map: the 2005 update. Obesity (Silver Spring). 2006;14(4):529–644.
22. Hainer V, Zamrazilova H, Spalova J, Hainerova I, Kunesova M, Aldhoon B, et al. Role of hereditary factors in weight loss and its maintenance. Physiol Res. 2008;57 Suppl 1:S1–15.
23. Thorleifsson G, Walters GB, Gudbjartsson DF, Steinthorsdottir V, Sulem P, Helgadottir A, et al. Genome-wide association yields new

sequence variants at seven loci that associate with measures of obesity. Nat Genet. 2009;41(1):18–24.
24. Meyre D, Delplanque J, Chevre JC, Lecoeur C, Lobbens S, Gallina S, et al. Genome-wide association study for early-onset and morbid adult obesity identifies three new risk loci in european populations. Nat Genet. 2009;41(2):157–9.
25. Willer CJ, Speliotes EK, Loos RJ, Li S, Lindgren CM, Heid IM, et al. Six new loci associated with body mass index highlight a neuronal influence on body weight regulation. Nat Genet. 2009;41(1):25–34.
26. Loos RJ, Lindgren CM, Li S, Wheeler E, Zhao JH, Prokopenko I, et al. Common variants near mc4r are associated with fat mass, weight and risk of obesity. Nat Genet. 2008;40(6):768–75.
27. Scuteri A, Sanna S, Chen WM, Uda M, Albai G, Strait J, et al. Genome-wide association scan shows genetic variants in the fto gene are associated with obesity-related traits. PLoS Genet. 2007;3(7):e115.
28. Hotta K, Nakamura M, Nakata Y, Matsuo T, Kamohara S, Kotani K, et al. INSIG2 gene rs7566605 polymorphism is associated with severe obesity in japanese. J Hum Genet. 2008;53(9):857–62.
29. Saunders CL, Chiodini BD, Sham P, Lewis CM, Abkevich V, Adeyemo AA, et al. Meta-analysis of genome-wide linkage studies in BMI and obesity. Obesity (Silver Spring). 2007;15(9):2263–75.
30. Franks PW, Jablonski KA, Delahanty LM, McAteer JB, Kahn SE, Knowler WC, et al. Assessing gene-treatment interactions at the FTO and INSIG2 loci on obesity-related traits in the diabetes prevention program. Diabetologia. 2008;51(12):2214–23.
31. Lappalainen TJ, Tolppanen AM, Kolehmainen M, Schwab U, Lindstrom J, Tuomilehto J, et al. The common variant in the fto gene did not modify the effect of lifestyle changes on body weight: the finnish diabetes prevention study. Obesity (Silver Spring). 2009;17(4):832–6.
32. Reinehr T, Hinney A, Toschke AM, Hebebrand J. Aggravating effect of INSIG2 and fto on overweight reduction in a one-year lifestyle intervention. Arch Dis Child. 2009;94(12):965–7. Epub 2009 Feb 17.
33. Jonsson A, Renstrom F, Lyssenko V, Brito EC, Isomaa B, Berglund G, et al. Assessing the effect of interaction between an fto variant (rs9939609) and physical activity on obesity in 15,925 swedish and 2,511 finnish adults. Diabetologia. 2009;52(7):1334–8.
34. Jonsson A, Franks PW. Obesity, fto gene variant, and energy intake in children. N Engl J Med. 2009;360(15):1571–2; author reply 1572.
35. Johnson L, van Jaarsveld CH, Emmett PM, Rogers IS, Ness AR, Hattersley AT, et al. Dietary energy density affects fat mass in early adolescence and is not modified by fto variants. PLoS One. 2009;4(3):e4594.
36. Stutzmann F, Cauchi S, Durand E, Calvacanti-Proenca C, Pigeyre M, Hartikainen AL, et al. Common genetic variation near mc4r is associated with eating behaviour patterns in european populations. Int J Obes (Lond). 2009;33(3):373–8.
37. Benzinou M, Creemers JW, Choquet H, Lobbens S, Dina C, Durand E, et al. Common nonsynonymous variants in pcsk1 confer risk of obesity. Nat Genet. 2008;40(8):943–5.

Medical Approach to a Patient with Postoperative Weight Regain

Robert F. Kushner and Kirsten Webb

Chapter Objectives

1. Summarize the current literature regarding the weight loss efficacy of surgical weight loss procedures.
2. Review the contributing surgical, biopsychosocial, and behavioral factors associated with weight regain following bariatric surgery.
3. Present a proposed evaluation and treatment algorithm for the medical management of weight gain following bariatric surgery.

Introduction

Weight loss surgery is considered to be the most efficacious treatment for individuals with clinically severe class III obesity (body mass index [BMI] ≥ 40 kg/m^2) or with moderate class II obesity (BMI ≥ 35–39.9 kg/m^2) when accompanied by an obesity-related comorbidity. Weight loss at 2–3 years following a variety of surgical procedures varies from 20 % to 34 % of total weight depending on the procedure performed. In general, weight loss is greatest following malabsorptive procedures (biliopancreatic diversion [BPD] and biliopancreatic diversion with duodenal switch [BPDDS]) followed by restrictive-malabsorptive (Roux-en-Y gastric bypass [RYGB]) and restrictive procedures (laparoscopic adjustable gastric banding [LAGB] and laparoscopic gastric sleeve [LGS]). Similarly, significant improvement in multiple obesity-related comorbid conditions has been reported including type 2 diabetes mellitus (T2DM), hypertension, dyslipidemia, obstructive sleep apnea (OSA), and quality of life. However, long-term durability of weight loss and improvement in comorbid conditions are less certain, and weight regain has been observed. Although the causative factors of weight regain have not been well characterized, clinicians are being asked to evaluate an increasing number of patients postoperatively. This chapter will review the current information regarding weight gain following bariatric surgery and the factors associated with weight regain and will present a proposed evaluation and treatment algorithm.

Estimating the Occurrence of Weight Regain

Analyzing outcome data for bariatric surgery suffers from many limitations. In general, published data is reported from case studies and case series stemming from single surgeons or single institutions. Often, surgical techniques such as pouch size and limb length as well as the surgical procedure performed will vary over time within and between surgical centers. Furthermore, definitions used to define weight loss outcomes have not been standardized. Whereas some studies report outcomes as percent excess weight lost (%EWL), other authors use change in BMI units (kg/m^2) or loss of total body weight measured in kilograms or percentage. Body weights are also often self-reported instead of measured. Additionally, since follow-up and reporting of patient outcomes is often incomplete, selection bias may occur. Realizing these limitations, cross-sectional data estimates that significant weight regain occurs in 20–35 % of patients, depending upon the procedure performed and duration of time following surgery [1–4]. This number is likely to be an underrepresentation of actual incidence rates.

In addition to uncertain rates of weight regain, it is also unclear what how much weight (actual or percentage) is regained among post-bariatric surgical patients. The Swedish

R.F. Kushner, MD
Division of General Medicine, Department of Medicine,
Northwestern University Feinberg School of Medicine,
750 North Lake Shore Drive, Rubloff 9-976,
Chicago, IL 60611, USA
e-mail: rkushner@northwestern.edu

K. Webb, MSN, CNP, CDE
Center for Lifestyle Medicine, Northwestern Medical Faculty Foundation, 675 N St Clair, 17-250, Chicago, IL 60611, USA
e-mail: kwebb1@nmff.org

Obese Subjects (SOS) study, the largest nonrandomized intervention trial comparing weight loss outcomes in a group of more than 4,000 surgical and nonsurgical subjects, has previously reported 10-year data [5]. Surgically treated subjects underwent fixed or variable banding, vertical banded gastroplasty (VBG, a procedure that is no longer performed), or RYGB. Total body weight change was maximal after 1 year in the three surgical subgroups (RYGB, −38±7 %; VBG, −26±10 %; and banding, −21±10 %). Weight regain was reported by the second year of follow-up. For the RYGB and banding subgroups, 10-year weight change was −25±11 % and −13.2±13 %, respectively. Thus, at 10 years, subjects who underwent RYGB experienced a mean weight regain of 12 % total body weight and those who underwent fixed or variable banding regained 8 % total body weight. This translates into regaining 34 % (for RYGB) and 38 % (for banding) of the maximal lost weight at 1 year. Categorical weight regain was not reported.

Other published studies are of shorter duration and include smaller numbers of subjects. For example, Himpens et al. [6] determined the long-term efficacy of LGS among 30 consecutive patients from a single center. Whereas 3-year mean %EWL was 77.5±19.8 %, 6-year mean %EWL was 53.3±28.3 %. Thus, among this cohort, mean %EWL between years 3 and 6 decreased by 24.2 %, representing a regain of 31 % of lost EWL. In a retrospective study from Christou et al. [7] of 161 patients who underwent a RYGB and followed for more than 10 years, %EWL diminished from a mean of 89.5 % after 2.5 years to 68.1 % at 12.3 years. The mean 21.4 % change in %EWL represents a regain of one-fourth of total %EWL.

In another historical cohort study of 93 patients who underwent RYGB and completed 5 years of follow-up, mean %EWL decreased from 83.0±21.7 % at 2 years to 74.3±23.7 % at 5 years. The 8.7 % reduction in %EWL represents a 10 % regain of lost EWL [8]. However, the authors note that the variation in change of %EWL between 2 and 6 years follow-up ranged from a minimum of −88.0 % to a maximum of 29.1 %. Finally, Nguyen et al. [9] conducted a prospective randomized trial comparing RYGB ($n=111$) to gastric banding ($n=86$). At 2 years, data was available for 84.6 % of RYGB patients and 91.9 % of gastric banding patients. Follow-up rates at 4 years were available for 83.1 and 93.3 % for the two surgical procedures, respectively. In contrast to other studies, there was no significant change in mean %EWL for the two procedures between years 2 and 4. However, the standard deviations were large suggesting wide variation in outcomes.

Using a different methodical design, Kofman et al. [10] conducted an Internet survey among individuals who had undergone RYGB surgery between 3 and 10 years prior to participation in the study. Weight regain, assessed using a series of self-report questions, was defined as the difference in pounds from the lowest postsurgical weight to present weight. Of the 497 individuals who responded, 25.6 % underwent surgery 3–4 years previously, 46.1 % between 4 and 5 years, and 16.9 % between 5 and 6 years before the survey. Mean maximum EWL of 81 % was achieved at 17.9 months after surgery. Eighty-seven percent of respondents reported gaining weight from their lowest postoperative weight; 33 % gained between 10 % and <20 % and 14 % gained 20 % or more of EWL. In summary, weight regain occurs following a variety of bariatric surgery procedure. However, current studies do not allow an accurate estimation of incidence rates.

Surgical, Biopsychosocial, and Behavioral Determinants of Weight Regain

It is reasonable to presume that weight regain following bariatric surgery may result from numerous causes, due to a combination of anatomical, physiological, behavioral, and psychological factors (Table 21.1). Thus, it is useful to classify the etiology of weight regain into distinct categorizes. Although not all of the factors are amenable to treatment when the patient presents with weight regain, this functional grouping provides an appreciation of the potential causative factors.

Table 21.1 Etiological factors for weight regain following bariatric surgery

Anatomical
LAGB malfunction or mismanagement
Band or port breakage, band too lose
RYGB
Pouch enlargement
Gastrojejunal anastomosis dilation
Gastro-gastric fistula
Physiological
Hormonal adaptation
Pregnancy
Menopause
Weight-gaining medications
Smoking cessation
Endocrine disorder: Cushing's disease, severe hypothyroidism
Behavioral
Dietary
Unhealthy eating patterns, grazing, nibbling, mindless eating
Consumption of high energy foods and beverages
Loss of dumping syndrome symptoms
Loss of control over urges, binges
Reduced vigilance
Excessive alcohol intake
Physical activity
Reduced leisure time activity
Increased sedentary behaviors
Insufficient moderate- and vigorous-intensity exercise
Development of physical limitations to exercise

Surgical Procedure Failure

Each type of bariatric procedure has its own potential mechanism of surgical failure that can lead to weight gain. In restrictive procedures such as LAGB, weight loss is based on the reduction of gastric volume due to the gastric band. Dilation of the band or insufficient tightening may result in a feeling of reduced restraint, leading to the ability to consume larger volumes of food and calorie-containing beverages as compared to the first months after surgery. This is supported by observations that suggest that restrictive procedures fail if the pouch and stoma are too large. In patients who have undergone RYGB, weight regain may occur as a result of breakdown of the surgical staple line and development of a gastro-gastric fistula, or enlargement of the gastric pouch or stoma outlet. A retrospective review from a bariatric center of excellence identified patients who underwent laparoscopic revisional surgery between 2001 and 2008. Of 384 secondary bariatric operations, 151 reoperative procedures were performed for complications such as pouch enlargements, strictures, and gastro-gastric fistulas with the major morbidity (13.2 %) related to leaks [11]. Similarly, another retrospective analysis identifies the major reasons for requiring surgical revision as weight regain (40.3 %), type-specific issues (27.8 %), dysphagia/reflux (25 %), and gastro-gastric fistula (6.9 %) [12]. Patients who experience these complications are generally appropriate candidates for a surgical revision procedure.

Biological

Hormonal Adaptations

The hormonal causes of weight regain after surgically induced weight loss are not fully understood. However, investigational data from nonsurgical weight loss suggest that there is a strong selection bias in favor of regulatory systems that vigorously defend against deficits in body weight. The regulatory changes with weight loss include significant reductions in levels of leptin and the gastrointestinal hormones peptide YY, cholecystokinin, and amylin and increase in the levels of ghrelin—a hormonal change that is associated with increased hunger and urges to eat. Ghrelin, an orexigenic or "hunger" hormone, is secreted by the stomach and is known to increase before meals and then fall after meals in humans. Multiple studies have shown that ghrelin levels are reduced following RYGB, though other clinical studies are conflicting [13]. The discrepancy in these findings may be due to the complexity of the ghrelin system or to the poor sensitivity of the techniques used to assess ghrelin levels [13]. PYY is an anorexigenic signal that suppresses appetite and is secreted after food intake. Glucagon-like protein-1 (GLP-1) is released into the circulation post meal by L cells in the small intestine to stimulate insulin secretion, inhibit glucagon release, and delay gastric emptying. Both anorexigenic hormones have been shown to increase after RYGB and LSG.

Although surgical revision of the gastrointestinal tract leads to alteration of gut hormones and the resultant changes in appetite and metabolism, it is unclear whether metabolic adaptation reoccurs to defend body weight. Surgically induced changes in ghrelin, PYY, and incretin hormone levels may diminish over time. Rodent studies have demonstrated that postsurgical weight regain is associated with failure to sustain elevated plasma PYY concentrations. The use of animal models for bariatric surgery should provide further clues into the mechanisms involving the hormonal causes of postsurgical weight regain.

Pregnancy

Weight gain associated with pregnancy is dependent upon many determinants, including physiological, psychological, and behavioral factors. Observational and cohort studies have shown that excessive gestational weight gain substantially increases the risk of weight retention at 1 year and future long-term weight gain at 15–21 years postpartum [14–16]. Weight retention is particularly more evident for women who are obese prior to pregnancy. Based on the existing literature, the Institute of Medicine published revised recommendations on appropriate weight gain during pregnancy. For underweight women, the recommended total weight gain is 12.5–18 kg; for normal weight women, 11.5–16 kg; for overweight women, 7–11.5 kg; and for obese women, 5–9 kg.

Among patients who have undergone bariatric surgery, counseling about pregnancy is important as almost half of all bariatric procedures are performed on women of reproductive age. Bariatric surgery is thought to improve fertility based on normalization of sex hormones, menstrual irregularities, and improvement in polycystic ovarian syndrome. Most authorities urge patients to delay conception for at least 1 year post-bariatric surgery to minimize complications from nutritional deficiencies and optimize weight loss. Maternal weight gain after bariatric surgery has not been well studied. In one prospective study of 79 consecutive first pregnancies following LAGB, mean maternal weight gain was 9.6±9.0 kg compared to 15.5±9.0 kg among 79 obese subjects matched for parity and maternal age [17]. The incidence of postpartum weight retention was not reported. Neonatal outcomes such as incidence of stillbirths, preterm deliveries, and birth weight have been shown to be consistent with community values [17, 18]. In one retrospective study, patients who conceived during the first postoperative year ($n=104$) had comparable short-term perinatal outcomes compared with patients who conceived after the first postoperative year ($n=385$) [18]. No significant differences were noted regarding hypertensive disorders, diabetes mellitus, or bariatric complications.

Menopause

The years surrounding menopause are associated with weight gain. Wing and colleagues [19] were among the first to observe this pattern in the Healthy Women's Study, a longitudinal investigation of biobehavioral factors during menopause in a cohort of 541 healthy and initially premenopausal women. Data published after the first 3 years of this study showed that the women gained on average 2.25 kg and about 20 % of subjects gained 4.5 kg [19]. Body composition studies demonstrate an increase in total body fat and visceral adipose tissue [20]. Change in weight and body fat is primarily due to decreased energy expenditure and physical activity along with loss of estrogen. Menopausal weight gain is associated with development of hyperlipidemia, hypertension, and insulin resistance. Literature on menopausal weight gain in patients who have undergone bariatric procedures is limited. However, it can be postulated that the same factors that contribute to weight gain in a nonsurgical menopausal woman can also affect a postsurgical menopausal patient.

Weight-Gaining Medications

It is well documented that many types of medications are associated with weight gain; these include antipsychotics, mood stabilizers, antidepressants, antidiabetics, and glucocorticoids. The degree of medication-induced weight gain varies by medication. Prescribed psychotropics may cause 2–17 kg of weight gain over the course of clinical treatment. In an analysis of four prospective trials of glucocorticoids in rheumatoid arthritis, the use of 5–10 mg/day of prednisone over 2 years was associated with an increase of mean body weight of 4–8 % [21]. Medication-induced weight gain can occur in individuals who have undergone bariatric procedures. However, currently there are no studies that have identified the effects of weight-gaining medications in this population.

Smoking Cessation

Tobacco use is a noteworthy health behavior to assess in bariatric candidates. One study found that 67 % of bariatric surgery candidates have a lifetime history of smoking and 27 % are current smokers [22]. Since current guidelines recommend smoking cessation at least 8 weeks prior to bariatric surgery, the effect of cigarette smoking on body weight may be an important factor. Longitudinal cohort data of 1,885 smokers from national surveys showed that mean weight gain after cessation of smoking was 2.8 kg in men and 3.8 kg in women; 9.8 % of men and 13.4 % of women gained more than 13 kg [23]. In the Lung Health Study of 5,887 smokers followed over 5 years, 33 % of sustained quitters gained ≥10 kg [24]. The etiology of weight gain is thought to be attributed to a reduction in energy expenditure and increased caloric intake. Smoking and smoking cessations rates have not been well characterized in the post-bariatric surgical population.

Medical Problems

As with any patient, individuals who have undergone bariatric procedures can develop medical conditions that are associated with weight gain. Although uncommon, medical causes of weight gain include Cushing's syndrome, acquired hypothalamic obesity syndromes, and myxedema from hypothyroidism. In a single-center study of 783 consecutive patients who were evaluated for endocrine disorders before bariatric surgery, Cushing's syndrome was diagnosed in six patients and ACTH-dependent hypercortisolism in an additional five [25]. A thorough clinical examination and biochemical work-up along with a heightened suspicion is necessary for diagnosis. Diagnosis of Cushing's syndrome can be challenging since obesity and hypercortisolism share many clinical features: central obesity, facial plethora, dorsocervical hump, and violaceous stria.

Musculoskeletal Disability

Obesity is associated with many health concerns, including impairments in physical function and mobility. Arthritis is the leading cause of disability among older adults in the United States owing to the increasing rates of obesity. Decreased physical activity related to arthritis is common, as evidenced by the 2007–2009 National Health Interview Survey in which 42.4 % of respondents reported activity limitations caused by arthritis [26]. The three most frequently found functional limitations among people with arthritis are bending or stooping, standing, and walking. These limitations can lead to decreased activities of daily living, which increase the risk of a sedentary lifestyle and weight gain. There is currently limited literature evaluating the role that bariatric surgery has on hip and knee osteoarthritis. No randomized controlled trials have been conducted assessing the impact that weight loss surgery has on hip and knee osteoarthritis. However, from the limited studies available, the general trend is that significant weight loss following bariatric surgery improves pain and function [27].

It is well established that participating in regular physical activity improves weight loss outcomes and is required to maximize postoperative results. When advising increased physical activity, real and perceived barriers to exercise should be individually evaluated and addressed. Staying mindful of possible orthopedic limitations, initial physical activity goals must be within the patient's tolerance.

Psychosocial

Several psychosocial characteristics have been proposed as risk factors for weight regain after bariatric surgery; these include depression, increased stress from changing life events, and disordered eating patterns. The presence of such factors may hamper long-term success.

Depression

Multiple studies have identified the relationship between obesity and depression as complex; raising the question of whether the causal pathway is bidirectional or reciprocal. The 10-year follow-up of the SOS study showed high rates of depression in both the surgically treated and conventionally treated groups and found that greater weight loss was associated with a greater reduction of depressive symptoms [28]. Other studies have shown an inverse relationship between the Beck Depression Inventory (BDI) score, a validated metric of depression, and the management of surgically mediated weight loss [29, 30]. Currently, no randomized controlled trials have been conducted on the long-term effects of bariatric surgery and depression. Therefore, the association between depression and weight changes following bariatric surgery is not completely understood.

Coping response to stressful life events can affect weight loss outcomes. A review of the literature by Elfhag et al. reveals factors associated with weight regain. These include poor coping strategies, psychosocial stressors, and eating in response to negative emotions and stress [31]. Personal crises such as bereavement, major illnesses, or even busy schedules can often lead to unhealthy coping mechanisms such as emotional eating. This habit can lead to the use of eating to regulate mood [31].

Disordered Eating

Two abnormal eating patterns have been described in obese patients: binge eating disorder (BED) and night eating syndrome (NES). Binge eating disorder was designated as an eating disorder in the fifth edition of Diagnostic and Statistical Manual of Mental Disorders (DSM-5) and is defined as the consumption of large quantities of food during a short amount of time (within any two-hour period) without being in control of this behavior. BED involves regular episodes of excessive, uncontrolled overeating and is strongly associated with psychological distress. Night eating syndrome is characterized by a circadian delay in the pattern of eating, defined by the main criteria of evening hyperphagia (i.e., the consumption of ≥ 25 % of the total daily caloric intake after the evening meal) and/or ≥ 2 nocturnal ingestions per week.

The prevalence rates at which bariatric candidates are affected by binge eating vary widely in the current literature. For example, de Zwaan et al. [32] used the Eating Disorder Examination Questionnaire, an instrument based on a structured interview widely considered the reference standard for the assessment of eating pathology. The authors found that 15 % of RYGB candidates met the diagnostic criteria for BED and 24 % reported features of the disorder but did not meet the full diagnostic criteria. In another study, Allison et al. [33] observed that <5 % of patients met the full diagnostic criteria for BED. Binge eating may be related to smaller weight loss or weight regain within the first two postoperative years [30]. However, this finding has not been reported consistently.

It has been established that patients who engaged in night eating preoperatively may continue this behavior postoperatively. This habit may be attributable to stretching of the gastric pouch, allowing for increased energy intake over time. Latner et al. found that more frequent nocturnal eating postoperatively was associated with a greater body mass index (BMI) and less satisfaction with bariatric surgery [34]. Much like binge eating, the prevalence of NES among bariatric candidates varies within the available literature. Regardless of the conflicting prevalence reports, the act of night eating presents a challenge to patients' compliance with the recommended postoperative diet and behavioral recommendations.

Behavioral

Weight loss surgery is commonly described as a tool to help patients lose and maintain weight loss. The surgical intervention imposes changes in dietary behavior that result in reduced caloric intake. At the same time, patients are counseled to increase physical activity and engage in programmed and structured exercise. Continued adherence to these recommendations is necessary for success.

Diet

Dietary caloric intake is reduced immediately following surgery due to a smaller gastric capacity, diminished hunger, and increased satiety brought about by altered gut hormones (discussed previously). The presence of dumping syndrome may also lead patients to reduce their intake of concentrated sweets and fatty foods to avoid associated postprandial symptoms, such as abdominal cramping, nausea, diarrhea, light-headedness, sweating, and tachycardia. In fact, over 60 % of patients report avoiding sweets and nearly 30 % avoid fatty foods after gastric bypass surgery [35]. Other food intolerances may occur as well. As a result, patients who have had RYGB may consume fewer fatty foods and sweets. However, over time, caloric intake is less restrained. In the SOS study, mean daily intakes of 2,900, 1,500, 1,700, 1,800, 1,900, and 2,000 kcal/day, respectively, were reported at baseline and 6 months, 12 months, 2 years, 3 years, and 4–10 years after surgery. These increases in caloric intake likely contribute to weight regain, which often begins in the second postoperative year [5]. These data suggest that some bariatric surgical patients have difficulties adhering to the postoperative diet.

Grazing, defined as the consumption of smaller amounts of food over extended periods of time, has been identified as a common high-risk eating pattern after bariatric surgery. Studies have shown that both preoperative and postoperative grazing behaviors independently predict poorer postsurgical weight loss [36]. In addition, dietary noncompliance, meaning the selection of high-calorie foods and beverages, can also add to higher calorie intake and weight regain. A recent postoperative behavioral survey identified a positive correlation of the magnitude of weight regain with dietary noncompliance which included consuming large quantities of food in the evening or night, eating large quantities of high-fat foods, and eating out more frequently [37]. These studies confirm the importance of diet quality and calorie control in any therapy for obesity.

Alcohol Use

Limited studies have looked at alcohol use disorder (AUD) before and after bariatric surgery. Suzuki et al. found that individuals undergoing bariatric surgery were found to have a prevalence of AUD comparable to the general population but that those with a lifetime history of AUD may be at an increased risk for elapsing after surgery, specifically after the RYGB [38]. No associations were found between weight loss following surgery and the development of AUD [38]. In another study, King et al. found a significantly higher prevalence of AUD in the second postoperative year overall and, specifically after RYGB, compared with the years immediately before and following surgery [39]. Future studies are needed to clarify if and how postoperative weight loss is related to alcohol use.

Physical Activity

Numerous studies suggest that self-reported levels of physical activity increase significantly after bariatric surgery [40, 41]. However, there is little objective data regarding changes in physical activity levels in the postoperative period. In one study, patients reported a large increase in moderate- to vigorous-intensity activity after surgery, but accelerometer data suggested that such an increase did not actually occur in most individuals [42]. In fact, data suggest that only 10–24 % of post-bariatric surgery patients meet national guidelines regarding minimal physical activity levels for general health promotion (i.e., ≥150 min/week or moderate-to-vigorous physical activity in bouts of 10 min or more) [43]. Data from the National Weight Control Registry indicate that patients who have lost weight through bariatric surgery tend to be less physically active than individuals who have lost similar amounts of weight through nonsurgical approaches [42].

In addition to hormonal changes, energy expenditure with weight loss is disproportionately reduced, largely attributable to increased skeletal muscle work efficiency and reduced physical activity. Due to these underlying adaptive physiological factors and the behavioral challenges of balancing caloric intake and expenditure, weight loss maintenance is difficult.

Support/Follow-Up

Obesity is a chronic, progressive disease that requires continual follow-up. The need for regular follow-up was demonstrated in the Weight Loss Maintenance Trial. In this randomized controlled trial of subjects who lost >4 kg in the initial weight loss phase, individuals were randomized to 1 of 3 interventions: (1) self-directed control group, (2) personal contact intervention that provided brief monthly or face-to-face contact, and (3) interactive technology intervention. All three groups were able to maintain some of the weight they lost, however, those who received personalized contact maintained significantly greater weight loss compared with the other two treatment groups at 24 and 30 months [44].

Despite the significant weight loss achieved through bariatric surgery, close follow-up is also recommended postoperatively to promote continued weight loss and/or maintenance. According to the AACE/TOS/ASMBS guidelines (2009), follow-up visits are recommended within 2 weeks after surgery, at 6 months, at 12 months postoperatively, and then annually. These postoperative visits are used to monitor patient's weight loss as well as counsel patients on issues related to dietary and exercise adherence. Even though regular postoperative follow-up is advised, clinical reports have suggested that follow-up is often suboptimal and can negatively affect weight loss. A recent study showed only 40 % of patients returned for each of their first 4 annual follow-up visits with the surgeon. Those who returned for all of their annual follow-up visits lost significantly more weight than did those who did not return [45]. This data suggests that lack of follow-up may be a determinant of weight regain after bariatric surgery.

Clinical Approach to Evaluating and Managing Postoperative Weight Regain

As discussed in the preceding section, the etiology of weight regain may have multiple determinants. Thus, patients should undergo a comprehensive evaluation to assess all potential causative factors. A proposed evaluation algorithm for assessment and treatment of postoperative weight gain is shown in Fig. 21.1. Several predictors of weight regain have been identified in selective studies. However, due to differences in methodology, patient populations studied, and

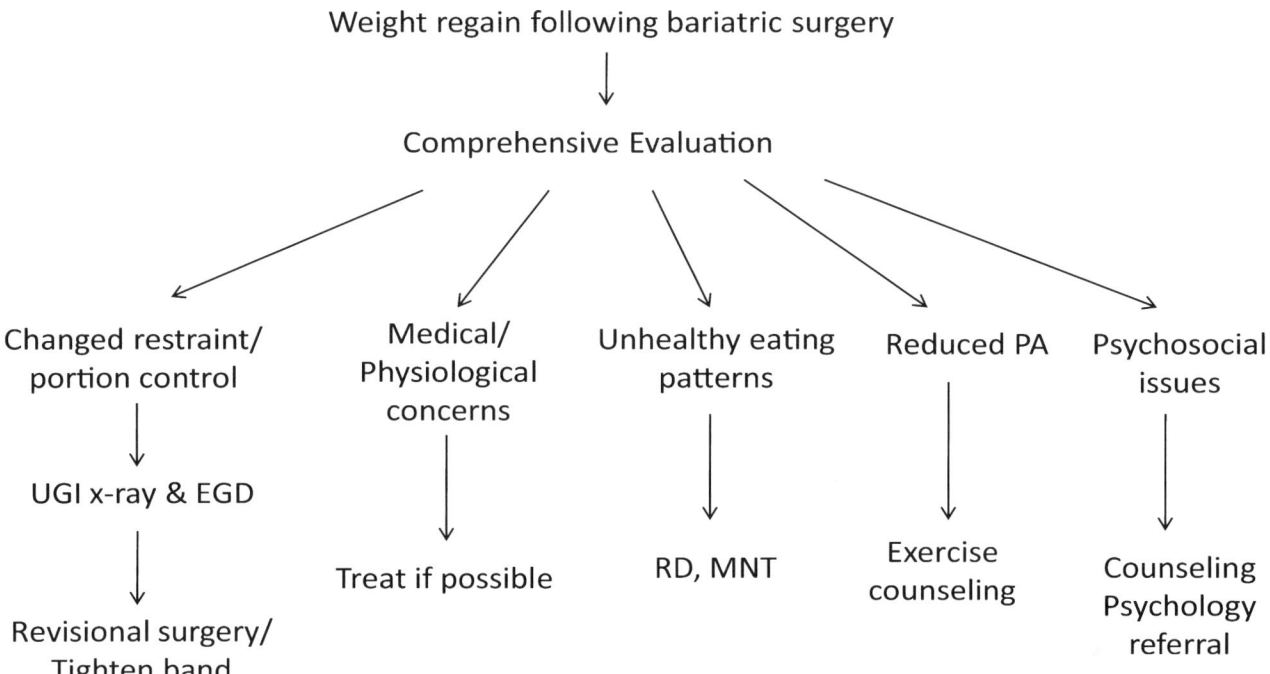

Fig. 21.1 Evaluation and treatment pathway for weight regain following bariatric surgery. *RD* registered dietitian, *MNT* medical nutrition therapy, *PA* physical activity

length and completion of follow-up, the predictive variables differ among publications. For example, Odom et al. [29] surveyed 203 patients (24.8 % response rate) from a single center after a mean follow-up of 28.1±18.9 months after RYGB. Seventy-nine percent of patients reported weight regain; 15 % regained ≥15 % of total weight lost, which they considered "significant weight regain." Independent predictors of significant weight regain were lack of control of food urges (odds ratio [OR]=5.1), concerns over alcohol or drug use (OR=12.74), lowest self-reported well-being scores (OR=21.5), and no follow-up visits (OR=2.60). In another survey of 497 patients who previously underwent RYGB after a mean of 4.2 years, participants who regained >10 % EWL reported significantly higher frequencies of binge eating, grazing, and loss of control [10]. Freire et al. [46] conducted a cross-sectional study among 100 patients who underwent open RYGB after a mean of 45.5±32.6 months. The incidence of weight regain was 69.7 % and 84.7 % at 2 and 5 years postsurgery, respectively (weight regain calculated as the increase from the lowest weight reported at any time after surgery). Factors associated with weight regain were poor diet quality, lack of physical exercise, and poor nutritional counseling [46]. Although the studies reviewed provide an indication of factors that have been associated with weight regain following bariatric surgery, we believe that a more comprehensive approach is indicated.

Anatomical Factors

Patients presenting with loss of restraint or reduced restriction of food volume may require an evaluation of the surgical procedure. An upper GI X-ray is a reasonable first step to assess pouch enlargement, anastomotic dilation, or formation of a gastro-gastric fistula among patients who underwent RYGB and for inadequate band restriction for patients who had LAGB performed. Depending on initial results, an esophagogastroduodenoscopy (EGD) will provide a more accurate delineation of the anatomy and intraluminal measurements. Subject to other biopsychosocial factors discussed below, patients can be considered as candidates to undergo a surgical revisional procedure.

Medical and Physiological Considerations

Patients identified to have an endocrinologic disorder, such as Cushing's syndrome or hypothyroidism, should be medically treated. However, the most common treatable medical reason for weight gain is prescription of weight-gaining medications. Therefore, all patients should have a thorough medication history reviewed. If possible, weight-gaining medications should be substituted for either

Table 21.2 Drugs that produce weight gain and alternatives

Category	Drugs that cause weight gain	Possible alternatives
Neuroleptics	Thioridazine; olanzapine; quetiapine; risperidone; clozapine	Molindone; haloperidol; ziprasidone
Antidepressants		
Tricyclics	Amitriptyline; nortriptyline	Protriptyline
Monoamine oxidase	Imipramine; phenelzine	Bupropion; nefazodone
Inhibitors	Mirtazapine	
Selective serotonin	Paroxetine	Fluoxetine; sertraline
Reuptake inhibitors		
Anticonvulsants	Valproate; carbamazepine; gabapentin	Topiramate; lamotrigine; zonisamide
Antidiabetic drugs	Insulin	Acarbose
	Sulfonylureas	Miglitol; metformin; orlistat
	Thiazolidinediones	DPP-4 inhibitors; GLP-1 analogs; SGLT-2 inhibitors
Anti-serotonin	Pizotifen	
Antihistamines	Cyproheptadine	Inhalers; decongestants
β (beta) adrenergic blockers	Propranolol	ACE inhibitors; calcium channel blockers
α (alpha) adrenergic blockers	Terazosin	
Steroid hormones	Contraceptives	Barrier methods
	Glucocorticoids	Nonsteroidal antiinflammatory agents
	Progestational steroids	

weight-neutral or weight-losing medications. A list of medications by disease category and effect on body weight is shown in Table 21.2. Substitutions will often need to be coordinated with the patient's other healthcare providers, particularly for the psychotropic medications.

Behavioral Factors

Among all of the determinants of weight regain, recidivism of behavioral patterns or developments of new maladaptive patterns are the most common. All patients should undergo a comprehensive dietary, physical activity, and behavioral and psychological assessment. Depending on clinic staffing and patient needs, the evaluations can be performed by a physician, registered nurse, nurse practitioner, physician assistant, registered dietitian (RD), and a mental healthcare professional. Diet can be assessed by either a 24-h dietary recall or food frequency with particular attention to total caloric intake, meal and snack patterns, presence of grazing or nibbling, binging behavior, and consumption of high-calorie foods and beverages. Physical activity is assessed by time spent in daily activities, sedentary time, and frequency, intensity, and duration of any planned exercise. Mental health is assessed for presence of stressors, affective disorders, substance abuse, and coping response. Concerns identified in any of these categories should be directly treated.

Physical Activity

Physical activity has been a focus among multiple investigators. In epidemiologic studies of postoperative patients, increased self-reported physical activity has been repeatedly associated with improved weight loss, mood, and psychosocial functioning [40, 43]. Similarly, in a cross-sectional study, which used armband accelerometers to measure activity in patients who had undergone gastric bypass 2–5 years earlier, higher levels of moderate-to-vigorous physical activity were associated with greater postoperative weight loss [47]. However, data from intervention studies are lacking. In one small, nonrandomized, prospective study, participation in a postoperative exercise program (including 75 min of supervised aerobic exercise and resistance training 3 times a week) for 3 months did not significantly increase weight loss after RYGB surgery [48]. However, the intervention did prevent the observed decrease in dynamic muscle strength that was seen in postoperative patients who did not exercise, and it was also associated with an increase in functional and aerobic capacity. In a small, randomized, controlled trial, Shah and colleagues randomly assigned 33 obese (BMI ≥ 35.5 kg/m^2) postoperative patients to either high-volume exercise (with a goal of expending $\geq 2,000$ kcal/week in moderate intensity aerobic exercise) or a usual activity control for 12 weeks [49]. Subjects assigned to the exercise intervention reported a greater than threefold increase in time spent in moderate physical activity and a nearly twofold increase in recorded step counts. In this small study, intervention group subjects did not have greater weight loss or greater improvements in body composition; however, they did have significantly greater improvements in physical fitness. Additional data are needed to further characterize the benefits of exercise in postoperative bariatric surgery patients and to determine the optimal physical activity levels in this group.

Additional concerns regarding prescription of exercise in the bariatric surgery patient are physical and cognitive barriers. Before bariatric surgery, an individual's ability to exercise is often limited due to musculoskeletal pain. Walking capacity of severely obese patients is on average 55 % of normal values and is inversely related to BMI [50]. Cognitive barriers to physical activity include lack of time, social stigma, lack of motivation, reduced awareness of the health benefits of exercise, fear of injury, a lack of confidence in the ability to participate in physical activity, and self-consciousness or embarrassment. Treatment strategies that address these barriers may help patients become more physically active.

Psychological Counseling and Peer Support in the Postoperative Period

Data suggest that patients with postoperative depression experience poorer weight loss than those who are not depressed. Similarly, postoperative patients who exhibit disordered eating patterns, such as grazing and loss of control over eating, have poorer weight loss and greater weight regain [10, 36]. Patients who are found to have mood disorders, disordered eating behavior, or substance abuse after bariatric surgery should be offered professional psychological counseling and support. It is not known, however, whether such treatment improves weight loss or other outcomes.

For unclear reasons, patients who exhibit disordered eating patterns may be more receptive to a behavioral intervention after surgery than before surgery. In one small nonrandomized prospective study, preoperative and postoperative bariatric surgical patients with binge eating or other disordered eating patterns were referred to a 10-week cognitive behavioral therapy program designed to address and improve the maladaptive eating patterns. Patients who were referred to the program postoperatively were much more likely to attend the initial session and to complete the program than patients referred preoperatively.

In epidemiologic studies, attendance at postoperative support groups is associated with improved weight loss outcomes [51, 52]. There is a lack of data regarding the effects of other types of postoperative psychological support, such as group or individual therapy, on weight loss and other outcomes.

Comprehensive Lifestyle Interventions After Bariatric Surgery

There is limited data regarding the benefits of comprehensive lifestyle interventions in the postoperative period. However, several pilot studies have been published over the past several years. In one small, randomized controlled trial, subjects who were assigned to a multifaceted lifestyle intervention after vertically banded gastroplasty reported improved dietary habits, increased physical activity levels, and reduced television viewing, as compared to subjects assigned to usual care [53]. Furthermore, subjects in the lifestyle intervention group lost significantly more weight at 1, 2, and 3 years after surgery than subjects in the usual care group.

Sarwer et al. [54] randomized 84 postoperative patients to either dietary counseling (brief: 15 min) every other week, in-person dietary counseling by a registered dietitian for the first 4 postoperative months, or standard care (no formal nutrition counseling sessions scheduled). Patients who received dietary counseling lost more total weight (20.7 ± 1.1 %) than those who received standard care (18.5 ± 1.1 %) at the end of 4 months. Total weight loss at 24 months was 32.4 ± 2.0 % versus 33.6 ± 2.5 %, respectively [54]. Although none of these weight loss differences reached statistical significance, the dietary counseling group reported greater improvements in eating behavior.

In a further study, Kalarchian and colleagues [55] reported the results of a small randomized, controlled study ($n=36$) involving patients who had undergone bariatric surgery at least 3 years earlier but who had failed to lose 50 % or more of their excess weight. Participants were randomly assigned to a comprehensive lifestyle intervention, including 12 weekly group education sessions and five individual telephone coaching sessions over 6 months, or a waitlisted control group. Subjects randomized to the intervention group lost slightly more weight (3.3 ± 8.1 kg) than those in the control group (1.3 ± 6.8 kg), but the difference was not statistically significant [55]. Interestingly, in this study, the presence of depressive symptoms at the beginning of the study was associated with greater weight loss in the intervention group but not the control group, suggesting that the behavioral component of the intervention may have been helpful for patients with depression.

These few pilot studies suggest that currently designed lifestyle interventions are modestly effective in enhancing further weight loss among post-bariatric surgery patients. Multiple factors appear to influence outcome results, including patient selection, timing and intensity of the intervention, comprehensiveness of counseling provided, and selection of outcome measurements. Furthermore, the influence of other determinants of weight loss or weight regain (discussed earlier) may need to be addressed.

Pharmacotherapy

There are no published studies describing the use of adjunctive pharmacotherapy for management of weight regain following bariatric surgery. This is due, in part, to a paucity of anti-obesity medication available and the prevailing paradigm of not combining surgical and pharmacologic modalities for treatment. However, with the recent approval by the US Food and Drug Administration (FDA) of lorcaserin (Belviq™) and phentermine/topiramate (Qsymia™) for chronic weight management, the use of drug therapy can be anticipated.

Conclusion

The incidence of weight regain following bariatric surgery is not well defined. However, the current literature suggests that a significant percentage of patients will experience regain beginning several years following surgery. There are multiple determinants of weight regain that include biological, surgical, behavioral, social, and psychological factors. However, the extent and significance of these factors is currently uncertain. Patients who present with significant weight regain following bariatric surgery should undergo a comprehensive evaluation for determination of remedial factors. Additional clinical research is needed to further delineate this long-term postoperative problem.

Question and Answer Section

Questions

1. Cross-sectional data from the literature suggests that weight regain after bariatric surgery occurs in what percentage of patients?
   A. 5–15 %
   B. 15–30 %
   C. 20–35 %
   D. 50 %
2. A 45-year-old female who underwent Roux-en-Y gastric bypass (RYGB) 4 years previously presents with 27 lb. weight gain. Medical history includes depression and gastroesophageal reflux disease (GERD). She states she has been very busy recently due to job and family stressors. She has not had any time to exercise or prepare meals. She feels depressed and guilty secondary to the weight gain. Current medications include omeprazole/sodium bicarbonate, sertraline, and a multivitamin-mineral supplement. On exam, BP 122/80, pulse 70, weight 220 lb., and height 5′6″. Surgical preop weight was 275 lb. Which of the following management plans would be the most beneficial to this patient?
   A. Refer to a health psychologist for counseling and support. Discontinue sertraline and prescribe paroxetine to improve depressive symptoms.
   B. Refer to a health psychologist for counseling and support. Order a UGI X-ray and EGD to assess integrity of RYGB.
   C. Refer to a health psychologist for counseling and support and a registered dietitian for education on healthy eating patterns. Provide counseling during her visit to further assess causes of weight gain.

Answers

1. Answer **C**.
2. Answer **C**.

References

1. O'Brien PE, McPhail T, Chaston TB, Dixon JB. Systematic review of medium-term weight loss after bariatric operations. Obes Surg. 2006;16:1032–40.
2. Shah M, Simha V, Garg A. Long-term impact of bariatric surgery on body weight, comorbidities, and nutritional status. J Clin Endocrinol Metab. 2006;91(11):4223–31.
3. Heber D, Greenway FL, Kaplan LM, Livingston E, Salvador J, Still C. Endocrine and nutritional management of the post-bariatric surgery patient: an endocrine society clinical practice guideline. J Clin Endocrinol Metab. 2010;95:4823–43.
4. Sjöström L, Narbro K, Sjöström CD, Karason K, Larsson B, Wedel H, et al. Swedish obese subjects study: effects of bariatric surgery on mortality in Swedish obese subjects. N Engl J Med. 2007;357:741–52.
5. Sjöström L, Lindroos AK, Peltonen M, Torgerson J, Bouchard C, Carlsson B, et al. Lifestyle, diabetes, and cardiovascular risk factors 10 years after bariatric surgery. N Engl J Med. 2004;351:2683–93.
6. Himpens J, Dobbeleir J, Peeters G. Long-term results of laparoscopic sleeve gastrectomy for obesity. Ann Surg. 2010;252:319–24.
7. Christou NV, Look D, MacLean LD. Weight gain after short and long limb gastric bypass in patients followed for longer than 10 years. Ann Surg. 2006;244:734–40.
8. Barhouch AS, Zardo M, Padoin AV, Colossi FG, Casagrande DS, Chatkin R, et al. Excess weight loss variation in late postoperative period of gastric bypass. Obes Surg. 2010;20:1479–83.
9. Nguyen NT, Slone JA, Nguyen XMT, Hartman JS, Hoyt DB. A prospective randomized trial of laparoscopic gastric bypass versus laparoscopic adjustable gastric banding for the treatment of morbid obesity. Ann Surg. 2009;250:631–41.
10. Kofman MD, Lent MR, Swencionis C. Maladaptive eating patterns, quality of life, and weight outcomes following gastric bypass: results of an internet survey. Obesity. 2010;18(10):1938–43.
11. Patel S, Szomstein S, Rosenthal RJ. Reasons and outcomes of reoperative bariatric surgery for failed and complicated procedures (excluding adjustable and gastric banding). Obes Surg. 2011;21:1209–19.
12. Deylgat B, D'Hondt M, Pottel H, Vansteenkiste F, Van Rooy F, Devriendt D. Indications, safety, and feasibility of conversion of

failed bariatric surgery to Roux-en-Y gastric bypass: a retrospective comparative study with primary laparoscopic Roux-en Y gastric bypass. Surg Endosc. 2012;26:1997–2002.
13. Scott WR, Batterham RL. Roux-en-y-gastric bypass and laparoscopic sleeve gastrectomy; understanding weight loss and improvements in type 2 diabetes after bariatric surgery. Am J Physiol Regul Integr Comp Physiol. 2011;301:R15–27.
14. Vesco K, Dietz PM, Rizzo J, Stevens VJ, Perrin NA, Bachman DJ, et al. Excessive gestational weight gain and postpartum weight retention among obese women. Obstet Gynecol. 2009;114:1069–75.
15. Amorim A, Rossner S, Neovius M, Lourenco PM, Linne Y. Does excess pregnancy weight gain constitute a major risk for increasing long-term BMI? Obesity. 2007;15:1278–86.
16. Manum AA, Kinarivala M, O'Callaghan MJ, Williams GM, Najman JM, Callaway LK. Associations of excess weight gain during pregnancy with long-term maternal overweight and obesity: evidence from 21 y postpartum follow-up. Am J Clin Nutr. 2010;91:1336–41.
17. Dixon JB, Dixon ME, O'Brien PE. Birth outcomes in obese women after laparoscopic adjustable gastric banding. Obstet Gynecol. 2005;106(part 1):965–72.
18. Sheiner E, Edri A, Balaban E, Levi I, Aricha-Tamir B. Pregnancy outcome of patients who conceive during or after the first year following bariatric surgery. Am J Obstet Gynecol. 2011;204(50):e1–6.
19. Simkin-Silverman LR, Wing RR. Weight gain during menopause. Is it inevitable or can it be prevented? Postgrad Med. 2000;108(3):47–50.
20. Lovejoy JC, Champagne CM, de Jonge L, Xie H, Smith SR. Increased visceral fat and decreased energy expenditure during the menopausal transition. Int J Obes. 2008;32:949–58.
21. Da Silva JA, Jacobs JW, Kirwan JR, Boers M, Saag KG, Inês LB, et al. Safety of low dose glucocorticoid treatment in rheumatoid arthritis: published evidence and prospective trial data. Ann Rheum Dis. 2006;65(3):285.
22. Levine MD, Kalarchian MA, Courcoulas AP, Wisinski MS, Marcus MD. History of smoking and post cessation weight gain among weight loss surgery candidates. Addict Behav. 2007;32:2365–71.
23. Williamsom DF, Madans J, Anda RF, Kleinman JC, Giovino GA, Byers T. Smoking cessation and severity of weight gain in a national cohort. N Engl J Med. 1991;324:739–45.
24. Ohara P, Connett JE, Lee WW, Nides M, Murray R, Wise R. Early and late weight gain following smoking cessation in the Lung Health study. Am J Epidemiol. 1998;148:821–32.
25. Fierabracci P, Pinchera A, Martinelli S, Scartabelli G, Salvetti G, Giannetti M, et al. Prevalence of endocrine diseases in morbidly obese patients scheduled for bariatric surgery; beyond diabetes. Obes Surg. 2011;21:54–60.
26. Centers for Disease Control and Prevention. Prevalence of doctor-diagnosed arthritis and arthritis-attributable activity limitation—United States, 2007–2009. MMWR Morb Mortal Wkly Rep. 2010;59(39):1261–65.
27. Gill RS, Al-Adra DP, Shi X, Sharma AM, Birch DW, Karmali S. The benefits of bariatric surgery in obese patients with hip and knee osteoarthritis: a systematic review. Obes Rev. 2011;12:1083–9.
28. Karlsson J, Taft C, Rydén A, Sjöström L, Sullivan M. Ten year trends in health related quality of life after surgical and conventional treatment for severe obesity: the SOS intervention study. Int J Obes. 2007;31:1248–61.
29. Odom J, Zalesin KC, Washington TL, Miller WW, Hakmeh B, Zaremba DL, et al. Behavioral predictors of weight regain after bariatric surgery. Obes Surg. 2010;20:349–56.
30. Hsu LK, Benotti PN, Dwyer J, Roberts SB, Saltzman E, Shikora S, et al. Nonsurgical factors that influence the outcome of bariatric surgery: a review. Psychosom Med. 1998;60:338–46.
31. Elfhag K, Rossner S. Who succeeds in maintaining weight loss? A conceptual review of factors associated with weight loss maintenance and weight regain. Obes Rev. 2005;6:67–85.
32. de Zwaan M, Mitchell JE, Howell LM, Monson N, Swan-Kremeier L, Crosby RD, et al. Characteristics of morbidly obese patients before gastric bypass surgery. Compr Psychiatry. 2003;44(5):428–34.
33. Allison KC, Wadden TA, Sarwer DB, Fabricatore AN, Crerand CE, Gibbons LM, et al. Night eating syndrome and binge eating disorder among persons seeking bariatric surgery: prevalence and related features. Surg Obes Relat Dis. 2006;2(2):153–8.
34. Latner JD, Hildebrandt T, Rosewall JK, Chisholm AM, Hayashi K. Loss of control over eating reflects eating disturbances and general psychopathology. Behav Res Ther. 2007;45:2203–11.
35. Silver H, Torquati A, Jensen G, Richards W. Weight, dietary and physical activity behaviors two years after gastric bypass. Obes Surg. 2006;16:859–64.
36. Colles SL, Dixon JB, O'Brien PE. Grazing and loss of control related to eating: two high risk factors following bariatric surgery. Obesity. 2008;16(3):615–22.
37. Zalesin KC, Franklin BA, Miller WM, Nori Janosz K, Veri S, Odom J, et al. Preventing weight regain after bariatric surgery: an overview of lifestyle and psychosocial modulators. Am J Lifestyle Med. 2010;4(2):113–20.
38. Suzuki J, Haimovici F, Chang G. Alcohol use disorders after bariatric surgery. Obes Surg. 2012;22(2):201–7.
39. King WC, Chen JY, Mitchell JE, Kalarchian MA, Steffen KJ, Engel SG, et al. Prevalence of alcohol use disorders before and after bariatric surgery. JAMA. 2012;307(23):2516–25.
40. Jacobi D, Ciangura C, Couet C, Oppert JM. Physical activity and weight loss following bariatric surgery. Obes Rev. 2011;12(5):366–77.
41. Wouters E, Larsen J, Zijlstra H, van Ramshorst B, Geenen R. Physical activity after surgery for severe obesity: the role of exercise cognitions. Obes Surg. 2011;21(12):1894–9.
42. Bond DS, Jakicic JM, Unick JL, Vithiananthan S, Pohl D, Roye GD, Ryderet BA, et al. Pre- to postoperative physical activity changes in bariatric surgery patients: self report vs. objective measures. Obesity. 2010;18(12):2395–7.
43. Rosenberger P, Henderson K, White M. Physical activity in gastric bypass patients: associations with weight loss and psychosocial functioning at 12-month follow-up. Obes Surg. 2011;21(10);1564–69.
44. Svetkey LP, Stevens VJ, Brantley PJ, Appel LJ, Hollis JF, Loria CM, et al. Comparison of strategies for sustaining weight loss: the weight loss maintenance randomized controlled trial. JAMA. 2008;299(10):1139–48.
45. Gould JC, Beverstein G, Reinhardt S, Garren MJ. Impact of routine and long term follow up on weight loss after laparoscopic gastric bypass. Surg Obes Relat Dis. 2007;3:627–30.
46. Freire RH, Borges MC, Alverez-Leite JI, Correia MITD. Food quality, physical activity, and nutritional follow-up as determinants of weight regain after Roux-en-Y gastric bypass. Nutrition. 2012;28:53–8.
47. Josbeno DA, Kalarchian M, Sparto PJ, Otto AD, Jakicic JM. Physical activity and physical function in individuals post-bariatric surgery. Obes Surg. 2011;21:1243–9.
48. Stegen S, Derave W, Calders P. Physical fitness in morbidly obese patients: effect of gastric bypass surgery and exercise training. Obes Surg. 2011;21:61–70.
49. Shah M, Snell PG, Rao S, Quittner B, Adams-Huet C, Livingston HE, et al. High-volume exercise program in obese bariatric surgery patients: a randomized, controlled trial. Obesity. 2011;9:1826–34.

50. Tompkins J, Bosch PR, Chenowith R, Tiede JL, Swain JM. Changes in functional walking distance and health related quality of life after gastric bypass surgery. Phys Ther. 2008;88:928–35.
51. Livhits M, Mercado C, Yermilov I, Parikh JA, Dutson E, Mehran A, et al. Behavioral factors associated with successful weight loss after gastric bypass. Am Surg. 2010;76(10):1139–42.
52. Sogg S. Alcohol misuse after bariatric surgery: epiphenomenon or "Oprah" phenomenon? Surg Obes Relat Dis. 2008;3(3):366–8.
53. Papalazarou A, Yannakoulia M, Kavouras SA, Komesidou V, Dimitriadis G, Papakonstantinou A, et al. Lifestyle intervention favorably affects weight loss and maintenance following obesity surgery. Obesity. 2010;18(7):1348–53.
54. Sarwer DB, Moore RH, Spitzer JC, Wadden TA, Raper SE, Williams NN. A pilot study investigating the efficacy of postoperative dietary counseling to improve outcomes after bariatric surgery. Surg Obes Relat Dis. 2012;8(5):561–8.
55. Kalarchian MA, Marcus MD, Courcoulas AP, Cheng Y, Levine MD, Josbeno D. Optimizing long-term weight control after bariatric surgery: a pilot study. Surg Obes Relat Dis. 2012;8(6):710–5.

The Role of Physical Activity in Optimizing Bariatric Surgery Outcomes

Dale S. Bond and Wendy C. King

Chapter Objectives

1. Discuss the importance of habitual physical activity in relation to health outcomes, weight loss, and weight loss maintenance.
2. Review evidence regarding the role of physical activity in bariatric surgery outcomes.
3. Describe the physical activity patterns of preoperative and postoperative patients.
4. Explain how to formulate an appropriate physical activity prescription and apply behavioral counseling strategies to facilitate patient engagement in habitual physical activity preoperatively and postoperatively.

Introduction

Engagement in habitual physical activity (PA) (i.e., planned or structured PA that is performed on a daily or near daily basis) is associated with numerous health benefits, is a critical component of lifestyle interventions for weight loss, and plays a key role in maintenance of nonsurgical weight loss [1–3]. Additionally, mounting evidence from both observational studies and recent small randomized controlled trials suggests that adherence to habitual PA may provide similar benefits within the context of bariatric surgery [4]. While initial research consistently suggested that bariatric surgery patients make large increases in their PA postoperatively [5], findings were largely derived from self-report measures, which are prone to bias and inaccuracies [6]. More recent studies using objective PA measures indicate that most patients have low levels of habitual PA and are highly sedentary preoperatively and fail to make substantial changes in their PA postoperatively [4]. Based on these data, it appears that adoption and maintenance of habitual PA poses a considerable challenge to many patients, despite experiencing substantial weight loss and improvements in physical function postoperatively. Given the difficulties faced by many patients in adhering to habitual PA, appropriate strategies for increasing preoperative and postoperative PA should be offered within the context of a multidisciplinary surgical treatment approach to optimize postoperative outcomes. We begin this chapter by describing the different components of PA and reviewing PA recommendations. Next, we discuss the health benefits of habitual PA, with particular focus on its role in nonsurgical weight loss and weight loss maintenance, and assess evidence regarding the role of PA in the context of bariatric surgery. Then, we describe objectively assessed PA patterns of preoperative and postoperative patients. Finally, we explain how to develop an appropriate PA prescription and apply behavioral counseling strategies to promote engagement in habitual preoperative and postoperative PA.

D.S. Bond, PhD (✉)
Department of Psychiatry and Human Behavior, The Weight Control and Diabetes Research Center, Brown Alpert Medical School, The Miriam Hospital, Providence, RI, USA
e-mail: dbond@lifespan.org

W.C. King, PhD
Department of Epidemiology, University of Pittsburgh, Pittsburgh, PA, USA
e-mail: kingw@edc.pitt.edu

Definition of Physical Activity and Its Components

Physical activity (PA) refers to any bodily movement produced by the skeletal muscles that produces an increase in energy expenditure above rest. Of the different major components of total daily energy expenditure (basal metabolic rate, physical activity, and metabolic response to food), PA is the most variable and is the second largest after basal metabolic rate, accounting for about 25 % of daily energy expenditure in a sedentary person and up to 50 % in a highly active person [1].

Total PA encompasses a broad range of occupational, transportation (walking, bicycling), domestic (household, yardwork, childcare, and other chores), and leisure-time (PA and exercise performed during "free" time and involving elements of personal choice, enjoyment, etc.) activities. PA also includes non-exercise activity thermogenesis (NEAT), such as fidgeting. Traditionally, increasing leisure-time PA has been the focus of PA interventions, although more recent efforts have targeted activities across multiple domains given that the average person only has 3–4 h of leisure time per day [1, 7].

Exercise is a specific form of leisure-time PA involving planned or structured repetitive bodily movement performed to improve or maintain one or more components of health-related physical fitness, including cardiorespiratory fitness, motor fitness, musculoskeletal fitness, body composition, and metabolism. It is important to note that some health benefits can still be obtained through being physically active even with little or no related gains in fitness [1]. This may be particularly relevant for some preoperative bariatric surgery patients who may have insufficient time before undergoing surgery or physical capacity to achieve significant fitness gains, but still can obtain health benefits by starting to incorporate more PA into their daily routine.

Intensity

The extent to which PA is health enhancing and increases energy expenditure is influenced in large part by the intensity or effort with which it is performed. The intensity of activities can be viewed along a continuum with sedentary activities at the lowest end of the continuum and vigorous-intensity activities at the highest end [7]. Sedentary activities are waking behaviors performed in a sitting or reclining posture (e.g., watching television, using a computer, driving a car, etc.), typically for extended periods of time, which require very low levels of energy expenditure. Mounting epidemiological evidence suggests that greater time spent in sedentary behaviors, independent of PA level, is associated with higher risk of obesity, cardiometabolic disease, and mortality [8]. Consequently, it is important to evaluate daily time spent in both sedentary and PA behaviors, given that an individual could meet PA recommendations yet still be very sedentary [9].

Light-intensity PA is performed at an intensity that is higher than sedentary behaviors, but lower than moderate-intensity physical activity, and includes activities such as standing, walking slowly, lifting lightweight objects, and light housework. Moderate-intensity PA is performed at an intensity that approximates a brisk walk. However, due to carrying extra weight, and potentially a lack of fitness, severely obese individuals may achieve moderate-intensity walking at 1.5 or 2 mph, while a "brisk" walk (i.e., 3 or 4 mph) may be a vigorous-intensity PA [10]. Other examples of activities that may be done at moderate intensity include low-impact aerobics, weight lifting, doubles tennis, house painting, and packing boxes. Finally, vigorous-intensity PA produces a substantial elevation in heart rate and breathing. Examples of activities that may be done at vigorous intensity include jogging, swimming laps, singles tennis, biking, and lifting heavy loads.

Methods of measuring PA intensity can be grouped under two general categories: (1) relative intensity and (2) absolute intensity [7]. Relative intensity methods assess the level of effort involved in performing a specific exercise or activity. Precise measurement of the relative intensity of a specific exercise or activity involves use of objective physiological indicators, such as heart rate. For example, moderate-intensity activity can be defined as 60–80 % of maximum heart rate estimated as (220-age) or 50–70 % of one's heart rate reserve (maximum heart rate – resting heart rate). Other methods to assess the relative intensity of PA are more subjective and rely on individual perceptions of heart rate, breathing, and body temperature. The talk test, based on the ability to talk and sing during PA, and the Borg Rating of Perceived Exertion (RPE) scale, based on how heavy and strenuous exercise feels, are two useful methods to help patients gauge PA intensity. For example, engagement in brisk walking or another moderate-intensity exercise would be indicated when a patient can talk, but cannot carry on a full conversation or sing (i.e., talk test), and reports working "somewhat hard" or a score of 12–14 on the RPE scale.

The intensity of a given activity can also be classified based on absolute intensity (i.e., the amount of energy that the body uses to perform the activity). Metabolic equivalents (METs) provide an objective means to express the energy cost and absolute intensity of physical activities. The MET level of an activity is defined as the ratio of an individual's metabolic rate (energy consumed) during an activity to their resting metabolic rate (equivalent to 1 MET). Activities requiring 3 to <6 times more energy than sitting (i.e., 3<6 METS) are moderate-intensity activities, while activities that require six or more METs are vigorous-intensity activities. Published MET values or energy expenditure tables based on MET values of well-defined physical activities may be helpful for estimating the intensity of various activities. However, often the MET values are based on small study samples of nonobese adults and may be less accurate in obese individuals who often expend more energy than lean individuals during physical activity due to the extra mass that they carry [7]. Thus, when communicating with patients, it is important to help them understand that they should pay attention to physiological sensations and potentially use a couple of methods (e.g., talk test and heart rate) to monitor their PA intensity when exercising.

Frequency and Duration

The frequency and duration of physical activity bouts are also very important components of what makes PA health enhancing. While there is a dose–response relationship

Table 22.1 Evidence-based physical activity guidelines for healthy and overweight/obese adults

Agency	Target population	Benefit	Recommendation
US Department of Health and Human Services (USDHHS)	Healthy adults	General health benefits	≥150 min of aerobic moderate-intensity physical activity (PA) or 75 min of aerobic vigorous-intensity PA per week in episodes of ≥10 min, plus muscle-strengthening activities for major muscle groups ≥2 days per week
Institute of Medicine (IOM)	Adults	Prevention of weight gain; Weight-independent health benefits	60 min of moderate-intensity PA per day
American College of Sports Medicine (ACSM)	Overweight and obese adults	Weight loss; Prevention of weight regain	≥250 min of moderate-intensity PA per week
International Association for the Study of Obesity (IASO)	Formerly obese adults	Prevention of weight regain	60 to 90 min of moderate-intensity PA per day (or lesser amounts of vigorous-intensity PA) on most days of the week

Table reprinted with permission from King and Bond [4]
PA physical activity, *min* minutes

between PA and many health outcomes, such that the more PA that is performed, the greater the benefit, researchers have worked to determine the minimum amount of PA needed to obtain many of the health benefits of PA, which has led to various PA guidelines and recommendations.

Physical Activity Recommendations

Habitual PA is an essential component of a healthy lifestyle. As shown in Table 22.1, evidence-based guidelines for the general population of adults and those who are overweight and obese generally recommend engaging in at least 150 min per week of PA that is of at least a moderate intensity to promote health and weight control, whereas higher doses of PA are recommended to achieve greater weight loss and prevent significant weight regain.

Despite the fact that PA is widely recognized as an important component of a multidisciplinary bariatric surgery program, formal evidence-based guidelines for preoperative and postoperative PA have not yet been developed. However, a number of informal guidelines have been put forth that track with the PA recommendations for improving health and long-term weight control. The American Society for Metabolic and Bariatric Surgery (ASMBS), the Obesity Society (TOS), and the American Association of Clinical Endocrinologists (AACE) identifies accumulating 30 min of exercise per day as one of many healthful behaviors that should be performed to achieve optimal body weight and improve body composition postoperatively [11]. Less rigorous preoperative recommendations have been made by the 2007 Expert Panel on Weight Loss Surgery [12] as well as the American Heart Association [13] to improve cardiorespiratory fitness, reduce risk of surgical complications, facilitate healing, and enhance postoperative recovery. Specifically, they recommend that patients be encouraged to adopt a preoperative exercise program consisting of low-to-moderate-intensity PA for at least 20 min per day on 3–4 days per week.

One of the reasons that evidence-based PA guidelines for the bariatric surgery population have been lacking is that examination of PA within the context of bariatric surgery is still a relatively new topic of study. However, in response to the rapid accumulation of evidence in this area, an expert panel from the ASMBS and the American College of Sports Medicine (ACSM) has been formed to develop formal preoperative and postoperative PA guidelines.

Assessment of Physical Activity

In order to determine dose–response relationships between PA and health outcomes and specify which aspects of PA are important for particular health outcomes, PA must be measured accurately and reliably. Unfortunately, measuring all aspects of PA (i.e., the frequency and duration of each type of PA at various intensities) is challenging, as is determining how best to quantify it. Large studies most frequently use PA surveys, or questionnaires, because the methodology is relatively inexpensive and participant burden is low. In addition, surveys are well suited for measuring "habitual" PA. The major limitation in using PA surveys is that they rely on study participants to accurately report intensity, frequency, and duration of PA. Thus, results are prone to being influenced by misinterpretation (e.g., a study participant may believe that their low-intensity PA is in fact moderate intensity or confuse improvement in physical function with an increase in PA) as well as social desirability (i.e., the desire of study participants to report socially favorable behaviors) [6].

The most accurate PA assessment methods (i.e., quantitative assessment of total energy expenditure via direct or indirect calorimetry) are generally not suitable for use in large studies due to researcher and participant burden and cost. However, several types of activity monitors allow for objective assessment of free-living PA (i.e., PA performed in normal daily life as opposed to an exercise laboratory). Four different types of activity monitors have been employed in this area of research: pedometers, accelerometers, step activity monitors, and multisensor devices. Pedometers are small, relatively inexpensive devices worn on the hip that estimate the number of steps taken and distance traveled typically via an internal spring lever that responds to vertical motion of the hips during walking, jogging, and running activity. Newer pedometers use an electronic sensor to detect motion, and some provide additional capabilities such as calculation of energy expenditure and positioning via global positioning system satellite networks. Accelerometers are small, battery-operated devices typically worn on the waist that employ microelectronic sensors to continuously record minute-by-minute changes in velocity across multiple planes of movement (vertical, anteroposterior, and lateral planes). Stored data can be downloaded to a computer and converted using proprietary software to activity counts and/or METs, thus allowing for quantification of time spent being sedentary and performing light-, moderate-, and vigorous-intensity physical activity. A step activity monitor, such as Orthocare Innovations' StepWatch™ Activity Monitor (Orthocare Innovations, Oklahoma City, OK) is a cross between a pedometer and an accelerometer, in that it continuously records the number of steps per time interval (i.e., 1 min) over extended monitoring periods. This allows for quantification of daily steps, as well as many other PA parameters, such as total time spent ambulating and in various PA intensities, as defined by cadence, as well as frequency of PA bouts. There are also multisensor monitors, such as the SenseWear Mini Armband (BodyMedia, Pittsburgh, PA), which simultaneously integrates motion data from a triaxial accelerometer and various physiological parameters (i.e., skin temperature and near body temperature, galvanic skin response, and heat flux) to provide estimates of energy expenditure. Data are used to estimate time spent in different intensities of physical activity and sedentary behaviors during waking hours. While the cost for high-quality activity monitors, burden of retrieving monitors from participants, and required technical expertise to process the data have prohibited their use in many studies, there is a growing body of literature with activity monitor use. However, just like PA surveys, there is great variability in the validity and reliability of activity monitors, with some of the less expensive pedometers being particularly prone to problems, so even studies reporting PA based on activity monitor use should be interpreted with caution [4, 6].

Relationship of Physical Activity to Health Outcomes

Despite the difficulty in accurately assessing PA, there is overwhelming evidence that PA is protective against many negative health outcomes. As summarized in the US Department of Health and Human Services 2008 report, regular PA improves health, independent of weight loss, by improving flexibility, strength, and balance, which reduces stiffness, joint pain, and risk of injury; helping build and maintain healthy bones; reducing risk of developing cardiovascular disease, stroke, type 2 diabetes, breast cancer, and colon cancer; improving cardiometabolic risk factors like blood pressure, blood cholesterol levels, insulin sensitivity, and C-reactive protein; improving immunity; reducing feelings of depression and anxiety; promoting psychological well-being; improving or maintaining some aspects of cognitive function; enhancing quality of sleep; and delaying all-cause mortality [14].

The Role of Physical Activity in Nonsurgical Weight Loss and Weight Loss Maintenance

Weight Loss

PA is an important contributor to weight management. Excess body fat develops from an imbalance of energy intake and expenditure. As mentioned earlier, PA accounts for the most variability in total energy expenditure. In addition to increasing energy expenditure directly, PA enhances metabolic rate via its effect on increasing fat-free mass and stimulating metabolic rate following PA. Regular PA also alters fat distribution by improving the body's ability to burn fat as fuel and reducing fat cell size [1, 15].

Research suggests a vicious cycle between inactivity and weight gain, such that a low PA level leads to weight gain, which leads to decreased PA. Conversely, increasing PA improves weight loss in overweight and obese adults, even during diet restriction [16], although as we will show later in this chapter, data to support a relative increase in PA to the decrease in weight following bariatric surgery is lacking. To date, most studies that have investigated the effect of increasing PA during diet restriction have been limited to overweight or class 1 obese adults. However, in a recent randomized clinical trial of 130 class 2 (body mass index [BMI] $35 \leq 40.0$ kg/m^2) and 3 (BMI ≥ 40 kg/m^2) obese adults, Goodpaster et al. [17] showed that participants randomized to a PA program (progressed to 60 min, 5 days per week) plus dietary counseling had greater weight loss and improvements in waist circumference and hepatic steatosis than those randomized to dietary counseling alone.

Weight Loss Maintenance

Habitual physical activity is an important contributor to long-term weight maintenance [3]. Clinical studies have reliably shown that obese participants who report engagement in higher levels of PA (approximately ≥250 min per week) are better able to maintain their weight losses, compared to participants who do not achieve this level of PA [16]. Additionally, participation in high levels of PA is a common characteristic of participants in the National Weight Control Registry (NWCR), who on average have lost almost 32 kg and kept it off for nearly 6 years. Accelerometer data has shown that NWCR participants engage in significantly higher levels of sustained moderate-to-vigorous physical activity (MVPA) than overweight controls matched to the NWCR participants' pre-weight-loss BMI (41.5 ± 35.1 min/day versus 19.2 ± 18.6; $p<.01$) and there is a trend toward more PA than never obese normal-weight controls matched to the NWCR participants' current BMI (25.8 ± 23.4; $p=0.08$) [18].

Participants in the aforementioned clinical study by Goodpaster et al. as well as those in the NWCR who have been successful at weight loss maintenance also report low levels of overall energy and dietary fat intake. Thus, high doses of PA operate in conjunction with positive changes in eating behaviors to promote optimal weight control after nonsurgical weight loss [2, 3, 16]. While clearly PA can be a significant component of weight loss maintenance, it is important to recognize that there is considerable variation in the amount of MVPA required to maintain weight loss. For example, while 25 % of NWCR participants averaged at least 57 min/day, 25 % averaged less than 19 min/day [18].

The Role of Physical Activity in Surgical Weight Loss and Weight Loss Maintenance

Weight Loss

Two systematic reviews published in 2010 concluded that PA is positively associated with greater weight loss following bariatric surgery [5, 19]. The vast majority of studies included in the reviews supported this conclusion. However, all of the reviewed studies were observational and many were cross-sectional. In addition, with the exception of one study [20], all studies relied exclusively on self-reported PA, often from self-developed surveys. A few more recent studies offer stronger evidence. In a sample of 277 participants of the Longitudinal Assessment of Bariatric Surgery-2 (LABS-2) study who wore the StepWatch™ Activity Monitor both before and 1 year following bariatric surgery, King et al. found that an increase in PA from preoperatively to 1 year postoperatively was independently related to a greater percentage weight loss at 1 year [21]. Specifically, an additional increase of 3,000 steps per day from preoperatively to 1-year postsurgery above the mean change in steps was significantly associated with an additional 1.5 kg decrease in weight ($p=0.04$) and an additional 1.1 % decrease in percentage body fat ($p=0.02$). Also in 2011, Egberts et al. reported on a randomized clinical trial of 50 laparoscopic adjustable gastric banding (LAGB) patients. Participants were randomized to either usual care or 12 weeks of aerobic and strength-building exercises with a personal trainer for 45 min/3 times a week. Those in the exercise group had better excess weight loss (37 %) and change in percentage body fat (3.6 %) compared to the usual care group (27 and 1.6 %, respectively) at the end of the intervention [22]. Given that loss of lean body mass (e.g., muscle, bone density) can be higher than desirable during the first postoperative year when weight loss is most rapid, PA's role in maintaining lean body mass may be even more important than PA's direct effect on weight loss.

Weight Loss Maintenance

No studies have yet to directly examine how PA relates to weight loss maintenance following bariatric surgery. However, a recent cross-sectional study by Josbeno et al. examined past-week PA and postoperative weight loss in a sample of 40 participants who were likely in the weight loss maintenance phase (i.e., 2–5 years post-op) following Roux-en-Y gastric bypass (RYGB) [23]. In this study, weekly minutes of MVPA at 2–5 years post-op, measured with the SenseWear Pro Armband, accounted for 18 % of the variance in percentage of excess weight loss (%EWL) at that same time point, after controlling for time since surgery, age, and daily caloric intake. In addition, those who participated in at least 150 min/week of MVPA (35 %) had significantly greater % EWL (68.2 ± 19.0 versus 52.5 ± 17.4; $p=.01$). A case-control study finally, in a case-control study, Bond and colleagues [24] found that postoperative NWCR participants ($n=105$) reported expending fewer calories through PA and, specifically, calories from vigorous-intensity PA, compared to nonsurgical NWCR participants ($n=210$), who were matched on gender, entry weight, maximum weight loss, and weight-maintenance duration. Together these studies suggest that many postoperative patients do not take advantage of the weight loss maintenance benefits of exercise.

Relationship of Physical Activity to Other Postoperative Outcomes

To date, very few studies have examined whether PA level or physical fitness influences outcomes of bariatric surgery other than weight loss. In a sample of 109 preoperative patients, McCullough et al. found that higher aerobic fitness at time of surgery was related to decreased, short-term complications after bariatric surgery [25]. Shah et al. [26] performed a randomized clinical trial supporting the role of PA in postoperative glucose control. Thirty-three postoperative patients were randomized to 12 weeks of either high-volume exercise + dietary counseling ($n=21$) or dietary counseling alone ($n=12$). Over the first 4 weeks of the program, participants in the exercise + diet group were progressed to expending $\geq 2,000$ kcal/week via moderate-intensity exercise on 5 or more days of the week. After 12 weeks, participants in the exercise + diet group had significantly greater improvements in self-reported PA, cardiorespiratory fitness, and glucose control compared to those who only received dietary counseling. In addition, three observational studies have found significant associations between PA and the mental health of postoperative patients. Using the International Physical Activity Questionnaire-Short Form to assess PA, Bond et al. [27] found that both patients who went from inactive (<200 PA minutes/week) preoperatively to active (≥ 200 PA minutes/week) 1 year postoperatively ($n=68$) and those who were active at both time points ($n=83$) reported greater preoperative to postoperative improvements in mental health functioning, as measured by the SF-36 Mental Component Summary (MCS) score than patients who remained inactive postoperatively ($n=39$). Using the 4-item Godin Leisure-Time Questionnaire, Rosenberger et al. [28] found that PA frequency and intensity of 131 RYGB patients were independently associated with better mental health functioning (i.e., SF-36 MCS score) and fewer depressive symptoms, as measured with the Beck Depression Inventory (BDI), 1 year postoperatively. Finally, Larson et al. [29] found a significant positive association between a composite physical exercise score from the Sport Index of the Baecke Questionnaire and mental health functioning (SF-36 MCS score) in 157 adults who were 1–6 years post-laparoscopic adjustable gastric banding. Future studies are needed to determine whether PA contributes to increased remission and long-term resolution of comorbidities, such as type 2 diabetes.

Objectively Assessed Levels of Physical Activity and Sedentary Behaviors

While the majority of studies assessing the PA behaviors of bariatric surgery patients have relied on self-report, in the last few years the use of objective monitors to quantify patterns of PA and sedentary behaviors in bariatric surgery patients has increased. Given the considerable advantages they offer over more traditional subjective measures, as discussed previously, our summary of patients' physical activity behaviors will focus on studies that have employed objective monitoring methods.

Preoperative Levels of Physical Activity and Sedentary Behaviors

Two studies using pedometers found that preoperative patients averaged $4,621 \pm 3,701$ [30] and $6,061 \pm 2,740$ [20] steps/day respectively, thereby placing most patients in the sedentary (<5,000 steps/day) or "low active" (5,000–7,499 steps/day) categories [31]. However, these findings may be limited by small sample sizes; poor adherence to completion of pedometer diaries, which may have been related to PA level; self-reporting of pedometer steps; and potential underestimation of steps due to slow walking speeds and abnormal gaits of severely obese individuals [4].

Studies using more accurate step activity monitors and accelerometers address many of the aforementioned limitations associated with pedometers. Using the StepWatch™ Activity Monitor, King et al. [32] examined PA levels of preoperative patients in the LABS-2 using the ankle-mounted StepWatch™ Activity Monitor from which minute-by-minute step count data from a one week assessment period was analyzed. Participants ($n=757$) averaged $7,569 \pm 3,159$ steps/day, higher than reported in the aforementioned pedometer studies, although more than half of the sample was either categorized as sedentary or low active. Bond et al. [33] used the RT3 accelerometer to compare PA levels in 38 preoperative patients and 20 normal-weight controls. Patients spent one-half as much time in MVPA compared with controls (26 min/d versus 52 min/d). Additionally, more than two-thirds (68 %) of patients did not accumulate any weekly MVPA in bouts ≥ 10 min, which are indicative of planned or structured physical activity, compared with only 13 % of controls. Similarly, in another report of the LABS-2 cohort, King et al. [21] found that the majority (61 %) of participants ($n=310$) did not perform any bout-related MVPA preoperatively.

Bond and colleagues [34] also used the multisensor SenseWear Pro Armband to assess the amount of time that preoperative patients spend in sedentary behaviors, defined as percentage of time spent performing activities <1.5 METs, excluding sleep. Participants, on average, were sedentary during the vast majority (79–81 %) of their waking time, a percentage much higher than that observed in the general adult population (57 %). The above findings suggest that preoperative patients are generally highly sedentary and rarely engage in structured or bout-related MVPA.

Preoperative to Postoperative Changes in Physical Activity Levels

The majority of studies that have assessed PA via self-report questionnaires indicate that patients report preoperative to postoperative increases of 100–500 %, whereas studies using pedometers show that patients report average increases in daily steps of 43–9 % [5, 20, 28]. However, recent work conducted by Bond et al. and King et al. involving the use of objective monitor methods demonstrates a much smaller magnitude of preoperative to postoperative change in PA levels [4]. Bond et al. [35] compared self-reported (via the Paffenbarger Physical Activity Questionnaire) and RT3 accelerometer estimates of preoperative to 6-month postoperative MVPA changes in 20 patients. While self-reported average weekly minutes of MVPA increased nearly 500 % from 45 to 212 min/week, there were no significant changes in objectively measured total and bout-related MVPA. Moreover, preoperatively, the percentage of participants who achieved ≥150 weekly minutes of MVPA based on the subjective and objective measures was identical (10 %). By contrast, at 6 months postoperatively, 55 % reported meeting this recommendation compared to 5 % according to the objective measure. In contrast, King et al. [21] reported that participants of the LABS-2 cohort were significantly more active 1 year after surgery. However, the magnitude of preoperative to 1-year postoperative changes was small (i.e., mean increase of 19 % for daily steps and 16 % for bout-related MVPA). Additionally, 25 % of participants reduced their PA by ≥5 % postoperatively.

Postoperatively, LABS-2 participants accumulated a median of only 23 (interquartile range, 0–76) minutes per week of bout-related MVPA, as measured by the StepWatch™ Activity Monitor, and only 11 % achieved the 150 min/week recommendation. Postoperative bout-related MVPA was estimated to be higher when measured with the RT3 accelerometer in Bond's study [33] ($n=20$; mean of 40 ± 71 min/week at 6 months) as well as the previously described study by Josbeno et al. [23] of participants who wore the SenseWear Pro Armband 2–5 years postsurgery ($n=40$; mean = 49 ± 69 min/week). However, all three studies estimated that, on average, postoperative patients' PA level is well below recommendations. Thus, it appears that despite experiencing substantial weight loss and other positive surgical outcomes, many patients still experience difficulty in adhering to habitual PA postoperatively. Consequently, there is a need to offer appropriate preoperative and postoperative PA prescriptions, guidance, and counseling within the context of a multidisciplinary care program.

Developing Appropriate Exercise and Physical Activity Prescriptions for the Preoperative and Postoperative Bariatric Surgery Patient

Rationale for Prescribing Exercise and PA Preoperatively

While preoperative patients may be particularly prone to PA barriers (to be described later), there are several reasons that support the implementation of exercise prescriptions preoperatively versus delaying until the postoperative period [4, 15]. First, most patients do not meet PA recommendations and are highly sedentary preoperatively. Thus, increasing PA preoperatively may improve health and health-related quality of life, reduce short-term surgical complications, and accelerate recovery. Second, many patients are both ready and able to change their PA behavior preoperatively. For example, preliminary findings from the ongoing National Institutes of Health (NIH)-funded Bari-Active randomized controlled trial involving a 6-week preoperative PA counseling intervention suggest that patients with initial low PA levels can achieve large increases in objectively measured bout-related MVPA, consistent with national guidelines [36]. Third, most patients fail to substantially increase their PA postoperatively despite experiencing rapid and significant weight loss, reporting the majority of the same barriers to PA as preoperative patients. Thus, addressing exercise barriers preoperatively may help patients establish healthy exercise attitudes and develop effective coping strategies that carry over into the postoperative period.

Preoperative Exercise and PA Prescription

Components of the preoperative exercise prescription include mode, frequency, duration, intensity, and progression. Traditionally, the three modes of activities that comprise a balanced exercise prescription include: (1) aerobic or endurance activities that are repetitive and increase breathing and heart rate over an extended period of time (e.g., brisk walking, jogging, swimming); (2) strength or resistance activities that work major muscle groups against some type of resistance (body weight, machines, free weights) to augment muscle tissue; and (3) flexibility activities that lengthen muscles and improve range of motion around a joint (e.g., stretching, yoga, T'ai Chi). Implementing a prescription that integrates all of these activities may overwhelm preoperative patients, however, who tend to be novice exercisers. Consequently, it is appropriate to begin by focusing on aerobic exercises, which provide the greatest health benefits (e.g., reduced cholesterol, increased metabolism, improved muscular endurance, etc.).

Consistent with the national recommendations and informal preoperative PA guidelines discussed previously, patients should gradually progress to performing at least 30 min of structured aerobic exercise at a moderate intensity (which patients can measure using methods such as the "talk test" and the RPE scale discussed earlier) on at least 5 days during the week. To achieve health benefits, structured PA should be accumulated either in a single daily long bout or in multiple shorter bouts of at least 10 min in duration throughout the day. Prescribing exercise in shorter bouts may serve as an efficacious strategy to counter barriers such as inadequate fitness level and perceived lack of time. Whether one daily long bout or several shorter bouts is planned, encouraging patients to find consistent times to exercise on a daily basis may better help to establish this behavior as a habit.

In addition to structured bouts of PA, patients should also be encouraged to increase their lifestyle-related PA, which involves making more "active choices" throughout the day (e.g., taking the stairs instead of the elevator, walking into buildings versus using drive-through windows, manually opening doors, etc.). While these activities are typically of shorter duration and thus may not contribute to improvements in endurance, they can reduce the amount of time spent being sedentary, increase overall energy expenditure, and possibly improve mobility, strength, and balance. Patients should also be advised to reduce the amount of time that they spend performing sedentary behaviors such as watching TV and using the computer, as these activities, independent of PA level, can potentially undermine achievement of optimal postoperative outcomes [8].

Postoperative Exercise and PA Prescription

The components of the preoperative and postoperative PA prescription are identical. However, in the immediate postoperative period, patients may have to "restart" gradually to allow for adequate recovery time. For example, patients who have undergone RYGB might be encouraged to get up and walk in the hospital for brief 1–2 min periods to improve circulation, walk around the house during the first 1–4 postoperative weeks, and then slowly start to increase PA in weeks 5–6. After progressing beyond the initial recovery period, patients should be advised to gradually progress to levels of PA that are consistent with guidelines to enhance weight loss and prevent significant weight regain (i.e., accumulation of 250–300 weekly minutes of moderate-intensity PA in bouts of at least 10 min in duration). Patients can start with 10 min of continuous moderate-intensity activity each day and then increase this amount by 5 min every 1–2 weeks until the goal is achieved.

Given their larger size and the greater volume of sweat that their bodies produce, bariatric surgery patients will require more fluid during PA than nonobese individuals. However, fluid consumption is limited postoperatively. Thus, patients should be advised to take frequent sips of water and exercise in cool temperatures when possible. Postoperative patients should also be encouraged to integrate strength activities into their routine to better preserve lean body mass and improve balance and coordination. However, given the potential for rapid weight loss to alter the body's center of gravity, patients should be especially careful when performing exercises that employ a higher degree of balance and coordination and/or perform these exercises under supervision until weight has stabilized. Strength training exercises that target the abdominal and lower back regions should also be avoided for the first few postoperative months to allow for sufficient healing. Finally, similar to the prescribed preoperative regimen, patients should continue to focus on increasing their lifestyle activity and decreasing sedentary behaviors [4, 15].

Individualizing Exercise and PA Prescriptions

PA prescriptions should be individualized or tailored to patients to address differences in health status, disease risk factors, physical capacity, personal goals, and exercise preferences. As shown in Table 22.2, the five As (*assess*, *advise*, *agree*, *assist*, and *arrange*) provide a useful organizational framework for this purpose [37]. Clinicians can begin by conducting an interview with a patient to *assess* PA-related knowledge, beliefs, and values, past PA experiences, PA mode preferences, readiness and confidence to change PA behavior, and potential obstacles to adherence to the exercise prescription. It is important to appreciate that engaging in a habitual PA program is not easy. Common barriers reported by adults include lack of time, childcare, and safe and affordable facilities or outdoor environments. In addition to overcoming these "run of the mill" barriers, severely obese adults may have additional barriers to PA that are unique to their size and health status. For example, they may lack confidence to go to a gym or fitness facility because they are unable to keep up in regular group exercise classes, they are too heavy to use much of the equipment and/or do not know how to use it, or they are simply too embarrassed to exercise in front of others. Due to low cardiorespiratory fitness or poor sleep quality, they may have excessive fatigue, such that they feel they lack sufficient energy to exercise. They may also suffer from osteoarthritis, chronic back pain, or other conditions that make many types of exercise painful or difficult to do. Finally, a history of activity-related injuries, impaired balance, or misinterpretation of normal side effects from exercising (e.g., muscle soreness or heavy breathing) may cause them to fear that exercise is dangerous to their health. Thus, it is very important to assess patients' confidence in their ability to increase their PA, as well as to objectively assess patients' ability to safely engage in and increase PA. For example, patients with symptoms and/or history of heart disease and other conditions may require formal testing before initiating habitual PA and will likely have to be progressed at a slower rate than patients without these conditions. Additionally, patients who are taking heart medications that can lower resting heart rate such as beta-blockers and angiotensin-converting enzyme (ACE) inhibitors should be given a lower heart rate target or instructed to use the talk test to monitor their PA intensity [4, 15].

After conducting the initial assessment, clinicians should *advise* the patient on the benefits of habitual PA, how to

Table 22.2 Clinician's guide to providing physical activity counseling to the bariatric surgery patient

Assess	Patient's knowledge, beliefs, and values regarding physical activity (PA)
	PA history, current PA level, and PA preferences
	Readiness to change, motivation, self-confidence, and barriers to implementing a PA program
	PA, physical function, and general health goals
	Physical limitations and pain associated with PA; refer to physical therapy as needed
	Patient's ability to safely increase PA; refer high-risk patients for exercise testing
Advise	Enhance motivation by summarizing the benefits of PA
	Help patient develop realistic expectations
	Discuss safety-related issues and provide guidance on how to minimize risks
	Provide strategies on how to overcome barriers to PA
	Teach patients how to gauge their PA intensity
	Tailor PA recommendations to the patients' capabilities and readiness
Agree	Collaborate with patient to determine specific PA goals (including type, duration, frequency, and intensity) and the time frame for goal evaluation and modification
	Provide written exercise contract including short-, mid- and long-term goals (include copies in medical file)
Assist	Teach patient behavioral strategies to be successful
	Provide printed material and online resources that support counseling messages
	Provide tools for self-monitoring PA such as pedometers and PA diaries
	Provide list of community resources for participating in PA, including safe walking paths
	Refer patients to exercise specialists as needed
Arrange	Share patient's PA plan with clinic staff/members of the bariatric team to establish team consensus and commitment
	Schedule follow-up contacts (in person or over the phone) to answer questions, discuss attainment of goals, provide positive reinforcement for progress toward goals, and revise treatment plan as needed
	Provide ongoing PA counseling at future appointments

Table reprinted with permission from King and Bond [4]

exercise safely, and physiological sensations such as dull muscle aches that typically occur when first initiating an exercise program versus physical symptoms that signal an exercise session should be terminated and medical attention should be sought (e.g., nausea, light-headedness, difficulty breathing, cold or clammy skin, angina). Given all of the barriers to PA, it is also critical that patients are not just told what to do, but are given ideas for overcoming barriers to adopting and maintaining a habitual PA routine. For example, while walking serves as a convenient and practical endurance exercise for most patients, some patients may have greater physical limitations or require mobility aids that necessitate introduction of alternative activities. Patients with sensory, balance, or gait deficits should be referred to physical therapy where they will be given specific rehabilitative exercise to address their specific problems. Other patients with knee, hip, or back pain may benefit from using a stationary bike or elliptical machine that better supports their weight and thus are lower impact. These patients may also benefit from physical therapy. Adults who lack confidence to exercise at a gym should be encouraged to try exercising at home with exercise videos, which are often available for free at local libraries, or to start out with a walking program. They should also be informed that many gyms and fitness facilities offer orientation programs to help new members become familiar with the various types of equipment and classes that are available and appropriate. Many community-oriented gyms offer lower intensity classes that are very welcoming of all ability levels, such as restorative yoga, arthritis aqua classes, and chair aerobics. Patients should also be taught problem-solving strategies. For instance, after a patient describes a barrier, the patient should be asked to brainstorm several possible solutions and then choose and implement what sounds like the best solution. After a week, the patient should be told to evaluate that choice and reconsider other options if the barrier persists [4, 15].

Based on the patients' capabilities and readiness, the clinician should *advise* the patient on appropriate short-, intermediate-, and long-term PA goals that are clearly defined in terms of mode, duration, frequency, and intensity. However, the relationship between the clinician and patient should be collaborative, such that both parties *agree* on the patient's PA goals, the expected goal achievement, and a plan for modification if goals prove too challenging and are not met. Goals should be realistic and attainable to enable the patient to develop a sense of confidence and mastery and should ultimately provide reinforcement and motivation for continued engagement in habitual PA. One way to help make these objectives more concrete for the patient is for the clinician and patient to develop a written behavioral contract. The contract should include short-, mid-, and long-term goals, a timeline and rewards for achievements, reasons for committing to an active lifestyle, and a list of persons who can provide support to the patient as they strive to change their PA behavior [4, 15].

Clinicians can *assist* patients to fulfill the components of their contract by teaching them PA behavioral change strategies. For example, once goals are clearly set, clinicians should help patients become active participants of the action planning and tailoring process by asking them to plan when, where, and how they will accumulate PA throughout each day according to their schedule of activities. Patients may also benefit from learning to establish specific incremental weekly goals that will help them reach their longer-term goals and can help them stay motivated and improve their self-efficacy. Learning to celebrate "small successes" on the way to PA goals is also a great way to stay motivated, especially when external rewards for goal achievement support PA (e.g., new workout outfit). Patients should also be taught to pay attention to internal rewards from PA, such as having more energy and feeling stronger. Other important behavioral strategies for adopting and maintaining a habitual PA routine include stimulus control and social support. Stimulus control involves adding cues to the external environment to promote PA, such as leaving an extra pair of walking shoes at work and setting up a reminder in one's calendar, and removing cues that promote sedentary behavior, such as avoiding the TV room and turning off the computer after each use. Social support involves recruiting family and friends to support one's PA goals. Having a walking partner, someone to carpool with to the gym, or a workout buddy to meet at the gym can be especially helpful. Patients should also be encouraged to enlist friends or family members to help with childcare or call, text, or email to ask about progress toward PA goals. Clinicians can also *assist* patients by providing self-monitoring tools (e.g., PA diaries and inexpensive pedometers); printed material, such as lists and/or maps with local health/fitness facilities; parks; walking paths; and online resources for education and motivational material (see Appendix at the end of this chapter for a list of online resources that may be helpful to both clinicians and patients) [4, 15].

Finally, clinicians should *arrange* ongoing contact and support to patients. This may involve periodic phone calls and additional face-to-face, individual sessions to evaluate progress toward goals, make necessary modifications, and provide additional reinforcement. Patients should be made aware that experiencing slips along the way is a normal part of the behavior change process and that the strategies they have learned can help to get them back on track [4, 15]. Patients with persistent barriers to habitual PA participation should be referred to appropriate specialists as per ASMBS's Allied Health Nutritional Guidelines.

Conclusion

PA has long been a cornerstone of lifestyle treatments for obesity. Research has demonstrated that adding a habitual PA program to a prescribed caloric-restricted diet yields greater weight loss, compared to caloric restriction alone. There is a growing body of evidence that higher levels of PA may also play a role in optimizing weight loss and other outcomes after bariatric surgery. However, recent research using objective monitoring methods indicates that many bariatric surgery patients are both inactive and highly sedentary preoperatively and postoperatively. Consequently, there is a need to integrate preoperative and postoperative PA counseling within a multidisciplinary patient care approach. The five As (*assess*, *advise*, *agree*, *assist*, and *arrange*) provide a useful organizational framework for effective PA counseling. PA prescriptions should be individualized to patients to address differences in health status, disease risk factors, physical capacity, personal goals, and exercise preferences.

Future Work

Research is needed to determine how type, intensity, frequency, and duration of PA are related to clinically significant improvements in outcomes of bariatric surgery and the most efficacious strategies to increase preoperative and postoperative PA within treatment-controlled designs.

Question and Answer Section

Questions

1. Research has shown that higher levels of physical activity are associated with improvements in all of the following postoperative outcomes except:
   A. Weight loss
   B. Body composition
   C. Health-related quality of life
   D. Long-term weight loss maintenance
2. Recent studies using objective monitors to assess physical activity in bariatric surgery patients have shown all of the following except:
   A. More than half of preoperative patients do not accumulate any moderate-to-vigorous-intensity physical activity in structured bouts of at least 10 min in duration.
   B. Most bariatric surgery patients make substantial increases in their physical activity postoperatively.

C. Most bariatric surgery patients do not meet physical activity recommendations for US adults (i.e., 150 min of moderate-intensity PA/week) postoperatively.

D. Preoperative bariatric surgery patients spend, on average, 80 % of their time in sedentary behaviors.

3. When a patient comes to a medical appointment at the surgical center, how can the bariatric team help encourage that patient to increase their physical activity? (Select all that apply.)

   A. Assess a patient's fitness, physical limitations, barriers to physical activity, and motivation to determine an appropriate physical activity goal.
   B. Help the patient identify specific physical activities that he/she can do, prefers (i.e., is not adverse to), and has the necessary resources to perform (e.g., pool, safe walking path, home videos with chair exercises, etc.).
   C. Tell the patient that they should walk for at least 150 min/week to improve their health.
   D. Have all members of the bariatric team mention the importance of physical activity during their interaction with the patient.
   E. Increase motivation by discussing how physical activity impacts health outcomes, especially those that are important to the individual patient (e.g., diabetes, sleep quality).

Answers

1. Answer is **D**. Although several studies suggest that engagement in higher levels of physical activity during the period of active weight loss after bariatric surgery may contribute to enhanced weight loss, no studies to date have directly examined whether physical activity contributes to improved long-term maintenance of weight loss.
2. Answer is **B**. While previous research indicates that patients report large increases in their physical activity postoperatively, studies using objective monitors do not support these findings and show that most patients fail to make significant changes in their physical activity postoperatively, despite experiencing marked weight loss.
3. Answers are **A**, **B**, **D**, and **E**. While ideally all patients will work toward a goal of accumulating at least 150 min/week of moderate-intensity physical activity, it is not appropriate to assume all patients can walk at this level when they start a physical activity program, and it is important to teach patients that they can achieve health benefits by increasing their physical activity level and doing various forms of exercise (even if they cannot walk or walk for 150 min/week at the start of their physical activity program).

Appendix: Online Resources

The National Physical Activity Plan by Centers for Disease Control and Prevention: http://www.cdc.gov/physicalactivity/index.html

- A comprehensive set of policies, programs, and initiatives aimed at increasing physical activity in all segments of the American population. There are sections aimed at health professionals as well as the general public, and specifically for older adults.

Physical Activity Guidelines for Americans by US Department of Health and Human Services: http://www.health.gov/paguidelines/

- In 2008, the federal government issued these evidence-based guidelines, described in detail and more briefly, along with material for individuals (i.e., "Be Active Your Way").

Be Active Your Way: A Guide for Adults by US Department of Health and Human Services: http://www.health.gov/paguidelines/adultguide/activeguide.aspx

- Sections include: getting started, making physical activity part of your life, keeping it up, stepping it up, and being active for life, which includes a physical activity diary. In addition to the guide information is summarized in a shorter fact sheet.

Get Active by US Department of Health and Human Services: http://www.healthfinder.gov/prevention/ViewTopic.aspx?topicID=22&cnt=1&areaID=0

- This site offers a background section, "The Basics," which provides educational information on physical activity and a "Take Action" section, which provides advice on how to be more active, tailored to individual's current physical activity level.

Get Moving by American Heart Association: http://www.heart.org/HEARTORG/GettingHealthy/PhysicalActivity/Physical-Activity_UCM_001080_SubHomePage.jsp

- Physical activity and inactivity information and advice on how to start an exercise program.

The Health Care Providers Action Guide by Exercise is Medicine: http://exerciseismedicine.org/physicians.htm

- A thorough exercise guide for health-care providers that includes information on providing prescriptions and referrals and assessment tools that can be used with patients.

The Public Action Guide by Exercise is Medicine: http://exerciseismedicine.org/documents/PublicActionGuide_HR.pdf

- A thorough exercise guide for individuals that includes a pre-exercise health assessment, a barrier to exercise assessment, an exercise time finder, and other motivational tools.

Walking, A Step in the Right Direction, by the Weight-control Information Network: http://win.niddk.nih.gov/publications/walking.htm

- An online brochure that describes how to create and follow a walking plan. Sections include: walking for your health, know before you go, start walking now, walking safely, stretch it out, and step right this way.

Walking Guide by the American Heart Association: http://www.startwalkingnow.org/home.jsp
- This walking guide includes a quiz that can be used to get a personalized walking plan, an activity tracker, and information on walking clubs and walking paths throughout the country.

Walking Works by BlueCross BlueShield Association: http://www.bcbs.com/why-bcbs/walkingworks/
- This walking guide provides information on how to start a walking program and a walking log.

Tips for Increasing Physical Activity by US Department of Agriculture: http://www.choosemyplate.gov/physical-activity/increase-physical-activity.html
- Tips for increasing physical activity at home, at work, and at play. The Website www.choosemyplate.gov also has sections on physical activity, its importance, how much is needed, and how many calories are used.

Tips for Family Fitness Fun in Shape Up America by Health Weight for Life: http://www.shapeup.org/children/tips_index.html
- Provides several handouts in English and Spanish, on tips for being more active with your family. The Website www.shapeup.org also has health messages on the importance of maintaining a healthy weight and increasing physical activity.

Workout descriptions in Get Fit and Moving by American Council on Exercise: http://www.acefitness.org/getfit/default.aspx
- Descriptions of various types of workouts (high/thigh, core, total body, at home, lunch time) are provided. This site may be more helpful for postoperative patients who have some exercise experience.

Exercise While Traveling by American College of Sports Medicine: http://www.acsm.org/docs/current-comments/exercisewhiletraveling.pdf
- Ideas for how to stick with an exercise routine even when traveling.

Public Information from the American College of Sports Medicine: http://www.acsm.org/access-public-information/search-by-topic
- Provides publications, audiotapes, and videotapes on physical fitness and weight loss for health professionals and the general public.

When to see a physician before exercising by American College of Sports Medicine: http://www.acsm.org/docs/current-comments/whentoseeadoctortemp.pdf
- Describes a risk stratification scheme physicians can use to determine which patients need to undergo exercise testing before initiating a new exercise program.

Patient-Centered Assessment and Counseling for Exercise (PACE) program: http://rtips.cancer.gov/rtips/programDetails.do?programId=199774
- Information on PACE, an individually adapted health behavior change intervention to increase physical activity of patients, suitable for implementation in a physician's office.

Energy Expenditure in Different Modes of Exercise by American College of Sports Medicine: http://www.acsm.org/docs/current-comments/energyexpendindifferentexmodes.pdf
- Describes energy expenditure from different modes of exercise as well as several other factors that should be considered when selecting an exercise mode.

Exercise for Persons with Cardiovascular Disease by American College of Sports Medicine: http://www.acsm.org/docs/current-comments/exercise-for-persons-with-cardiovascular-disease.pdf
- Describes how exercise in an integral component of a comprehensive approach to treating heart disease, while describing risks of exercise relevant to patients with cardiovascular disease, as well as compliance issues and behavioral strategies to help patients meet their exercise goals.

Resistance Training and Injury Prevention by American College of Sports Medicine: http://www.acsm.org/docs/current-comments/rtandip.pdf
- Describes the effect resistance training has on the bone, connective tissue, and muscle and advocates for patients to see an exercise physiologist or sports trainer to develop a safe and effective program.

References

1. Bouchard C, Blair SN, Haskell W. Why study physical activity and health? In: Bouchard C, Blair SN, Haskell WL, editors. Physical activity and health. Champaign: Human Kinetics; 2007. p. 3–19.
2. Jakicic JM, Davis KK. Obesity and physical activity. Psychiatr Clin N Am. 2011;34:829–40.
3. Wing RR. Physical activity for weight loss maintenance. In: Bouchard C, Katzmarzyk PT, editors. Physical activity and obesity. 2nd ed. Champaign: Human Kinetics; 2010. p. 245–8.
4. King WC, Bond DS. The importance of pre- and postoperative physical activity counseling in bariatric surgery. Exerc Sport Sci Rev. 2013;41(1):26–35.
5. Jacobi D, Ciangura C, Couet C, Oppert JM. Physical activity and weight loss following bariatric surgery. Obes Rev. 2011;12:366–77.
6. Thomas JG, Bond DS, Sarwer DB, Wing RR. Technology for behavioral assessment and intervention in bariatric surgery. Surg Obes Relat Dis. 2011;7:548–57.
7. Warburton D. The physical activity and exercise continuum. In: Bouchard C, Katzmarzyk PT, editors. Physical activity and obesity. 2nd ed. Champaign: Human Kinetics; 2010. p. 7–12.
8. Thorp AA, Owen N, Neuhaus M, Dunstan DW. Sedentary behaviors and subsequent health outcomes in adults a systematic review

of longitudinal studies, 1996–2011. Am J Prev Med. 2011 Aug;41(2):207–15. doi:10.1016/j.amepre.2011.05.004. Review
9. Owen N, Healy GN, Matthews CE, Dunstan DW. Too much sitting: the population health science of sedentary behavior. Exerc Sport Sci Rev. 2010;38:105–13.
10. King WC, Hames K, Goodpaster B. BMI predicts walking speed at which moderate-intensity physical activity is achieved. Med Sci Sports Exerc. 2010;42:S514.
11. Mechanick JL, Kushner R, Sugerman HJ, Gonzalez-Campoy JM, Collazo-Clavell ML, Spitz AF, et al. American association of clinical endocrinologists; obesity society; american society for metabolic and bariatric surgery. american association of clinical endocrinologists, the obesity society, and american society for metabolic and bariatric surgery medical guidelines for clinical practice of the perioperative nutritional, metabolic, and nonsurgical support of the bariatric surgery patient. Obesity (Silver Spring). 2009;17 suppl 1:S1–70.
12. Blackburn GL, Hutter MM, Harvey AM, Apovian CM, Boulton HR, Cummings S, et al. Expert panel on weight loss surgery: executive report update. Obesity (Silver Spring). 2009;17:842–62.
13. Poirier P, Cornier MA, Maazone T, Stiles S, Cummings S, Klein S, et al. American Heart Association Obesity Committee of the Council on Nutrition, Physical Activity, and Metabolism. Bariatric surgery and cardiovascular risk factors: a scientific statement from the American Heart Association. Circulation. 2011;19:1683–701.
14. U.S. Department of Health and Human Services (USDHHS). Physical activity guidelines and advisory committee report, 2008. http://www.health.gov/pagguidelines/report/ Accessed 7 Aug 2012.
15. Zunker C, King WC. Physical activity pre- and post bariatric surgery. In: Mitchell JE, de Zwaan M, editors. Psychosocial assessment and treatment of bariatric surgery patients. London: Psychology Press and Routledge, part of the Taylor and Francis Group; 2011. p. 131–58. ISBN-10: 0415892198.
16. Donnelly JE, Blair SN, Jakicic JM, Manore MM, Rankin JW, Smith BK. Appropriate physical activity intervention strategies for weight loss and prevention of weight regain in adults. Med Sci Sports Exerc. 2009;41:459–71.
17. Goodpaster BH, DeLany JP, Otto AD, Kuller L, Vockley J, South-Paul JE, et al. Effects of diet and physical activity interventions on weight loss and cardiometabolic risk factors in severely obese adults: a randomized trial. JAMA. 2010;304:1795–802.
18. Catenacci VA, Grunwald GK, Ingebrigsten JP, Jakicic JM, McDermott MD, Phelan S, et al. Physical activity patterns using the accelerometry in the national weight control registry. Obesity (Silver Spring). 2011;19:1163–70.
19. Livhits M, Mercado C, Yermilov I, Parikh JA, Dutson E, Mehran A, et al. Exercise following bariatric surgery: a systematic review. Obes Surg. 2010;20:657–65.
20. Colles SL, Dixon JB, O'Brien PE. Hunger control and regular physical activity facilitate weight loss after laparoscopic adjustable gastric banding. Obes Surg. 2008;18:833–40.
21. King WC, Hsu JY, Belle SH, Courcoulas AP, Eid GM, Flum DR, et al. Pre- to postoperative changes in physical activity: report from the longitudinal assessment of bariatric surgery-2. Surg Obes Relat Dis. 2012;8(5):522–32.
22. Egberts K, Brown WA, O'Brien PE. Optimising lifestyle factors to achieve weight loss in surgical patients. Surg Obes Relat Dis. 2011;7:368.
23. Josbeno DA, Kalarchian M, Sparto PJ, Otto AD, Jakicic JM. Physical activity and physical function in individuals post-bariatric surgery. Obes Surg. 2011;21:1243–9.
24. Bond DS, Phelan S, Leahey TM, Hill JO, Wing RR. Weight-loss maintenance in successful weight losers: surgical vs non-surgical methods. Int J Obes. 2009;33:173–80.
25. McCullough PA, Gallagher MJ, Dejong AT, Sandberg KR, Trivax JE, Alexander D, et al. Cardiorespiratory fitness and short-term complications after bariatric surgery. Chest. 2006;130:517–25.
26. Shah M, Snell PH, Rao S, Adams-Huet B, Quittner C, Livingston EH, et al. High-volume exercise program in obese bariatric surgery patients: a randomized, controlled trial. Obesity (Silver Spring). 2011;19:1826–34.
27. Bond DS, Phelan S, Wolfe LG, Evans RK, Meador JG, Kellum JM, et al. Becoming physically active after bariatric surgery is associated with improved weight loss and health-related quality of life. Obesity. 2009;17:78–83.
28. Rosenberger PH, Henderson KE, White MA, Masheb RM, Grilo CM. Physical activity in gastric bypass patients: associations with weight loss and psychosocial functioning at 12-month follow-up. Obes Surg. 2011;21(10):1564–9.
29. Larsen JK, Geenen R, van Ramshorst B, Brand N, Hox JJ, Stroebe W, van Doornen LJ. Binge eating and exercise behavior after surgery for severe obesity: a structural equation model. Int J Eat Disord. 2006;39(5):369–75.
30. Josbeno DA, Jakicic JM, Hergenroeder A, Eid GM. Physical activity and physical function changes in obese individuals after gastric bypass surgery. Surg Obes Relat Dis. 2010;6:361–6.
31. Tudor-Locke C, Bassett DR Jr. How many steps/day are enough? Preliminary pedometer indices for public health. Sports Med 2004;34:1–8.
32. King WC, Belle SH, Eid GM, Dakin GF, Inabnet WB, Mitchell JE, et al. Longitudinal assessment of bariatric surgery study. physical activity levels of patients undergoing bariatric surgery in the longitudinal assessment of bariatric surgery study. Surg Obes Relat Dis. 2008;4:721–8.
33. Bond DS, Jakicic JM, Vithiananthan S, Thomas JG, Leahey TM, Sax HC, et al. Objective quantification of physical activity in bariatric surgery candidates and normal-weight controls. Surg Obes Relat Dis. 2010;6:72–8.
34. Bond DS, Unick JL, Jakicic JM, Vithiananthan S, Pohl D, Roye GD, et al. Objective assessment of time spent being sedentary in bariatric surgery candidates. Obes Surg. 2011;21:811–4.
35. Bond DS, Jakicic JM, Unick JL, Vithiananthan S, Pohl D, Roye GD, et al. Pre- to postoperative physical activity changes in bariatric surgery patients: self-report vs. objective measures. Obesity (Silver Spring). 2010;18:2395–7.
36. Bond DS. Bari-active: a preoperative behavioral intervention to increase physical activity. Obes Surg. 2011;21:1042.
37. Meriwether RA, Lee JA, Lafleur AS, Wiseman P. Physical activity counseling. Am Fam Physician. 2008;77:1129–36.

Index

A
Accelerometers
 and cameras, 57
 and EMA, 61
 physical activity, 57
Acceptance and Commitment Therapy (ACT), 152
Achieving, new normal lifestyle
 behaviors and ways of thinking, 138
 description, 136
 dietary lifestyle, 136–138
 physical activity, 138
ACT. *See* Acceptance and Commitment Therapy (ACT)
Adherence
 bariatric surgery, 49
 dietary and behavioral recommendations, 49
 medical/psychological treatment, 37
 memory, 50
 multivitamin infusion, 115
 postoperative guidelines, 49–50
 preoperative eating disorders, 50
 smartphones, 60
 vitamin and mineral supplementation, 87
Adjustable gastric banding (AGB), 135
Aills, L., 81, 82, 85, 135
Alcohol
 blood alcohol content (BAC), 47–48
 consumption, 167
 preoperative assessment and treatment recommendations, 48
 prevalence, 47
 and substance use, 46
 use/abuse, 70
Alcohol use disorder (AUD), 210
Alger-Mayer, S., 27
Allison, K.C., 3–8, 209
American Association of Clinical Endocrinologists (AACE), 219
American Society for Metabolic and Weight Loss Surgery (ASMBS). *See* Bariatric surgery
American Society of Parenteral and Enteral Nutrition (ASPEN), 86
Amino acids
 dietary and endogenous proteins, 101
 nitrogen-containing compounds, 102
 and postprandial protein synthesis, 103
Anastomotic leak detection, 180
Anemia
 etiologies, postoperative, 116
 megaloblastic, 115
 and myelodysplastic changes, bone marrow precursors, 112
 and myelopathy, 116

Anorexia, 122, 124–125
Anorexia nervosa (AN), 30, 46
Antidepressant/mood-altering medications, 179
Anxiety
 clinicians, patients normalization, 34
 and depression, 11, 44
 and mood disorder, 36
Apovian, C., 157–162
Appel, L., 150
Applegate, K.L., 33–41
ASPEN. *See* American Society of Parenteral and Enteral Nutrition (ASPEN)
Aspirin and ibuprofen products, 179
Astrup, A., 107
Ataxia
 and paresthesias, 116
 thiamin deficiency identification, 114
 Wernicke's encephalopathy, with risks of, 112
AUD. *See* Alcohol use disorder (AUD)

B
B12, 119, 120
Bailer, B.A., 3–8
Bandura, A., 96
Bariatric surgery. *See also* Educational and counseling needs; Medical approach, postoperative weight regain; Physical activity (PA)
 combined restrictive and malabsorptive procedures, 119–120
 eating disorders (*See* Eating disorders)
 habitual postoperative PA program, 151
 lower mean consumption of, 152
 medical management (*see* Medical management)
 medical preparation (*see* Medical preparation)
 morbidity and mortality, 151
 NCP (*see* Nutrition care process (NCP))
 post hoc analysis, 152
 postoperative dietary regimen/adaptive eating behaviors, 151
 postoperative nutrition assessment and follow-up (*see* Postoperative nutrition assessment and follow-up)
 preoperative nutrition assessment and follow-up (*see* Preoperative nutrition assessment and follow-up)
 psychological assessment (*see* Psychological assessment)
 psychopathology (*see* Psychopathology)
 psychosocial status (*see* Psychosocial status)
 quality of life (*see* Quality of life)
 registered dietitian, 151
 restrictive procedures, 119
Beck depression inventories (BDI), 38, 209, 222

BED. See Binge eating disorder (BED)
Behavior
   AUD, 210
   depression and suicidal, 45
   description, 209
   diet and eating, 148
   diet and exercise, 158
   dietary caloric intake, 209–210
   dietary intake and eating, 151
   dysfunctional sexual, 22
   eating disorders (see Eating disorders)
   maladaptive, 149
   physical activity, 210
   support/follow-up, 210
Behavioral assessment
   food in response, emotional stress, 167
   long-term surgical outcomes, 168
   mental health evaluation, 168
   patient evaluation/selection process, 168
   psychopathology, 168
Behavioral health specialist, 186
Benotti, P.N., 165–172
Beriberi, thiamin deficiency, 112
BID. See Body image dissatisfaction (BID)
Bi-level positive airway pressure (BiPAP)
   laparoscopic RYGB patients, 177
   noninvasive positive pressure devices, 177
Binge eating disorder (BED)
   alcohol abuse, 39
   behavior pre-and postsurgery, 26, 27
   and depression, 44
   diagnostic criteria, 45
   EDE, 26
   and LOC, 15, 28–29, 46
   mood disorders, 67
   and NES, 36, 45
   pre-and postsurgery, weight loss/regain postsurgery, 26, 27
   preoperative patients, 26, 45
   prevalence rates, 25, 67
   screening measurement, 39
   syndrome, 26
BiPAP. See Bi-level positive airway pressure (BiPAP)
Bishop-Gilyard, C.T., 19–23
Blackstone, R., 177
Boan, J., 27
Bocchieri-Ricciardi, 27
Body image
   appearance-enhancing behaviors, 21
   body shape questionnaire (BSQ), 22
   description, 21
   plastic surgical procedures, 22
   in postoperative patients, 49
   weight loss, 21, 49
Body image dissatisfaction (BID)
   description, 68
   obesity, 23
Bond, D.S., 55–63, 217–227
Bone metabolism
   fat-soluble vitamins, 125
   hyperoxaluria, 125–126
   malabsorptive procedures, 125
   vitamin D and calcium, 125
Bone reabsorption, 125
Borkgren-Okonek, M.J., 178
Bradley, L.E., 147–153

Brunault, 27
Buchwald, H., 91
Bupropion plus naltrexone, 161
Burgmer, 27
Busetto, L., 27
Butryn, M.L., 147–153

C
Calcium
   supplements, 125
   and vitamin D, 125
Carbohydrates
   amylose and amylopectin, 104
   dextrins, 105
   digestion and absorption, 104
   disaccharides and polysaccharides, 104
   glucose and galactose, 105
   requirements, 105
   triacylglycerol-raising effects, sucrose, 105
   WLS, 105
Cardiac
   bariatric surgery, impact on, 169–170
   cardiovascular physiology, obesity, 170
   exercise testing, 170
   guidelines, 170
   maladaptive remodeling, 169
   "reverse remodeling", 170
   risk factors, 170
   stress echocardiography, 170
Carvajal, R., 19–23
Cash, T.F., 21
CBT. See Cognitive behavior therapy (CBT)
Child maltreatment, 6
Christou, N.V., 206
Clinical domain
   altered GI function, 81
   biochemical category, 81
   defined, 81
   weight category, 81–82
Clinical predictors
   description, 196
   preoperative BMI, 196
   preoperative weight loss, 197
   variables, 197
   weight loss, bariatric surgery, 195–196
Cognitive behavior therapy (CBT)
   to bariatric surgery patients, application, 97, 98
   components, 97
   internal/external cues, 96
   weight management, 96
Collazo-Clavel, M., 168
Colles, S.L., 27, 176
Colonic preparations, preoperative bariatric surgery, 176
Competency
   assignment process, 188
   domains, JCAHO, 188
Comprehensive medical evaluation, 168
Continuous positive airway pressure (CPAP)
   after laparoscopic RYGB, 177
   obstructive sleep apnea postoperatively, 177–178
Counseling. See Educational and counseling needs
Cox, T.L., 21
CPAP. See Continuous positive airway pressure (CPAP)
Crowley, 27

D

DAA. *See* Dispensable amino acids (DAA)
Dalencourt, G., 165–172
Dansinger, M.L., 104
Dehydration, 121, 123
De Man Lapidoth, 27
DeMaria, E.J., 171
Depression
    and anxiety, 12, 44
    and BED, 44
    diagnosis, 44
    and excess weight, 5
    features, 44
    Hamilton rating scale, 38
    LSG, 43–44
    and mood disorders, 44
    and obesity, 43
    preoperative, 44
    and suicide, 45
    symptoms, 5
Depressive symptoms
    obesity, 5
    psychotherapeutic care, 5
    weight and depression, 5
Determinants, weight regain. *See* Medical approach, postoperative weight regain
DEXA. *See* Dual-energy X-ray absorptiometry (DEXA) scans
de Zwaan, M., 11–16, 25–31, 124, 209
Diabetes
    adverse hypoglycemic effect, 177
    comorbid medical problems, obesity, 176
Diabetes medications, weight loss
    GLP-1 agonists, 161
    metformin, 161
    pramlintide, 162
Diabetes prevention program, 149
Diabetes support and education (DSE), 149–150
Diet
    evaluation and instruction, 82
    and nutrition, 96
    and physical activity, 59
    progression recommendations, 85–86
    quality, 94
    stages, 92
    weight loss, 77
Dietary lifestyle
    AHA recommendations, weight loss surgery patient, 136
    American society, metabolic and bariatric surgery, 136
    description, 136
    meal replacements and eating frequency, 137–138
    "my plate" tools, 136–137
    nutrition and dietetics academy, 136
    satiety, 138
Diet-progression recommendations
    bariatric surgeries, stages, 85
    blenderized/pureed diet, stage III, 86
    full-liquid diet, stage II, 85–86
    "mechanically soft diet", stage IV, 86
    regular bariatric diet stage, stage V, 86
    surgical procedure, 85
    weight loss surgery, stage I, 85
Disease management, 181
Dispensable amino acids (DAA), 101
Drug absorption
    intestinal pH, 178
    pharmacokinetic studies, 178
DSE. *See* Diabetes support and education (DSE)
Dual-energy X-ray absorptiometry (DEXA) scans, 87
Dumping syndrome
    and excess calories, 123
    gastrointestinal and vasomotor symptoms, 181
    "late dumping", 123
    protein supplements, 121
    with RNYGB, 123
DVT prevention, 178
Dymek, 27
Dyslipidemic medications, 179

E

Early nutrition
    constipation, 123–124
    dehydration, 121
    Dumping syndrome, 123
    flatulence, 122
    gastroesophageal reflux disease (GERD), 121–122
    gastrointestinal complications, 120
    halitosis, 123
    lactose intolerance, 122
    nausea and vomiting, 121
    pregnancy, 124
    protein energy malnutrition (PEM), 122–123
    soft foods, 121
Eating behavior
    dietary counseling, 83
    long-term success, bariatric patient, 77
    and preoperative psychosocial characteristics, 77
    tolerance and adherence, stage IV, 86
Eating disorders
    after, bariatric surgery
        AN, 30
        BED and LOC, 28–29
        caloric intake, 28
        chewing and spitting out food, 30
        EDE-BSV, 28
        grazing, 30
        night eating, 30
        sweet eating, 30
        vomiting, 29–30
    prior, bariatric surgery
        BED, 25–27
        description, 25
        grazing, 26
        NES, 26
        sweet eating, 28
    substance abuse, 196, 197
Ecological momentary assessment (EMA)
    accelerometers, 57
    alcohol consumption, 57
    bariatric surgery patients, 57
    protocol, 56
Educational and counseling needs
    The Academy of Nutrition and Dietetics, 95
    CBT, 96–97
    components, 95
    "forced behavior modification", 91
    health belief model, 96
    healthcare setting, 95
    language and cultural factors, 96
    learning needs assessment, 95
    literacy, numeracy and cognitive capacity, 95–96
    long-term postoperative (*see* Long-term postoperative)

Educational and counseling needs (cont.)
  motivational interviewing, 97
  NCP (see Nutrition Care Process (NCP))
  preferred learning styles, 95
  preoperative nutrition (see Preoperative nutrition educational and counseling)
  readiness to learn, 95
  registered dietitian (RD), 91–92
  safe and effective outcomes, 92
  short-term postoperative (see Short-term postoperative)
  social learning theory, 96
  transtheoretical model of change, 96, 97
Egberts, K., 221
EIM. See Exercise is Medicine® (EIM)
Elfhag, K., 209
Emotional eating, 94
Empathy, 187, 188, 190
Ernst, B., 111
Ethicon Endo-Surgery, 62
Excess weight loss (EWL), 48, 198, 206
Exercise
  individualizing and PA prescriptions, 224–226
  PA preoperatively, 223–224
  postoperative PA, 224
Exercise is Medicine® (EIM), 136
Exercise specialist, 187
Extreme obesity
  in adolescence, 66
  bariatric surgery, 4–5
  cardiac structure and function, 169, 170
  cardiovascular disease, 170
  cardiovascular physiology, 170
  development and maintenance, 5
  HRQOL, 20
  leg edema, 167
  literature, 25
  obesity, 4
  physical and emotional, 20
  pulmonary hypertension, 169
  resting pulse rates, 167
  thallium scanning, 170
  weight loss, 171

F
Fabricatore, A.N., 6
Family functioning, 66, 68, 69, 71
Faria, S., 151
Faria, S.L., 105
Fat macronutrients
  bile salts absorption, 106
  description, 105
  lingual lipase, 106
  lipolysis and lipogenesis, 106
  recommendations, intake, 106–107
  surgical bypass, malabsorption, 106
  in WLS, 107
Fatty acids
  and glycerol, 106
  hexose monophosphate shunt, 105
  and monoglycerides, 106
  saturated short-, medium- and long-chain, 106
Faulconbridge, L.F., 3–8
FDA-approved drugs
  lorcaserin, 160
  orlistat (xenical), 158–159
  phentermine/diethylpropion, 159
  phentermine plus topiramate, 159–160
Folate, 120
Food/nutrition-related history, 79
Forman, E., 147–153
Franceschelli, J., 175–182
Frank, L.L., 77–88, 135
Freire, R.H., 211
Friedman, K.E., 33–41
Fujiko, 27
Furtado, M.M., 111–117

G
Gastroesophageal reflux disease (GERD)
  chronic, 122
  comorbidities, morbid obesity, 121
Gehrer, S., 115
Geisinger RYGB Predictors Project
  active substance abuse, 197
  research-based clinic, 197
  RYGB program, 197–199
  statistical modeling, 199
Genetic factors
  genes and response, bariatric surgery, 200
  GWAS SNPs, 199
  and obesity, 199–200
  obesity GWAS SNPs, 200
  postoperative weight loss, association with, 201
  surgicogenomics, weight loss, 200–201
  and weight loss, 200
Genome wide association studies (GWAS)
  description, 199
  obesity, 200
GERD. See Gastroesophageal reflux disease (GERD)
Gerhard, G.S., 195–202
Glucagon-like peptide-1 (GLP-1) agonists, 161
Goodman, E., 67
Goodpaster, B.H., 220, 221
Gorin, A.A., 27, 124
Grazing
  eating, 94
  and emotional eating, 152
  LOC, 46
  postoperative, 30
  preoperative, 26
Green, 27
Greenberg, I., 39
Guisado, 27
Gut hormones, 138
GWAS. See Genome wide association studies (GWAS)

H
Hamilton, M.A., 38
Healing nutrition. See Nutritional recovery
Health belief model, 96
Health-related quality of life (HRQOL)
  excess weight, 20, 48
  generic measures, 66
  IWQOL, 20
  mental health summary scores, 48
  obesity, 19, 66
  quality-of-life domains, 66–67
  SF-36, 19
  and weight, 49
  and WRQOL, 66

Heinberg, L.J., 34, 39, 43–52
High-risk behaviors, 66, 69, 70
Himpens, J., 206
The "Honeymoon phase", 191
The "Hope phase", 191
Horchner, R., 20
Hospital stay, preoperative bariatric surgery
    day of surgery, 177
    intraoperatively, 177
HRQOL. See Health-related quality of life (HRQOL)
Hsu, 27

I
IAA. See Indispensable amino acid (IAA)
Impact of weight on quality of life (IWQOL)
    description, 15
    obesity, 20
Indispensable amino acid (IAA)
    negative nitrogen balance, 102
    PDCAAS, 102
    and protein requirement, 101
Informed consent, 167
Intake domain, 81
The Integrated health team approach, 185, 186
Internet
    computers and mobile smartphones, 55
    telephone counseling, 155
Iron
    citrate, acidic environment, 125
    dehydration/deficiency, 123
IWQOL. See Impact of weight on quality of life (IWQOL)

J
Jeon, K.J., 107
Johnston, C.S., 131
Joint Commission on Accreditation of Healthcare Organizations (JCAHO), 188
Jones-Corneille, J., 13
Josbeno, D.A., 221, 223

K
Kalarchian, M.A., 13, 14, 27, 36, 151, 213
King, W.C., 210, 217–227
Kinzl, J.F., 27
Kofman, M.D., 27, 45, 206
Koilonychia (Spoon-shaped nails), 115
Kolotkin, R.L., 20
Kushner, R.F., 205–214

L
Laparoscopic adjustable gastric banding (LAGB), 195, 196
Laparoscopic sleeve gastrectomy (LSG), 43–44
Larsen, J.K., 27, 222
Late nutrition
    anorexia, 124–125
    eating disorders after weight loss surgery, 124
    weight gain/plateau, 125
Latner, J.D., 21, 209
Lavery, M.E., 43–52
LeBrun, C.M., 119–126
Lee, T., 170
Legenbauer, 27

Lifestyle modification, obesity treatment
    AHEAD, 149–150
    bariatric surgery (see Bariatric surgery)
    caloric restriction, 148
    cognitive-behavioral strategies, 149
    components, 147, 148
    developments, 152–153
    diabetes prevention program, 149
    efficacy, 149
    individuals, body mass index (BMI), 147
    long-term weight maintenance, 150–151
    physical activity, 148–149
    power-up trials, 150
    self-directed diets and commercial weight-loss programs, 147
    self-monitoring, 148
    social cognitive theory, 147
    structured treatment protocol, 147–148
Lindroos, A.K., 30
Lipolysis and lipogenesis, 106
Liquid diets, preoperative bariatric surgery, 176
Litchford, M.D., 101–108
Livhits, M., 26, 51
Long-term postoperative
    Dumping syndrome, 94
    early plateau and weight regain, 93–94
    inactivity, 94–95
    maladaptive eating, 94
    noncompliance, vitamin and mineral supplementation and nutrient deficiencies, 94
    unhealthy eating habits, 94
Long-term success, 190
Long-term weight maintenance
    environmental and behavioral factors, 150
    of lifestyle modification, 150
    patient and treatment provider, regular contact, 151
    The registry, 150
Look AHEAD (Action for Health in Diabetes) study, 149–150
Lorcaserin, 160
Loss of control (LOC) eating
    and binge episodes, 6
    prevalence rates, 29
LSG. See Laparoscopic sleeve gastrectomy (LSG)

M
Macronutrients
    carbohydrates (see Carbohydrates)
    fat (see Fat macronutrients)
    metabolic expenditure, 101
    protein (see Proteins)
Magro, D.O., 91
Maintenance nutrition. See Postsurgery weight regain management
The "Maintenance phase", 191–192
Major depressive disorder, 67
Malabsorption
    gastric restriction, 120
    of nutrients, 119
    nutritional complications, weight loss surgery, 120
Maladaptive eating
    disorders, 94
    eating behaviors, 94
    grazing and emotional, 94
    mindless, 94
Malone, 27

Martinez, T., 185–193
Marti-Valeri, C., 178
Mauri, M., 13
McCullough, P.A., 222
Mechanick, J.I., 135
Medical approach, postoperative weight regain
    anatomical factors, 211
    behavioral (see Behavior)
    depression, 209
    disordered eating, 209
    etiological factors, bariatric surgery, 206
    evaluation and treatment pathway, 210, 211
    hormonal adaptations, 207
    lifestyle interventions after bariatric surgery, 213
    medical problems, 208
    menopause, 208
    multiple obesity-related comorbid conditions, 205
    musculoskeletal disability, 208
    occurrence, 205–206
    pharmacotherapy, 214
    physical activity, 212–213
    physiological considerations, 211–212
    pregnancy, 207
    psychological counseling and peer support, 213
    psychosocial, 209
    RYGB and LAGB, 205
    smoking cessation, 208
    surgical procedure failure, 207
    weight-gaining medications, 208
Medical management
    postoperative, 178–181
    preoperative (see Preoperative bariatric surgery)
Medical nutrition therapy, 131
Medical preparation
    behavioral assessment, 167–168
    cardiac (see Cardiac)
    comprehensive medical evaluation, 168
    initial patient assessment, 167, 168
    insurance providers, 165
    patient education, 166
    patient informed consent, 167
    patients with refractory extreme obesity, 165
    physician education, 165–166
    preoperative, 165
    respiratory (see Respiratory)
    risk-benefit analysis, 171
    risk reduction strategies, 171–172
    thrombosis (see Thrombosis)
Medication adjustments
    ACE inhibitors, 176
    diabetic, 176
    NSAIDs/aspirin/antiplatelet, 176
Metabolic surgery
    beneficial eating behaviors, 84
    diet modifications, 84
    diet-progression recommendations, 85–86
Metformin, 161
Mindless eating, 94
Minnesota multiphasic personality inventory-2 (MMPI-2), 39
Mitchell, J.E., 11–16, 25–31, 47
MMPI-2. See Minnesota multiphasic personality inventory-2 (MMPI-2)
Mobile phone and smartphone technology, 59–60
Monitoring and evaluation, NCP, 82
Mori, D.L., 34
Motivational interviewing, 97

Mühlhans, B., 13
Multidisciplinary team approach
    bariatric team meetings, 187
    behavioral health specialist, 186
    equipment and environment, 192
    exercise specialist, 187
    integrated health, 185, 186
    management and success, bariatric patient, 187
    morbid obesity, 185
    nursing competencies, implementation, 188
    obesity medicine, 187
    patient education, 188–189
    program policies and procedures, 187
    registered dietitian, 186
    regularly scheduled team meetings, 187
    simple supportive behavior, 186
    skilled surgeon and well-trained, 185
    specialized nursing, 186
    staff development and education, 187–188
    support group (see Support group)
    type II diabetes mellitus (T2DM), 185
Multifactorial disease, 185, 189
Multivitamin infusion (MVI), 115
Muscle accretion utilization, 103
MVI. See Multivitamin infusion (MVI)

N
Nausea and vomiting, 121
NCP. See Nutrition care process (NCP)
Nguyen, N.T., 175, 206
Niemeier, H.M., 152
Night eating syndrome (NES)
    in bariatric surgery, 26
    and BED, 36
    characterisation, 26
    prevalence, 209
Noll, J.G., 69
Nonsurgical weight loss and maintenance
    contributor, PA, 220
    habitual, 221
    inactivity and weight gain, 220
    overall energy and dietary fat intake, 221
Nutritional recovery
    adequate protein and micronutrients, 135
    description, 135
    dietary strategies, food tolerance, 135
    physical activity, 135–136
Nutrition assessment
    anthropometric measurements, 79
    biochemical data, medical tests and procedures, 80–81
    description, 78
    domains, 78
    food and nutrition professional, 78
    food/nutrition-related history, 79
    nutrition-focused physical findings, 81
    obtain, verify and interpret needs, bariatric patient, 78, 79
    outpatient vs. inpatient bariatric patients, 79, 80
    patient/client history, 81
    percent excess weight loss (%EWL), 79–80
    protein malnutrition, 86–87
Nutrition care process (NCP)
    assessment, 78–81, 98
    components, 77, 78
    description, 97
    diagnosis, 81–82, 98

individualized care and predictability, 77
intervention, 82, 98–100
monitoring and evaluation, 82, 100
for weight loss surgery, 97, 99
Nutrition counseling. *See* Educational and counseling needs
Nutrition diagnosis
assessment and intervention, 81
behavioral/environmental domain, 82
clinical domain, 81–82
intake domain, 81
professionals, 81
RD, 82
Nutrition education. *See* Educational and counseling needs
Nutrition-focused physical findings, 81
Nutrition guidelines
and appropriate foods, 92
and exercise, 91
NIH, 96
Nutrition intervention strategy
healthy diet, exercise and behaviors, 130–131
"liver prep diet", 131
pre-weight loss surgery diets, 132–133

O

Obesity
in men, 22
pharmacotherapy (*see* Pharmacotherapy, obesity treatment)
quality of life, 19
and sexual functioning, 22
Obesity GWAS SNPs, 200
Obesity medicine, 187
Obstructive sleep apnea management
CPAP/BiPAP, 177
noninvasive positive pressure devices, 177
patients with respiratory conditions, 178
Odom, J., 211
Ogden, C.L., 27
Oral contraceptive agents, 180
Orlistat (xenical), 158–159

P

PA. *See* Physical activity (PA)
Paddon-Jones, D., 87
Padwal, R., 178
Pagophagia, 115
Papalazarou, A., 151
Paresthesias
copper deficiency, 116
thiamin deficiency, 114
vitamin B12 deficiency, 114
Parrott, J.M., 129–142
Parrott, J.S., 129–142
Patient/client history, 81
Patient education
appropriate education, surgery candidates, 166
bariatric surgery, 166, 188
education checklist, 189
eligibility criteria, 166
selection and preoperative preparation, 188
visual, verbal and written, 188–189
Patient informed consent, 167
Pawlow, L., 168
Pawlow, L.A., 40
PCSK1. *See* Proprotein convertase subtilisin/kexin type 1 (PCSK1) gene

PDCAAS. *See* Protein digestibility correct amino acid score methodology (PDCAAS)
Pekkarinen, 27
PEM. *See* Protein energy malnutrition (PEM)
Percent excess weight loss (%EWL), 79
PES. *See* Problem, etiology, signs/symptoms (PES)
Pharmacotherapy, obesity treatment
contraindications and goals, 158
diet, exercise and behavior modification, 158
health-care professionals, 157
medications, 157
US Food and Drug Administration (FDA), 157–158
waist circumference, 158
weight-promoting medications, 158, 159
Phentermine/diethylpropion, 159
Phentermine plus topiramate, 159–160
Physical activity (PA)
assessment of, 219–220
bariatric surgery, preoperative and postoperative, 223–226
behaviors, 55
counseling, 58
description, 217
eating, 55, 57–58
education, 59
EIM, 136
and energy expenditure, 62
evidence-based guidelines, healthy and overweight/obese adults, 219
and fiber intake, 93
frequency and duration, 218–219
to health, relationship, 220
intensity, 218
"lack of time", "too tired" and "pain and discomfort", 136
level and potential, 35
lifestyle, 138
measurement devices, 61–62
non-exercise activity thermogenesis (NEAT), 218
nutrition, 77
The 2008 Physical Activity Guidelines for Americans, US, 135–136
and postoperative dietary, 29
postoperative eating, 56
postoperative outcomes, 217, 221–222
preoperative to postoperative changes, 222–223
regular exercise, 94
and sedentary behaviors, 222
skeletal muscles, 217
strategies, managing weight regain, 140
weight loss (*see* Weight loss)
The 2008 Physical Activity Guidelines for Americans, US, 135–136
Physician education
obesity management, patients, 166
obesity treatment centers and primary care physicians, 166
primary care providers, 165
Piechota, T., 91–100
Pietrzykowska, N.B., 175–182
Pilone, V., 48
Postoperative medication administration
anastomotic leak detection, 180
antidepressant/mood-altering, 179
antihypertensive, 179
aspirin and ibuprofen products, 179
diabetic, 178–179
dyslipidemic, 179
nausea and vomiting, 180
oral contraceptive agents, 180
Roux-en-Y gastric bypass/duodenal switch procedures, 178

Postoperative medication administration (cont.)
    small pouch syndrome, 180–181
    thiamine deficiency, 181
    warfarin and antiplatelet, 179–180
Postoperative nutrition assessment and follow-up
    description, 83
    laboratory assessment values, pre-and post-bariatric patient, 84
    medical issues after bariatric surgery, 83–84
    patient–provider contact, 84
Postsurgery weight regain management
    contribution/prevention factors, 140, 141
    dietary strategies, 139–140
    food intake and behaviors, self-regulation, 138–139
    maladaptive behaviors, 139
    physical activity strategies, 140
Powell, A.G., 157–162
Powers, 27
Pramlintide, 162
Preoperative and postoperative nutrition, 120
Preoperative bariatric surgery
    colonic preparations, 176
    hospital stay, 177
    liquid diets, 176
    medication adjustments, 176
    NSAIDs, 175–176
    pulmonary training, 176–177
    weight loss and smoking cessation, 175
Preoperative consultation, 4, 188
Preoperative evaluation, 6, 7, 25
Preoperative micronutrient deficiencies, 111–112
Preoperative nutrition assessment and follow-up
    bariatric surgical patients, 81
    deficiencies, 83
    dietitians, 81
    nutrition professional, 81
    psychosocial–behavioral evaluation, 82
Preoperative nutrition educational and counseling
    description, 92
    diet stages, 92
    eating behaviors, 93
    hydration, 92
    protein, 93
    realistic weight loss with weight loss surgery, 92
Preoperative weight loss, 197
Pre-weight loss surgery diets, 132–133
Problem, etiology, signs/symptoms (PES), 81
Proprotein convertase subtilisin/kexin type 1 (PCSK1) gene, 200
Protein digestibility correct amino acid score methodology (PDCAAS), 102, 103
Protein energy malnutrition (PEM)
    clinical signs, protein malnutrition, 122–123
    malabsorptive procedures, 122
    post-bariatric patients, 123
    quality of protein, 122
Protein malnutrition
    after bariatric surgery, 86
    domains, RD, 86
    parenteral nutrition, 86
    post-BPD/BPD/DS patients, 87
Proteins
    dietary sources, 102
    and energy intake, 101–102
    insufficient intake, 102
    muscle accretion utilization, 103
    and nitrogen cycle, 102
    quality, 102
    requirements, 103
    surplus intake, 102–103
    turnover and metabolism, 102
    urea-N, 102
    WLS (see Weight loss surgery (WLS))
Psychiatric disorders, 11–14, 34, 43, 45, 50, 196, 197
Psychological assessment
    alcohol use, 37
    bariatric surgery, 37
    BDI, 38
    behavioral health, 34, 37
    CCBRS, 35
    clinician preparation, 40
    consultations, 33–34
    decision-making process, 34
    diagnostic, 33
    dieting/weight history, 35
    domains, 34–35
    eating pathology, 35–36
    medical/psychological treatment, 37
    physical activity level, 35
    psychopathology and treatment history, 36–37
    social support, 37–38
    stressors, 38
    treatment plan, 34
    WALI, 34
Psychopathology
    anxiety, 14
    bariatric surgery, 11–12, 15
    binge eating disorder, 15
    current psychiatric diagnoses, 13
    description, 11
    eating behavior, 7
    glucagon-like peptide-1 (GLP-1), 14
    lifetime psychiatric diagnoses, 13
    and obesity, 11–12
    postoperative outcomes, 14
    psychopharmacology, 15
    psychosocial interventions, 15
    and treatment history, 36–37
Psychosocial status
    adherence, 49–50
    alcohol, 46–48
    bariatric surgery, 43
    BID (see Body image dissatisfaction (BID))
    body image, 49
    characteristics, 209
    childhood maltreatment, 6
    childhood trauma, 69
    depression, 43–44
    depressive symptoms, 5
    disordered eating, 45–46
    eating and physical activity habits, 5–6
    family support, 6
    high-risk behaviors, 70
    HRQOL (see Health-related quality of life (HRQOL))
    intelligence (IQ) testing, 4
    interpersonal relations, 68
    knowledge, 3–4
    mental health treatment, 5
    organizational framework, 65–66
    parent/family functioning, 68–69
    personality characteristics, 4–5
    psychological characteristics and postoperative outcomes, 7
    psychopathology, 67
    quality of life, 48–49

self-concept, 67–68
self-esteem, 4
social support, 50–51
socioeconomic status, 69
stigma and discrimination, 6–7
stressors, 209
suicide, 45
timing of surgery, 7
weight and dieting, 4
weight loss treatment, 3
Pulmonary training, preoperative bariatric surgery, 176–177

Q

QEWP-R. *See* Questionnaire for eating and weight patterns-revised (QEWP-R)
QOL. *See* Quality of life (QOL)
Qsymia™, FDA-approved drugs, 159–160
Quality of life (QOL)
    bariatric surgery patients, 20
    body image, 21–22
    description, 19
    and excess weight loss (EWL), 48
    gastric bypass patients, 20
    HRQOL, 19–20, 48
    psychological and social, 20
    psychosocial functioning, 20
    sexual function, 22
    and weight-related, 20–21
Questionnaire for eating and weight patterns-revised (QEWP-R), 27, 39

R

Raftopoulos, I., 27
Ramanan, B., 171
Ramirez, A., 177
Ratcliff, M.B., 68, 70
RD. *See* Registered dietitian (RD)
The "Reality phase", 191
Registered dietitian (RD)
    assessment domains, 86
    bariatric "pathway", 79
    description, 77
    food and nutrition experts, 81
    nutrition screening process, 79
    patient's presurgical preparedness, surgery, 82
    preexisting nutrient deficiency, 83
Reiter-Purtill, J., 65–71
Respiratory
    BMI, 169
    chronic nicotine use, 169
    lung function changes, with obesity, 169
    obesity hypoventilation, 169
    problems and symptoms, 168
    pulmonary hypertension, 169
    sleep disordered breathing, 169
Restrictive
    and malabsorptive procedures, 119–120
    procedures, 119
Risk-benefit analysis, 171
Risk reduction strategies
    mobility and exercise tolerance, 171
    preoperative period, bariatric surgery, 171
    short-term preoperative weight loss, 172

Rosenberger, P.H., 13, 222
Roux-en-Y gastric bypass (RYGB)
    Geisinger RYGB Predictors Project (*see* Geisinger RYGB Predictors Project)
    and LAGB, 195, 196
    patients with preoperative weight loss, 197
Rowston, 27

S

Sabbioni, 27
Sallet, 27
Sarwer, D.B., 3–8, 19–23, 34, 43, 48, 50, 83, 87, 147–153, 213
Saunders, R., 30, 46
Scholtz, 27
SCL-90-R. *See* Symptoms checklist-90-R (SCL-90-R)
Sedentary behaviors and PA, 222–223
Segal, A., 125
Sexuality
    and obesity, 22
    quality of life, 19
    sexual functioning, 22
    weight loss, 22
Shah, M., 212, 222
Short-term postoperative
    complications, 93
    constipation, 93
    dehydration and inadequate protein intake, 93
    description, 93
    diarrhea, 93
    Dumping syndrome, 93
    nausea and vomiting, 93
    vitamin and mineral supplements, 93
Single nucleotide polymorphisms (SNPs)
    obesity GWAS, 200
    UCP2, 200
    weight loss after RYGB surgery, 201
Small pouch syndrome, 180–181
SMART. *See* Specific, measurable, attainable, realistic and time-bound (SMART)
Smoking cessation
    negative urine cotinine level, 175
    and weight loss, 175
Smolak, L., 21
SNPs. *See* Single nucleotide polymorphisms (SNPs)
Social learning theory, 96
Social support
    description, 50–51
    and EWL, 51
    and weight loss, 51
Sogg, S., 34, 40
S/P bariatric surgery
    calcium and vitamin D, 115
    calcium citrate *vs.* calcium carbonate, 115–116
    copper, 116
    folic acid, 114–115
    iron, 115, 116
    selenium, 116
    thiamin (vitamin B1), 112, 114
    vitamin B12, 114
    vitamins A, E, K and zinc, 116
Specific, measurable, attainable, realistic and time-bound (SMART), 82
Spitznagel, M.B., 50
Still, C., 172, 175–182
Suboptimal weight loss and weight regain, 87–88
Substance abuse, 196, 197

Suicide
    after bariatric surgery, 45
    and depression, 20
    risk factors, 45
    weight loss, 45
Support group
    education, 190
    facilitator, 191
    The "Honeymoon Phase", 191
    The "Hope Phase", 191
    The "Maintenance Phase", 191–192
    meetings, 190
    morbid obesity, 189
    postoperative and preoperative, 190
    protein intake and vitamin supplementation, 190
    psychological aspects, 189
    The "Reality Phase", 191
    traits, 190
Surgical weight loss and maintenance, 221
Suzuki, J., 210
Sweet eating
    postoperative, 30
    preoperative, 28
Symons, T.B., 87
Symptoms checklist-90-R (SCL-90-R), 39
Sysko, R., 67, 69

T
Technology. *See* Weight loss
Teenagers, 65
Thiamin (vitamin B1), 112, 114
Thomas, J.G., 55–63
Thrombosis
    adipose tissue secretion, 170
    chronic atrial fibrillation/prosthetic heart valves, 171
    coagulation factors, 170
    prothrombotic tendencies, 171
Tong, J., 121
Topiramate, 159–160
Toussi, R., 27, 49, 52
Transtheoretical model of change, 96, 97
Treatment planning
    behavioral, 40
    factors, 40
    pre-bariatric surgery, 39
    weight-loss intervention, 39–40
Turner, P., 171

V
Varela, J.E., 177
Vasquez, T.L., 177
Vaz, 27
Very-low-calorie diets (VLCDs), 131
Vincent, H.K., 48
Virtual reality (VR) technology, 60–61
Vitamin A, 120
Vitamin and mineral deficiencies
    description, 111
    preoperative micronutrient, 111–112
    risk after bariatric surgery, 112–114
    S/P bariatric surgery (*see* S/P bariatric surgery)
Vitamin and mineral supplementation, 87
Vitamin D deficiency
    OH-hydroxy D levels, 125
    pre-and postsurgery, 125
Vitamin E, 120
Vitamin K, 120
VLCDs. *See* Very-low-calorie diets (VLCDs)
Vomiting, 29–30, 36, 39, 46, 93, 121, 122

W
Wadden, T.A., 26, 27, 34
Walfish, S., 39
WALI. *See* Weight and lifestyle inventory (WALI)
Warfarin and antiplatelet medications, 179–180
Webb, K., 205–214
Weight and lifestyle inventory (WALI), 6, 34
Weight gain/weight plateau, 125
Weight loss
    bariatric-focused tools, 61
    behavioral treatment programs, 58–59
    description, 55
    eating and physical activity behaviors, 55–58
    EMA (*see* Ecological momentary assessment (EMA))
    Ethicon Endo-Surgery, 62
    healthcare intervention, 55
    human brain, 56
    leisure time activities, 55
    lifestyle modifications (*see* Lifestyle modification, obesity treatment)
    mobile phone and smartphone technology, 59–60
    nonsurgical (*see* Nonsurgical weight loss and maintenance)
    surgical, 221
    technology-based treatments, 58
    VR technology, 60–61
    Web-based intervention, 59
Weight loss maintenance
    nonsurgical, 220 221
    surgical, 221
Weight loss surgery (WLS)
    average percentage, 134
    behavioral changes, 134–135
    carbohydrate content, 105
    daily fat intake, 107
    description, 129
    diet progression, 85
    eating disorders, 124
    energy/VLCD, 131
    exercise, benefits, 134
    "forced behavior modification", 91
    high-protein diets, 104
    lean body mass loss with, protein, 103–104
    and managing comorbidities, 130
    medical nutrition therapy, 131
    NCP, 99
    nutrition intervention strategy, 130–133
    nutrition, recovery (*see* Nutritional recovery)
    patient for lifestyle changes, 131
    for patients, 104, 105
    phases, 129, 130
    preoperative, 92
    protein requirement, 131
    and realistic weight loss with, 92
    regaining, 134
Weight plateau, 125
Weight-promoting *vs.* weight-neutral medications, 158, 159
Weight regain. *See* Medical approach, postoperative weight regain; Postsurgery weight regain management

Weight Watchers diet, 104
Weineland, S., 153
Wernicke's encephalopathy, 112
West-Smith, L., 40
Wheeler, E., 50
White, M.A., 26, 27, 46
Wilson, J.A., 176
Wing, R.R., 208

WLS. *See* Weight loss surgery (WLS)
Wood, G.C., 27, 195–202

Z
Zeller, M.H., 65–71
Zonisamide/bupropion, 162